Heather McDick
15/5/87

IRON AND INFECTION

IRON AND INFECTION

Molecular, Physiological and Clinical Aspects

Edited by

J.J. Bullen
University of Miami School of Medicine

and

E. Griffiths
National Institute for Biological Standards and Control

A Wiley–Interscience Publication

JOHN WILEY & SONS
Chichester · New York · Brisbane · Toronto · Singapore

Library of Congress Cataloging-in-Publication Data:

Iron and infection.

'A Wiley Interscience publication.'
Includes index.
1. Bacterial diseases. 2. Iron—Metabolism.
3. Microbial metabolism. 4. Host–parasite relationships.
I. Bullen, J.J. II. Griffiths, E. (Elwyn),
1940– . [DNLM: 1. Bacterial Infections—
metabolism. 2. Iron—metabolism. WC 200 I71]
QR201.B34I76 616.9′2 86–13213

ISBN 0 471 91168 2

British Library Cataloguing in Publication Data:

Iron and infection : molecular,
physiological and clinical aspects.
1. Iron—Physiological effect
I. Bullen, J.J. II. Griffiths, E.
616.07′1 QP913.F4

ISBN 0 471 91168 2

Printed and bound in Great Britain.

Contents

List of contributors

A. Bezkorovainy
Department of Biochemistry, Rush-Presbyterian–St. Luke's Medical Center, 1753 West Congress Parkway, Chicago, Illinois 60612, USA

J.J. Bullen
Department of Surgery, University of Miami School of Medicine, Jackson Memorial Medical Center, PO Box 016310, Miami, Florida 33101, USA

J.H. Crosa,
Department of Microbiology and Immunology, School of Medicine, The Oregon Health Sciences University, 3181 SW Sam Jackson Park Road, Portland, Oregon 97201, USA

E. Griffiths
National Institute for Biological Standards and Control, Holly Hill, Hampstead, London NW3 6RB, England

M.J. Kluger
Department of Physiology, The University of Michigan Medical School, Ann Arbor, Michigan 48109, USA

Preface

The topic of iron and infection originates from the work of Schade and Caroline (1944, *Science*, **100**, 14–15) on the bacteriostatic properties of raw hen egg white and the effect of added iron. These observations were largely ignored for twenty years but since the late 1960s have been directly or indirectly responsible for a growing interest in the role that iron plays in bacterial virulence and host defence. We believe that the significance of this role cannot be fully appreciated unless all its aspects are taken into account.

The availability of iron for the essential metabolism of pathogenic organisms and the need of the host to bind and sequestrate the metal are the central issues. With this in mind we have attempted to set out the advances in chemistry, microbiology, molecular genetics and clinical science that have been made in this field in recent years. We hope this will stimulate interest in these subjects and encourage the development of further research.

In many respects iron occupies a unique position in biological systems. This does not mean that it is the only important factor in host–parasite relationships, but it is an essential ingredient that must be considered in many, and perhaps all aspects, of defence against infection.

JJB
EG

“But iron, cold iron, is master of them all.”

Rudyard Kipling: Rewards and Fairies*

Iron and Infection
Edited by J.J. Bullen and E. Griffiths

Chapter 1

Iron in biological systems

E. GRIFFITHS
National Institute for Biological Standards and Control,
Holly Hill,
Hampstead, London, NW3 6RB, England

1. INTRODUCTION

It is now forty years since Schade and Caroline first discovered that specific iron-binding proteins, present in blood and in the whites of eggs, would inhibit the growth of certain bacteria (Schade and Caroline, 1944, 1946). They concluded that these proteins bound iron so tightly that bacteria were unable to obtain a sufficient amount of the metal for growth; adding iron easily overcame the resulting bacteriostasis. The active component in egg white was later shown to be ovotransferrin (conalbumin) by Alderton, Ward and Fevold (1946), a protein which had already been isolated in 1900 by Osborne and Campbell; the active component in blood was found to be a similar iron-binding protein, now known as transferrin to indicate its importance in mammalian iron transport (Schade and Caroline, 1946; Holmberg and Laurell, 1945, 1947). Since interest in the role of transferrin as a transporter of iron predominated at the time, the significance of the bacteriostatic action of these iron-binding proteins was virtually forgotten and seems generally to have been considered as nothing more than an interesting *in vitro* observation.

However, interest was revived a decade or so later when it was discovered that animals injected with iron in various forms were much more susceptible to infection than the untreated controls. This enhanced susceptibility of iron-treated animals to infection is now well recognized and can be seen with a number of different organisms (Table 1). The ability of iron compounds to

Table 1 Bacteria whose virulence in experimental infections is enhanced by injecting iron compounds

Aeromonas hydrophila	Miles, Khimji and Maskell, 1979
Clostridium perfringens	Bullen, Cushnie and Rogers, 1967
Cl. oedematiens	Miles, Khimji and Maskell, 1979
Corynebacterium renale	Henderson, Kadis and Chapman, 1978
Escherichia coli	Bullen, Leigh and Rogers, 1968
Klebsiella pneumoniae	Miles, Khimji and Maskell, 1979
Listeria monocytogenes	Sword, 1966
Neisseria gonorrhoeae	Payne and Finkelstein, 1975
N. meningitidis	Calver, Kenny and Lavergne, 1976
Pasteurella multiocida	Bullen *et al.*, 1968
P. haemolytica	Chengappa, 1983
Pseudomonas aeruginosa	Forsberg and Bullen, 1972
Salmonella typhimurium	Kaye, Merselis and Hook, 1965
Staphylococcus aureus	Gladstone and Walton, 1971
Vibrio anguillarum	Crosa, 1980
V. cholerae	Ford and Hayhoe, 1976
V. vulnificus	Wright, Simpson and Oliver, 1981
Yersinia pestis	Jackson and Burrows, 1956
Y. enterocolitica	Robins-Browne and Prpic, 1985

abolish the antibacterial effects of body fluids *in vitro* is also now well established and only iron has been found to act in this way (Bullen, 1981; Finkelstein, Sciortino and McIntosh, 1983; Griffiths, 1983; Weinberg, 1984). Clearly, though, many pathogenic organisms can multiply very successfully in body fluids and cause infection in humans and animals in the absence of added iron, suggesting that they may have special attributes relating to the assimilation of iron. The investigation of these phenomena in detail, often at the molecular level, has now led not only to a better understanding of the mechanisms involved in microbial pathogenicity but also to an explanation of the changes in resistance to infection which sometimes accompany clinical alteration of the iron status of the host. Both of these aspects are considered in later chapters of this book where it will be seen that it is the lack of available iron that is the key to the peculiar importance of the element in infection. To understand why the availability of iron should be so limiting *in vivo*, it is necessary to know something about the properties of iron and about the essential role of iron complexes in biological systems.

2. THE AVAILABILITY OF IRON

It is now known that although there is plenty of iron present in the body fluids of humans and animals, the amount of free iron, which might be readily available to bacteria, is extremely small. Most of the body's iron is found intracellularly, in ferritin, haemosiderin or haem, and that which is extracellular in body fluids is attached to high affinity iron-binding proteins, transferrin in serum and lymph and another related protein called lactoferrin in external secretions and milk (Aisen, 1980; Bezkorovainy, 1980; Morgan, 1981; see also Chapter 2); the iron-binding protein present in avian egg white, ovotransferrin, has already been mentioned. These proteins have association constants for iron of about 10^{36} and they are normally only partly saturated; e.g. in humans the serum transferrin is usually only 30–40 per cent saturated. Thus, although there is an abundance of iron present in body fluids, the amount of free iron in equilibrium with iron-binding proteins can be calculated to be of the order of 10^{-18} *M*, which is virtually zero (Bullen, Rogers and Griffiths, 1978), a result confirmed by many experiments (discussed by Aisen 1980; Bezkorovainy, 1980; Morgan, 1981). Indeed, there is usually a reserve of free binding sites on circulating transferrin capable of binding iron, possibly during periods of rapid entry of the metal into plasma. This may be an important safeguard against the presence of free or loosely bound iron. More recently, Gutteridge and his colleagues (Gutteridge, Rowley and Halliwell, 1981, 1982; Gutteridge *et al.*, 1985) have developed an assay, based on the use of the antibiotic bleomycin, to detect the presence of low molecular weight iron complexes capable of taking part in free radical reactions. The assay depends on the fact that degradation of DNA by bleomycin requires the presence of traces of iron salts. Suitable calibration of the DNA degradation allows the 'free' iron content of body fluids

Table 2 Bleomycin-detectable iron in human extracellular fluids

Fluid tested	Concentration of non-protein bound iron (micromoles per litre)
Normal serum	0
Haemochromatosis serum (newly diagnosed patient)	19.4
Haemochromatosis serum (patient on maintenance venesection)	0.7
Haemochromatosis serum (highly venesected patient with haemochromatosis)	0
Synovial fluid (rheumatoid patients)	2.8
Cerebrospinal fluid (normal)	2.2
Sweat (trunk of athletes)	4.6

Data taken from Gutteridge, Rowley and Halliwell (1981, 1982) and Gutteridge *et al.* (1982, 1985).

to be determined; iron bound to ferritin, haemoglobin, lactoferrin or transferrin is unavailable and is not detected. No bleomycin-detectable, unbound iron has been found in serum or plasma from normal humans, as would be predicted from the low percentage saturation of transferrin (Table 2). However, serum from patients suffering from the inherited disease haemochromatosis, in which much more dietary iron than usual is absorbed from the gut (see below and Table 3), and who are well known to be overloaded with iron, have often been found to contain unbound iron in a form detectable by the bleomycin assay (Gutteridge *et al.*, 1985) (Table 2). Some other extracellular fluids from normal individuals also, surprisingly, have contained bleomycin-detectable iron (Table 2). The addition of apotransferrin to these fluids made the iron unreactive on subsequent assay by the bleomycin method.

Generally, it is true to say that in normal animals and in humans iron is almost always bound to proteins, leaving only an extremely low concentration of 'free' iron; indeed, in all biological systems iron is always found bound to complexing agents. The reason for this is that ferric iron under physiological conditions tends to oxidize, hydrolyse and polymerize, forming essentially insoluble ferric hydroxide and oxyhydroxide polymers (May and Williams, 1980). The solubility product constant for ferric hydroxide has been estimated to be about 10^{-36} and any 'free' Fe^{3+} in excess of 2.5×10^{-18} *M* would be precipitated as insoluble ferric hydroxides (Chaberek and Martell, 1959; Spiro and Saltman, 1969; Bullen, Rogers and Griffiths, 1978). Moreover, the more soluble ferrous iron is readily oxidized to ferric iron under the conditions found in the extracellular environment of most aerobic cells. A similar situation exists in the Earth's surface. Even though iron is abundant in the Earth's crust, indeed it is the second most common metal, it is, generally, biologically unavailable because under the oxidizing atmosphere surface iron exists as an insoluble oxyhydroxide polymer. The problems of dissolving iron and acquiring it from an insoluble source, as well as maintaining it in a soluble form *in vivo*, have been overcome during evolution by the development of iron-complexing agents which serve to dissolve iron in the media surrounding living organisms, deliver it to the cells and transport it within higher plants and animals. Bacteria synthesize a large number of different iron-chelating agents or siderophores

Table 3 Iron-overload conditions in humans

Dietary origin: (e.g. Bantu siderosis)
Inherited disorder of iron absorption: (idiopathic haemochromatosis)
Clinical consequence of regular blood transfusion used to control other haematological disorders

(Lankford, 1973; Neilands, 1981) and those produced by bacterial pathogens are considered in Chapter 3. In plants, iron is translocated in the sap in the form of complexes with low molecular weight chelators, such as citrate and malate. In addition, chelators may be secreted by the roots of plants to allow soil iron to be dissolved and utilized by the plant (Brown and Tiffin, 1965; Brown, 1966; Tiffin, 1970; Leong, 1986). In contrast, certain root-colonizing rhizobacteria can markedly increase the yields of potatoes, sugar beet and other plants they colonize by secreting siderophores which complex iron strongly and make it unavailable to other potentially harmful microorganisms (Kloepper *et al.*, 1980; Schroth and Hancock, 1982). Iron chelators in the form of proteins have been identified in the extracellular fluid of some invertebrates (Palmour and Sutton, 1971) and in all vertebrates examined. In the vertebrates the problem of the low solubility of ferric salts at neutral pH is overcome by the formation of specific protein complexes, such as transferrin, lactoferrin, ferritin and haem proteins. It is interesting to note that one of the most primitive members of this subphylum, the hag fish (class Agnatha), whose ancestors existed many millions of years before the appearance of mammals, possesses a transferrin that is remarkably similar to the human protein (Aisen, Leibman and Sia, 1972). It has been proposed that 'modern' transferrins are the descendants of a primitive transferrin which consisted of the N-terminal half of a present-day transferrin and had just one iron-binding site (Williams, 1982). The duplicate structure and two iron binding sites of 'modern' transferrins is thought to have arisen by gene duplication (Williams, 1982; see also Chapter 2). Although virtually all of the iron in vertebrates is bound to protein, some iron is also thought to be complexed to low molecular weight ligands, such as citrate or phosphate, and it has been suggested that these low molecular weight molecules may mediate the transfer of iron both inside and outside cells. For example, physiological concentrations of citrate do catalyse Fe^{3+} exchange between transferrin molecules (Aisen and Leibman, 1968). However, the concentration of such low molecular weight iron complexes in biological fluids of vertebrates is severely limited and their individual concentrations are almost invariably unmeasurable (May and Williams, 1980), as is indicated when serum is subjected to the bleomycin assay (Gutteridge, Rowley and Halliwell, 1981). One important reason for keeping the concentration of the low molecular weight iron complexes in body fluids low may be to avoid the toxic effects of iron.

3. THE TOXICITY OF IRON

Although iron is essential for a wide variety of metabolic processes in the body, the metal can also have deleterious effects. Like many other transition elements, iron is an important biological catalyst. This is because it possesses unfilled *d* atomic orbitals and is able to undergo changes in oxidation states

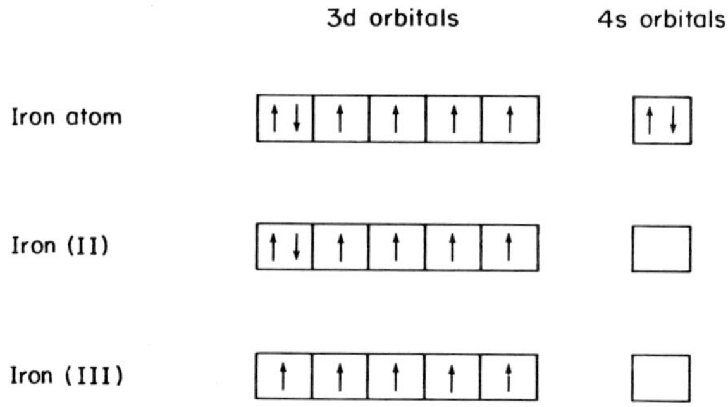

Figure 1 Arrangement of electrons in iron atoms and ions

involving one electron (Fig. 1). This easy access to two oxidation states, iron (II) (Fe^{2+}, ferrous iron) and iron (III) (Fe^{3+}, ferric iron), allows it to coordinate electron donors and to participate in redox processes. However, the very advantages that make iron an excellent catalyst also make it a potentially hazardous metal since reactions involving oxygen favour a univalent reductive pathway which can lead to the formation of unstable intermediates with unpaired electrons: i.e. to 'free radical' formation. The term 'free radical' has been broadly defined by Halliwell and Gutteridge (1985) as any species capable of independent existence that contains one or more unpaired electrons; an unpaired electron is one which occupies one atomic or molecular orbital by itself. By this definition iron itself with its unpaired electrons, like the oxygen molecule in the ground or triplet state, qualifies as a radical. The presence of one or more unpaired electrons causes the species to be attracted slightly to a magnetic field and to be what is called paramagnetic. The two unpaired electrons of the ground state O_2 molecule are to be found in each of the two different $\pi^* \pi^*$ antibonding orbitals, shown diagrammatically in Fig. 2(a), and have the same spin quantum number; this is the most stable configuration of the molecule. In practice it is found that the reaction of a compound having two unpaired electrons with parallel spins to give products having paired electrons with opposing spins is very slow. If O_2 attempts to oxidize another atom or molecule by accepting a pair of electrons from it, both new electrons must be of parallel spins so as to fit into the vacant spaces in the $\pi^* \pi^*$ orbitals. A pair of electrons in an atomic or molecular orbital would not meet this criterion since they would have opposite or antiparallel spins in accordance with Pauli's principle. This fact imposes a restriction on oxidations by O_2 and tends to make oxygen accept its electrons one at a time; in fact it slows down its reaction time with non-radical species. Transition metals are found at the active site of many oxidases and oxygenases because their ability to accept and donate single electrons can overcome this spin restriction (Hill, 1981). Uncatalysed reactions of molecular oxygen at room temperature are therefore very slow; if this was

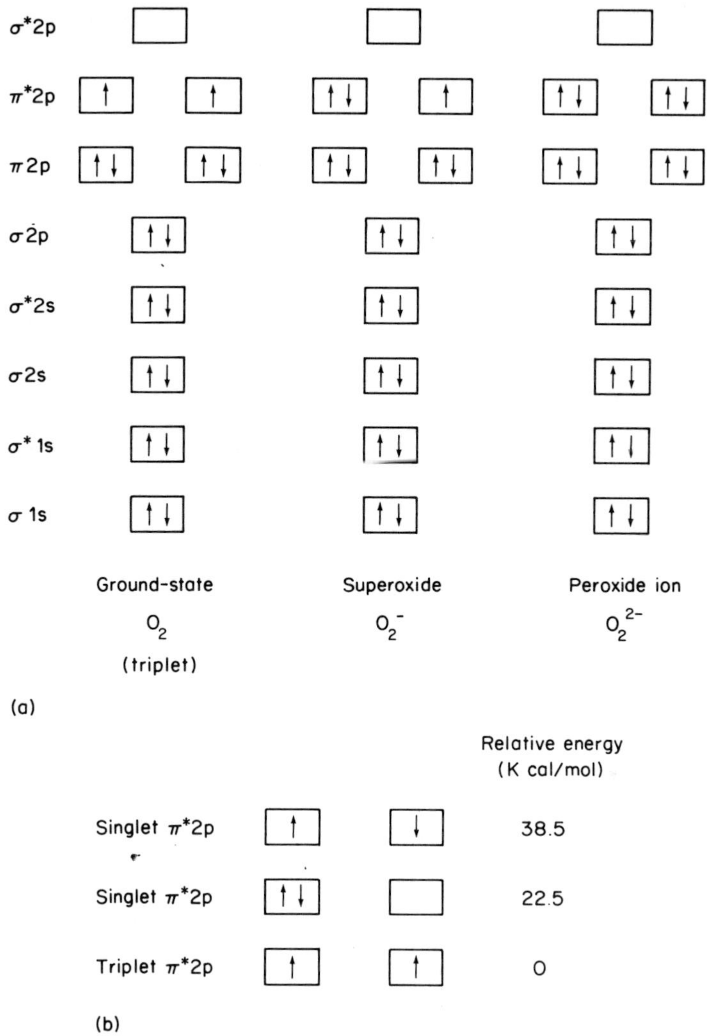

Figure 2 (a) Arrangement of electrons in the diatomic oxygen molecule. (b) Possible electron occupancy of the π* orbitals in molecular oxygen

not the case, there would be little free oxygen in the environment and aerobic life would not exist. More reactive forms of oxygen, called singlet oxygens, can, however, be generated by an input of energy, for example, by increasing temperature, where spin inversion takes place (Fig. 2b); in both forms of singlet oxygen the spin restriction is removed and so oxidizing ability is greatly increased.

When a single electron is accepted by the ground state O_2 molecule, it enters one of the $\pi^* \pi^*$ antibonding orbitals and the product is the superoxide radical O_2^- (Fig. 2a). Addition of a second electron to O_2^- gives the peroxide ion, O_2^{2-}, which has no unpaired electrons and is not a radical. At physiological pH the O_2^{2-} ion is immediately protonated to produce hydrogen peroxide, H_2O_2, and O_2; the overall reaction can be written:

$$2O_2^- + 2H^+ \rightarrow H_2O_2 + O_2 \quad (1)$$

Both the superoxide radical, O_2^-, and H_2O_2 can be detected during normal metabolism in many biological systems and there is ample evidence that they exist *in vivo* (Fridovich, 1975, 1978; Bhuyan and Bhuyan, 1977; Babior, 1978a, 1978b; Chance, Sies and Boveris, 1979; Takeshize and Minakami, 1979; Williams and Chance, 1983).

Since the O–O bond in H_2O_2 is relatively weak, homolytic fission readily converts H_2O_2 into two hydroxyl radicals, OH, a reaction which can be achieved by heat or by ionizing radiation. In addition, a mixture of H_2O_2 and Fe^{2+} also readily forms the OH· radical. The reaction, which is referred to as the Fenton reaction, can be expressed as follows:

$$Fe^{2+} + H_2O_2 \rightarrow OH\cdot + Fe^{3+} + OH^- \quad (2)$$

Traces of Fe^{3+} can also react with H_2O_2 to produce the Fe^{2+} required in reaction (2):

$$Fe^{3+} + H_2O_2 \rightarrow Fe^{2+} + O_2^- + 2H^+ \quad (3)$$

Iron (III) also reacts with O_2^-:

$$Fe^{3+} + O_2^- \rightarrow Fe^{2+} + O_2 \quad (4)$$

In addition, the following reactions may take place:

$$OH\cdot + H_2O_2 \rightarrow H_2O + H^+ + O_2 \quad (5)$$

$$OH\cdot + Fe^{2+} \rightarrow Fe^{3+} + OH^- \quad (6)$$

The overall sum of these reactions, unless some other reagent is present to intercept the OH· radical, is the iron-catalyzed decomposition of H_2O_2:

$$2H_2O_2 \underset{\text{Fe Catalyst}}{\rightarrow} 2H_2O + O_2 \quad (7)$$

Of the univalent reduction products derived from oxygen in the presence of iron, it is the hydroxyl radical, OH·, that is by far the most toxic. This free radical reacts with extremely high rate constants with most organic molecules found in cells. In particular, it attacks and destroys cell membranes, as well as DNA. Indeed, the reactivity of the OH· radicals is so great that if they are generated in living systems they will react immediately with whatever biological molecule is in their vicinity. This very reactivity also limits their biological lifetime. Since the OH· radical is so damaging, it is not surprising that aerobic organisms have evolved two enzymes to remove the two reactants, H_2O_2 and O_2^-, as fast as they appear to minimize the production of this radical. The enzyme superoxide dismutase scavenges the O_2^- and glutathione peroxidase (selenium enzyme) and catalase deal with H_2O_2. These enzymes are present in what appears to be relatively large amounts in all aerobic organisms and their role, as well as the role of other molecules, in protecting biological systems against oxygen radicals has been discussed in detail by Halliwell and Gutteridge (1985). Despite their presence, free superoxide anion and hydrogen peroxide can still be detected during normal metabolism in most biological systems. Since toxicity of the O_2^- and H_2O_2 involves their conversion to the OH· radical, a reaction which in turn will depend on the amount of catalytic iron available, it can be seen that it is also important that iron be chelated in a controlled way *in vivo* so that uncontrolled free radical reactions are avoided.

As mentioned above, most iron is tightly bound to proteins in vertebrates and would be unavailable for the Fenton reaction. The small pool of non-protein bound iron present could, however, conceivably provide iron for this reaction; physiological chelates, such as ferric citrate, have been shown to react with H_2O_2 *in vitro*. Normally this 'free iron' pool is kept extremely small, but 'free iron' has been detected in individuals with iron-overload disease. Normally the total amount of iron in the body is well controlled. In humans there is no obvious physiological route for the excretion of excess iron, although small amounts, about 1 mg daily, are lost from the body by, for example, desquamation from epithelial surfaces; in women, menstrual loss accounts for about 15–20 mg monthly (Jacobs, 1980). The capacity for iron excretion seems to be a little greater in other mammals (Finch *et al.*, 1978). Generally, iron balance depends on the regulation of iron absorption, and the amount of iron crossing the epithelial barrier in the small intestines is related to the iron status of the host. However, in certain situations the body does become overloaded with iron and the individuals concerned suffer from tissue damage or pathological siderosis. Increased iron absorption may arise through an increase in the amount of iron available in the diet or through an increase in the absorptive activity of the gut epithelium (Table 3). It is important to emphasize that an increase in the iron content of the diet alone does not necessarily result in iron loading; the availability of the iron in the diet also plays an essential role. Thus, Hofvander (1968) found that Ethiopian adults who had a diet containing 300–500 mg of iron daily did not suffer from iron overload, or pathological siderosis, while members of the African Bantu tribe, who had a somewhat lower dietary intake of iron, did suffer from the results of iron overload induced tissue damage. In the former case it is thought that much of the iron, which arises from contamination derived from iron-rich soil, is unavailable. In the latter case, most of the ingested iron comes from iron cooking pots and the availability of this iron is increased considerably when it is consumed in the form of an acid alcoholic drink called 'Kaffir beer'. This beer not only contains iron-complexing ligands such as fructose, but its acidity also helps to leach the iron from the containers (Walker and Arvidsson, 1953; DeBruin *et al*, 1968; Charlton, Bothwell and Seftel 1973). The degree of siderosis in the Bantu increased progressively with age in both males and females. A slower developing iron overload of dietary origin is seen in patients suffering from an inherited disease in which much more dietary iron than normal is absorbed from the gut (Table 3); this disease is called idiopathic haemochromatosis. The time taken for iron overload to develop in haemochromatosis depends to some extent on the patient's diet, but diagnosis is rarely made in patients under the age of 30 years. Although these patients are well known to be overloaded with iron, the nature of the biochemical lesion responsible for increased iron assimilation still remains unclear (Powell and Halliday, 1980). Iron-overload conditions can also result from medical treatment for other disorders, such as, for example, thalassaemias (Table 3). Thalassaemias are genetically inherited conditions in which the rate of synthesis of one of the haemoglobin chains is diminished, the prefix α or β being used to indicate the chain that is being synthesized abnormally slowly (Hoffbrand, 1980). Untreated patients with thalassaemia major, the homozygous state, die of anaemia in infancy but can be kept alive by regular blood transfusions. Since each unit of blood contains about 0.2 g of iron, these patients soon become overloaded with iron, leading to saturation of serum transferrin and often to the appearance of non-protein bound iron in the blood (Hershko *et al.*, 1978). This type of iron overload condition, where an underlying haematological disorder is complicated by excess iron, is often called transfusion siderosis, but in many respects it is similar to idiopathic haemochromatosis.

In all of these iron-overload conditions, ferritin, haemosiderin and transferrin become heavily loaded with iron. 'Free', non-protein bound iron, in the form of low molecular weight complexes, has been found in the serum of some individuals suffering from idiopathic haemochromatosis and transfusion siderosis (Hershko *et al.*, 1978; Gutteridge *et al.*, 1985). Iron accumulates in most organs of the body, but especially in the liver, spleen and heart, the latter organ being particularly sensitive. For example, many thalassaemics treated by transfusion die in their twenties and thirties from heart failure. The ultrastructural appearance of iron-loaded cells from iron-overloaded individuals is dominated by an accumulation of electron-dense ferritin cores, mainly in the cytoplasm and by the accumulation of electron-dense deposits of iron within the lysosomes (Iancu and Neustein, 1977; Jacobs, 1980). These iron deposits are thought to be responsible for damaging the organelles, and liposomal abnormalities are well recognized in experimental iron overload, as well as in human iron-overload conditions. Fibrosis also occurs in various tissues in patients with haemochromatosis and transfusion siderosis.

Much of the evidence concerning the toxicity of iron in these iron-overload conditions points strongly to the importance of free radical reactions, of which lipid peroxidation and the formation of OH· from iron salts and H_2O_2 are of major importance (for reviews see Jacobs, 1980; Halliwell and Gutteridge, 1984, 1985). Gutteridge *et al.* (1985) have not only shown that sera from patients with idiopathic haemochromatosis, unlike sera from normal adults, contain iron in a form detectable by the bleomycin assay but also that this 'free' iron is capable of stimulating lipid peroxidation and the formation of the OH· radical. The disruptive effects of lipid peroxidation on cellular systems have been discussed by Quinn and Williams (1978) and by Halliwell and Gutteridge (1985). Both lactoferrin and transferrin at physiological degrees of iron saturation are inhibitors of iron-dependent lipid peroxidation (Gutteridge, Rowley and Halliwell, 1981), and it has been suggested that one of the immediate benefits of continuous chelation therapy in transfusion siderosis is to remove the 'free', easily chelated, iron fraction (Propper and Marino, 1978). Another situation where the pathological accumulation of iron is thought to play a part in disease is in rheumatoid arthritis. It has been suggested that the iron which accumulates in rheumatoid synovial membrane and fluid contributes to the variable expression of rheumatoid disease by promoting the production of damaging free radicals (Blake, Hall and Bacon, 1981; Halliwell and Gutteridge, 1984). *In vitro* studies have shown that the OH· radical degrades the hyaluronic acid that is responsible for the lubricating properties of normal synovial fluid (Wong *et al.*, 1981). Synovial fluid appears to have little superoxide dismutase or catalase activity (McCord, 1974; Blake *et al.*, 1981). In addition to the damaging role of oxygen radicals in a number of pathologies, there is also accumulating evidence that peroxidation reactions may cause some of the dysfunctions associated with ageing (Cutler, 1985).

Although biological systems strive to minimize the production of free radicals, there is one case where free radicals are specifically generated to produce non-specific damage. This occurs in polymorphonuclear leukocytes during phagocytosis and is important for killing ingested bacteria. A great deal of attention has been focused on the ability of phagocytes to generate H_2O_2, O_2^- and OH·, and mechanisms are reviewed by Spitznagel (1983), Babior (1984) and Segal (1984). When phagocytes are exposed to certain stimuli they undergo marked changes in their oxygen metabolism known as the 'respiratory burst'. Their rates of oxygen uptake increases greatly and they produce large amounts of O_2^- and H_2O_2. This alteration results from the activation of a membrane-bound oxidase, dormant in resting cells, that catalyses the one-electron reduction O_2 to O_2^- at the expense of NADPH (Markert, Glass and Babior, 1985):

$$2O_2 + NADPH \rightarrow 2O_2^- + NADP \quad (8)$$

Most of this O_2^- reacts rapidly with itself, dismuting to produce oxygen and H_2O_2 according to equation (1). The H_2O_2 and O_2^- are then used as starting materials for the production of the bactericidal oxidants; these fall into two groups: oxidized halogens and oxidizing radicals like OH·. The production of the former involves myeloperoxidase which uses the H_2O_2 to form hypochlorite and other oxidized derivatives of chloride, which are potent antimicrobial agents. Recent work suggests that the myeloperoxidase – H_2O_2–halide system can oxidize the iron–sulphur centres in intact microorganisms such as *Escherichia coli*, and that this may be one of the killing mechanisms (Rosen and Klebanoff, 1985). The production of the other group of bactericidal oxidants, the oxidizing radicals, is considered to involve the iron–catalysed production of OH· from O_2^- and H_2O_2, as described before, as well as more obscure oxidizing radicals.

4. BIOCHEMICAL FUNCTIONS OF IRON

The electronic arrangement responsible for the excellent catalytic properties of the iron atom, perhaps the most versatile of all biocatalytic elements, has already been mentioned (Fig. 1), as has the reversible change in its oxidation state involving one electron. The main advantage of iron as a catalytic element, however, resides in the fact that the redox properties of the metal can be modified by its interaction with coordinating ligands so that the ease of electron acceptance can vary over a wide range; in fact, the redox potentials of enzymes containing iron cover a range of nearly 1,000 mV. Iron has six molecular orbitals available for bonding and these can form bonds along three axes of symmetry, giving the octahedral geometry commonly found in iron complexes (Spiro and Saltman, 1974). However, the actual bond lengths and bond angles of biological iron complexes vary not only with the different oxidation states of the iron but also with the nature of the interacting ligand. Iron (III) has a smaller ionic radius than iron (II) and it will, therefore, bond to reacting molecules with bond distances that are smaller than those of iron (II). The fact that each oxidation state has a characteristic geometry means that any redox change must be accompanied by appropriate changes in bonding to accommodate the new geometry. Since the ligands involved in bonding to the iron are usually linked to each other in some way, the configuration of a complex will be restricted and will tend to stabilize either the oxidized or reduced state of iron depending on which geometry is the more compatible; this will clearly affect the redox potential.

The nature of the coordinating ligand itself also affects the redox potential of the coordinating iron. When iron is coordinated in an octahedral geometry, the five orbitals are arranged into two sets with different energy levels, three of

	3d orbitals lower energy	Higher energy*	Unpaired electrons	Spin	Ligand field
Fe^{3+}	↑ | ↑ | ↑	↑ | ↑	5	High	Weak
Fe^{3+}	↑↓ | ↑↓ | ↑	|	1	Low	Strong
Fe^{2+}	↑↓ | ↑ | ↑	↑ | ↑	4	High	Weak
Fe^{2+}	↑↓ | ↑↓ | ↑↓	|	0	Low	Strong

* In a free iron ion in the gas phase, all five 3d orbitals have the same energy. When the ion is bound to a set of ligands, the 3d orbitals attain different energies by virtue of their spatial arrangement with respect to the ligands: this is called ligand field splitting (Cotton and Wilkinson, 1972).

Figure 3 Effect of weak and strong ligand field on the arrangement of electrons in Fe^{3+} and Fe^{2+} ions

one kind and two of another, the latter two having the higher energy (Fig.3). The energy difference between the two sets of orbitals will depend on the strength of the negative charges on the coordinating ligands. Strong electronegative ligands, described as 'strong field', such as oxygen, will tend to repel the *d* electrons and force them into spin-paired orbitals. In contrast, 'weak-field' ligands allow the *d* electrons to assume the maximum unpaired parallel spin arrangement. The arrangement of *d* electrons in their orbitals will in fact be governed by a balance between Hund's rules, which state that the most stable configuration is one with the maximum number of unpaired electrons arranged with parallel spins, and the energy effects of the coordinating ligand which make it energetically unfavourable to place electrons in the two higher energy levels. It can be seen from Fig. 3 that when the ligand field is strong, iron (II) (Fe^{2+}) will exist in a low spin state with all its electrons paired. Iron (III) (Fe^{3+}) will be strongly paramagnetic with many unpaired electrons. A change of ligand can thus produce a complex with different magnetic properties. Since a change in spin state is also accompanied by a change in the ionic radius of the iron atom and also by a change of iron–ligand bond length, changing the ligand will produce a different geometric arrangement. Only high spin Fe^{3+} and low spin Fe^{2+} have symmetrical arrangements of electrons, and the uneven distribution of electrons in the other states tends to distort the geometry of the complex. However, a suitable arrangement of coordinating ligands can stabilize a distorted geometry and so stabilize a particular spin state, thus affecting the redox value of the complex as a whole.

All these various properties of iron complexes affect the ease with which the iron can accept or lose an electron, i.e. affect its redox potential. The immediate environment of an iron atom within an iron protein will thus decide the redox activity and the function of the whole molecule. While the ligand atoms donating electrons to iron will mainly be O, N and S, the many different arrangements which exist are reflected in the enormously wide range of iron proteins found in nature. These proteins play essential roles in such fundamental reactions as ribonucleotide and dinitrogen reduction, as well as in energy-yielding electron transfer.

Metalloproteins containing iron fall into three main groups:

1. Proteins that form complexes with iron
2. Proteins characterized by their ability to bind oxygen reversibly
3. Proteins which function as enzymes concerned mostly with redox reactions

The first group of proteins, namely transferrin, lactoferrin, ovotransferrin and ferritin are discussed in detail in Chapter 2 of this book. The second group comprise proteins whose function it is to bind molecular oxygen reversibly, and several of these exist in nature. Most of them contain iron, usually but not always as haem (Table 4); the properties of haemoglobin and myoglobin are considered in detail in Chapter 2. In mammals, haemoglobin serves to transport bound oxygen within erythrocytes and myoglobin acts as an oxygen store in skeletal muscle tissue. *Leghaemoglobin* is a haem protein which is very similar to human haemoglobin but is found in the nodules of nitrogen-fixing plants; it is believed to play a role in modulating oxygen supply (Ellfolk, 1972). Quite apart from binding oxygen reversibly, haem proteins also participate in several other reactions with molecular oxygen. In fact, haem proteins participate in many types of, often, essential biochemical reactions including the

Table 4 Examples of proteins which bind molecular oxygen reversibly

Protein	Prosthetic group
Haemoglobin (blood)	Haem (Fe^{2+})
Myoglobin (muscle)	Haem (Fe^{2+})
Leghaemoglobin (root nodule)	Haem (Fe^{2+})
Haemerythrin (marine invertetrates)	Non-haem iron
Haemocyanin (anthropod/mollusc)	Cu^{+}

Table 5 Examples of mammalian and microbial iron enzymes and proteins

MAMMALIAN	
Oxygen-binding proteins	
Haemoglobin	Dickerson and Geis (1983)
Myoglobin	
Oxygen metabolism	
Haem type:	
Tryptophan-2,3-dioxygenase	Feigelson and Brady (1974)
Non-haem type:	
Cysteamine dioxygenase	Wrigglesworth and Baum (1980)
Prolyl hydroxylase	
Lysyl hydroxylase	
Phenylalanine hydroxylase	
Tyrosine hydroxylase	
Tryptophan hydroxylase	
Peroxide and superoxide metabolism	
Catalase	Halliwell and Gutteridge (1985)
Peroxidase	
Electron transfer enzymes	
Haem type:	
Cytochromes	Wrigglesworth and Baum (1980)
Sulphite oxidase	
Non-haem type:	
Iron–sulphur proteins (mitochondrial)	Wrigglesworth and Baum (1980)
Ribonucleotide reductase	Reichard and Ehrenberg (1983)
Flavoproteins	
Aldehyde oxidase	Wrigglesworth and Baum (1980)
Xanthine oxidase	
Xanthine dehydrogenase	
MICROBIAL	
Oxygen-binding proteins	
Haemoglobin-like proteins	Lascelles (1964)
Leghaemoglobin	Ellfolk (1972)
Oxygen metabolism	
Haem type:	
Tryptophan dioxygenase	Nozaki and Ishimura (1974)
Non-haem type:	
Catechol oxygenases	Nozaki and Ishimura (1974)
Peroxide and superoxide metabolism	
Superoxide dismutase	Halliwell and Gutteridge (1985)
Catalase	
Peroxidase	

Table 5 (contd.)

Electron transfer enzymes	
Haem type:	
Cytochromes	Yamanake and Okunuki (1974)
Sulphite reductase	Murphy and Siegel (1973)
Non-haem type:	
Iron–sulphur proteins (ferredoxin, rubredoxin)	Lovenberg (1974)
Nitrogenase	Streicher and Valentine (1974)
Glutamate synthase	Miller (1974)
Hydrogenase	Mortenson and Chen (1974)
Ribonucleotide reductase	Reichard and Ehrenberg (1983)
Flavoproteins	
Succinic dehydrogenase	Veeger, Dervartanian and Zeylemaker (1969)
Nitrate reductase	Forget and Dervartanian (1972)
Xanthine oxidase	Smith, Rajagopalan and Handler (1967)
NADH dehydrogenase	Dervartanian (1972)
Formate dehydrogenase	Hopner and Troutwein (1972)
NADPH sulphite reductase	Siegel, Faeder and Kamin (1972)
Other iron enzymes	
L(+)-Tartrate dehydrase	Hurlberg and Jacoby (1965)
3-Deoxy-D-arabino-heptulosonate-7-phosphate synthase	McCandless and Herrmann (1978)
Enzymes acting on amino acids, amines and acetyl phospate	Sagers (1974)
Iron-storage proteins	
Ferritin	David (1974)
Bacterioferritin	Yariv *et al.* (1981)

transfer of electrons to molecular oxygen in cellular respiration, the reduction of peroxides, oxygenation and hydroxylation of organic substrates, as well as the transfer of electrons between dehydrogenases and various electron acceptors. There are also non-haem iron enzymes in both mammalian and microbial systems that carry out similar, as well as other, functions (see Table 5).

It is not the intention here to provide a detailed discussion of all the various iron enzymes and proteins found in nature. Excellent reviews of the many functions of iron can be found in *Iron in Biochemistry and Medicine* (Jacobs and Worwood, 1974, 1980) and in *Microbial Iron Metabolism* (Neilands, 1974). In the context of the present book the aim is to emphasize the essential role iron plays in the life processes of both eukaryotic and prokaryotic cells. Table 5 shows a selection of iron-dependent enzymes and proteins involved in mammalian and microbial metabolism. Inspection of the table will show that iron plays a central role in the metabolism of prokaryotes, eukaryotes, aerobic, anaerobic, photosynthetic and nitrogen-fixing life forms. Indeed, in mammals and many prokaryotic systems, such as in *Escherichia coli*,

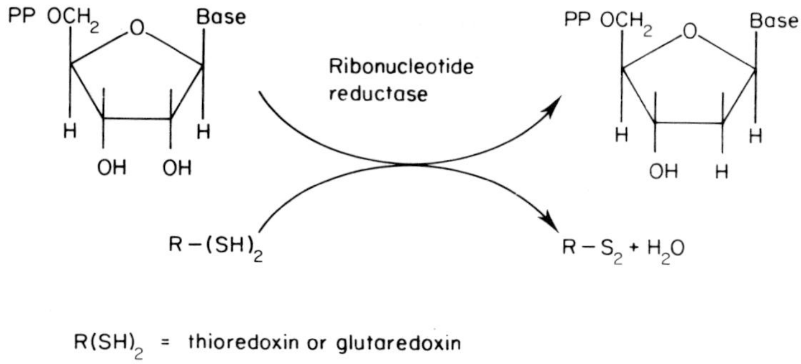

Figure 4 Ribonucleotide reductase catalysed formation of deoxyribonucleoside diphosphates

the very process of DNA replication depends on iron. Iron-containing ribonucleotide reductases catalyse the enzymatic conversion of ribonucleotides to the deoxyribo-nucleotides by substituting the OH at position 2^1 on the molecules in hydrogen (see Fig 4; Reichard and Ehrenberg, 1983); this is an obligatory step in DNA synthesis. The four common ribonucleoside diphosphates are all reduced by the same enzyme which maintains a balanced supply of deoxyribonucleoside triphosphates, needed for DNA synthesis, through allosteric control mechanisms. These controls regulate both the overall activity and substrate specificity of the enzyme in any one system (Thelander and Reichard, 1979; Holmgren, 1981; Follmann, 1982). There is a second class of ribonucleotide reductases which differs from the iron-dependent enzymes. These contain no iron but use the vitamin B12 coenzyme as a cofactor for the reduction of ribonucleoside triphosphates (Blakley and Barker, 1964; Orme-Johnson, Beinert and Blakley, 1974). They are found notably in lactic acid bacteria, some of which appear to be organisms which function either in the absence of iron or with a very limited supply of the metal (Neilands, 1974; Archibald, 1983).

Generally, it is true to say that iron is an essential element for all forms of life, although it seems that certain strains of lactobacteria have gone to some length to avoid a need for the element (Archibald, 1983). In view of the numerous and diverse functions of iron and iron enzymes, it is not surprising that iron deficiency has a profound effect on many biochemical processes in microorganisms; these have been thoroughly reviewed by Lankford (1973) and Light and Clegg (1974). For example, catalase activity is markedly reduced in many microorganisms in conditions of iron limitation (Waring and Werkman, 1944; Schade, 1963; Theodore and Schade, 1965). A similar reduction occurs in the cytochrome content of iron-deficient organisms (Waring and Werkman, 1944). The individual cytochromes, however, differ in their response to iron limitation (Ohnishi, Schleyn and Chance, 1969). In *Candida utilis*, cytochrome a and a_3

vary little over a wide range of iron concentration while cytochrome b varies considerably. Cytochrome c content also increases with increasing amounts of iron but over a much narrower range than in the case of cytochrome b. Waring and Werkman (1944) point out that when organisms are grown in iron-poor media, the iron requirements of the cytochromes are met first. Thus, iron-deficient *Aerobacter indologenes* have an almost normal cytochrome system although catalase and peroxidase activities are less than 5 per cent of normal and some other iron-containing enzymes are completely absent. It is clear, therefore, that some iron-containing enzymes are more sensitive to iron limitation than others. It is also clear that bacteria can survive and grow, although perhaps not so efficiently, without some of their iron enzymes, and it seems reasonable to assume that bacteria grown with an inadequate iron supply will sacrifice first any excess of iron-containing enzymes over that quantity essential for continued growth and survival. To predict which iron-dependent function might be crucial for bacterial multiplication in any particular situation is, therefore, not a simple matter. The effects of iron deficiency in higher animals have been reviewed by Beutler and Fairbanks (1980).

The vital role of iron in metabolism would suggest that living cells should have evolved specific mechanisms which ensure that sufficient iron is made available for essential physiological functions. The ways in which higher animals handle iron supply and demand have already been touched upon and details can be found in *Iron in Biochemistry and Medicine* (Jacobs and Worwood, 1980) and in *Iron Metabolism in Man* (Bothwell *et al.*, 1979). Microorganisms are also faced with the problem of extracting iron from the environment, where it mostly occurs in a highly insoluble form. In many cases their response to this environment has been to elaborate specific ligands, called siderophores, which are designed to solubalize and transport the metal. Two distinct iron transport systems, called 'low affinity' and 'high affinity', can be found in aerobic and facultative anaerobic organisms. In the case of enteric species, like *E. coli*, these two systems have been well defined. For example, strains of *E. coli* which are deprived of their 'high affinity' systems will still thrive on laboratory media containing excess available iron. Little is known about the low affinity pathway of iron assimilation, although the process is assumed to be widely distributed in microorganisms. The 'high affinity' systems have, however, been studied in great detail. They are made up of low molecular weight chelators, which are virtually ferric specific, the siderophores, and their corresponding membrane receptors; the ligand atoms linked to iron are predominantly oxygen, most often provided by hydroxamic acid or catechol moieties. Siderophores have been detected in very many aerobic and facultative anaerobic microorganisms, and their structures and synthesis, together with the mechanisms involved in assimilating iron in microbial species, have been extensively reviewed by Lankford (1973) and Neilands (1981, 1984). The fact that some bacteria can produce more than one type of chelator, as well as sometimes using ferric siderophores produced by other species, emphasize the great lengths bacteria have had to go to ensure their iron supply. The fact that vertebrates need to keep iron solubilized but not readily available for reacting in systems which produce toxic radicals means that the availability of 'free' iron is severely restricted in healthy animals. The mechanisms whereby a pathogen acquires iron *in vivo* thus become an essential component of the virulence or pathogenic properties of the organisms. The many ways that bacterial pathogens have adapted to the iron-restricted environment found *in vivo* and acquire iron are considered in Chapter 3.

REFERENCES

Aisen, P. (1980). The transferrins. In *Iron in Biochemistry and Medicine* (Eds. A Jacobs and M. Worwood), Vol. II, pp. 87–129. Academic Press, London.

Aisen, P., and Leibman, A. (1968). Citrate-mediated exchange of Fe^{3+} among transferrin molecules. *Biochemical Biophysical Research Communications*, **32**, 220–226.

Aisen, P., Leibman, A., and Sia, C.L. (1972). Molecular weight and subunit structure of hagfish transferrin. *Biochemistry*, **11**, 3461–3464.

Alderton, G., Ward, W.H., and Fevold, H.L. (1946). Identification of the bacteria-inhibiting iron-binding protein of egg white as conalbumin. *Archives of Biochemistry and Biophysics*, **11**, 9–13.

Archibald, F. (1983). *Lactobacillus plantarum*, an organism not requiring iron. *FEMS Microbiology Letters*, **19**, 29–32.

Babior, B.M. (1978a). Oxygen-dependent microbial killing by phagocytes. *New England Journal of Medicine*, **298**, 659–668.

Babior, B.M. (1978b). Oxygen-dependent microbial killing by phagocytes. *New England Journal of Medicine*, **298**, 721–725.

Babior, B.M. (1984). The respiratory burst by phagocytes. *Journal of Clinical Investigation*, **73**, 599–601.

Beutler, E., and Fairbanks, V.F. (1980). The effects of iron deficiency. In *Iron in Biochemistry and Medicine* (Eds. A. Jacobs and M. Worwood), Vol. II, pp. 393–425. Academic Press, London.

Bezkorovainy, A. (1980). *Biochemistry of Non-Heme Iron*. Plenum Press, New York.

Bhuyan, K.C., and Bhuyan, D.K. (1977). Regulation of hydrogen peroxide in eye humors: effect of 3-amino-IH-1,2,4-triazole on catalase and glutathione peroxidase of rabbit eye. *Biochimica et Biophysica Acta*, **497**, 641–651.

Blake, D.R., Hall, N.D., and Bacon, P.A. (1981). The importance of iron in rheumatoid disease. *Lancet*, **2**, 1142–1144.

Blake, D.R., Hall, N.D., Treby, D.A., Halliwell, B., and Gutteridge, J.M.C. (1981). Protection against superoxide and hydrogen peroxide in synovial fluid from rheumatoid patients. *Clinical Science*, **61**, 483–486.

Blakley, R.L., and Barker, H.A. (1964). Cobamide stimulation of the reduction of ribotides to deoxyribotides in *Lactobacillus leichmannii*. *Biochemical and Biophysical Research Communications*, **16**, 391–397.

Bothwell, T.H., Charlton, R.W., Cook, J.D., and Finch, C.A. (1979). *Iron Metabolism in Man*. Blackwell, Oxford.

Brown, J.C. (1966). Fe and Cu uptake as related to root-sap and stem-exudate citrate in soyabeans. *Physiologia Plantarum*, **19**, 968–976.

Brown, J.C., and Tiffin, L.O. (1965). Iron stress as related to the iron and citrate occurring in stem exudate. *Plant Physiology*, **40**, 395–400.
Bullen, J.J. (1981). The significance of iron in infection. *Reviews of Infectious Diseases*, **3**, 1127–1138.
Bullen, J.J., Cushnie, G.H., and Rogers, H.J. (1967). The abolition of the protective effect of *Clostridium welchii* type A antiserum by ferric iron. *Immunology*, **12**, 303–312.
Bullen, J.J., Leigh, L.C., and Rogers, H.J. (1968). The effect of iron compounds on the virulence of *Escherichia coli* for guinea pigs. *Immunology*, **15**, 581–588.
Bullen, J.J., Rogers, H.J., and Griffiths, E. (1978). Role of iron in bacterial infection. *Current Topics in Microbiology and Immunology*, **80**, 1–35.
Bullen, J.J., Wilson, A.B., Cushnie, G.H., and Rogers, H.J. (1968). The abolition of the protective effect of *Pasteurella sceptica* antiserum by iron compounds. *Immunology*, **14**, 889–898.
Calver, G.A., Kenny, C.P., and Lavergne, G. (1976). Iron as a replacement for mucin in the establishment of meningococcal infection in mice. *Canadian Journal of Microbiology*, **22**, 832–838.
Chaberek, S., and Martell, A.E. (1959). Organic Sequestering Agents, p.446. John Wiley, New York.
Chance, B., Sies, H., and Boveris, A. (1979). Hydroperoxide metabolism in mammalian organs. *Physiological Reviews*, **59**, 527–605.
Charlton, R.W., Bothwell, T.H., and Seftel, H.C. (1973). Dietry iron overload. *Clinical Haematology*, **2**, 383–403.
Chengappa, M.M. (1983). Hemoglobin enhancement of experimental infections of mice with *Pasteurella haemolytica*. *American Journal of Veterinary Research*, **44**, 1545–1546.
Cotton, F.A., and Wilkinson, G. (1972). *Advanced Inorganic Chemistry*, 3rd ed. Interscience, New York.
Crosa, J.H. (1980). A plasmid associated with virulence in the marine fish pathogen *Vibrio anguillarum* specifies an iron sequestering system. *Nature*, **284**, 566–568.
Cutler, R.G. (1985). Peroxide-producing potential of tissues: inverse correlation with longevity of mammalian species. *Proceedings of the National Academy of Sciences (USA)*, **82**, 4798–4802.
David, C.N. (1974). Ferritin and iron metabolism in phycomyces. In *Microbial Iron Metabolism: A Comprehensive Treatise* (Ed. J.B. Neilands), pp. 149–158. Academic Press, New York.
DeBruin, E.J.P., Mekel, R.C.P.M., Theron, J.J., and Jansen, C.R. (1968). An evaluation of the increase in the iron content of foodstuffs cooked in various utensils. *South African Medical Journal*, **42**, 108–110.
Dervartanian, D.V. (1972). NADH dehydrogenases from *Azobacter vinelandii*. *Zeitschrift fur Naturforschung*, **27b**, 1082–1084.
Dickerson, R.E., and Geis, I. (1983). *Haemoglobin Structure, Function, Evolution and Pathology*. The Benjamin Cummings Publishing Company, Menlo Park, California.
Ellfolk, N. (1972). Leghaemoglobin, a plant haemoglobin. *Endeavour*, **31**, 139–142.
Feigelson, P., and Brady, F.O. (1974). In *Molecular Mechanisms of Oxygen Activation* (Ed. O. Hayaishi), pp.87–133. Academic Press, London.
Finch, C.A., Ragan, H.A., Dyer, I.A., and Cook, J.D. (1978). Body iron loss in animals. *Proceedings of the Society for Experimental Biology and Medicine*, **159**, 335–338.
Finkelstein, R.A., Sciortino, C.V., and McIntosh, M.A. (1983). Role of iron in microbe–host interactions. *Reviews of Infectious Diseases*, **5**, 5759–5776.

Follmann, H. (1982). Deoxyribonucleotide synthesis and the emergence of DNA in molecular evolution. *Naturwissenschaften*, **69**, 75–80.

Ford, A., and Hayhoe, J.P.V. (1976). An investigation of alternatives to hog gastric mucin as virulence enhancing agents in the cholera vaccine potency assay. *Journal of Biological Standards*, **4**, 353–366.

Forget, P., and Dervartanian, D.V. (1972). The bacterial nitrate reductases: EPR studies on nitrate reductase A from *Micrococcus denitrificans*. *Biochimica et Biophysica Acta*, **256**, 600–606.

Forsberg, C.M., and Bullen, J.J. (1972). The effect of passage and iron on the virulence of *Pseudomonas aeruginosa*. *Journal of Clinical Pathology*, **25**, 65–68.

Fridovich, I. (1975). Superoxide dismutases. *Annual Review in Biochemistry*, **44**, 147–159.

Fridovich, I. (1978). The biology of oxygen radicals. *Science*, **201**, 875–880.

Gladstone, G.P., and Walton, E. (1971). The effect of iron and haematin on the killing of staphylococci by rabbit polymorphs. *British Journal of Experimental Pathology*, **52**, 452–464.

Griffiths, E. (1983). Availability of iron and survival of bacteria in infection. In *Medical Microbiology* (Eds. C.S.F. Easmon, M. Brown and P.A. Lambert), Vol. **3**, pp.150–177. Academic Press, London.

Gutteridge, J.M.C., Rowley, D.A., and Halliwell, B. (1981). Superoxide-dependent formation of hydroxyl radicals in the presence of iron salts. *Biochemical Journal*, **199**, 263–265.

Gutteridge, J.M.C., Rowley, D.A., and Halliwell, B. (1982). Superoxide-dependent formation of hydroxyl radicals and lipid peroxidation in the presence of iron salts. *Biochemical Journal*, **206**, 605–609.

Gutteridge, J.M.C., Rowley, D.A., Griffiths, E., and Halliwell, E. (1985). Low-molecular weight iron complexes and oxygen radical reactions in idiopathic haemochromatosis. *Clinical Science*, **68**, 463–467.

Gutteridge, J.M.C., Rowley, D.A., Halliwell, B., and Westermarck, T. (1982). Increased non-protein-bound iron and decreased protection against superoxide radical damage in cerebrospinal fluid from patients with neuronal ceroid lipofuscinoses. *Lancet*, **2**, 459–460.

Halliwell, B., and Gutteridge, J.M.C. (1984). Oxygen toxicity, oxygen radicals, transition metals and disease. *Biochemical Journal*, **219**, 1–14.

Halliwell, B., and Gutteridge, J.M.C. (1985). *Free Radicals in Biology and Medicine*. Oxford University Press, Oxford.

Henderson, L.C., Kadis, S.,and Chapman, Jr., W.L. (1978). Influence of iron on *Corynebacterium renale*-induced pyelonephritis in a rat experimental model. *Infection and Immunity*, **21**, 540–545.

Hershko, C., Graham, G., Bates, G.W., and Rachmilewitz, E.A. (1978). Non-specific serum iron in thalassaemia: an abnormal serum iron fraction of potential toxicity. *British Journal of Haematology*, **40**, 255–264.

Hill, H.A.O. (1981). Oxygen, oxidases and the essential trace metals. *Philosophical Transactions of the Royal Society, London*, Series B, **294**, 119–128.

Hoffbrand, A.V. (1980). Transfusion siderosis and chelation therapy. In *Iron in Biochemistry and Medicine* (Eds. A. Jacobs and M. Worwood), Vol II, pp. 499–527. Academic Press, London.

Hofvander, Y. (1968). Hematological investigations in Ethiopia with special reference to a high iron intake. *Acta Medica Scandinavica*, **185**, Supplement 494.

Holmberg, C.G., and Laurell, C.B. (1945). Studies on the capacity of serum to bind iron. A contribution to our knowledge of the regulation mechanism of serum iron. *Acta Physiologica Scandinavica*, **10**, 307–319.

Holmberg, C.G., and Laurell, C.B. (1947). Investigations in serum copper. I. Nature of serum copper and its relation to the iron-binding protein of human serum. *Acta Chemica Scandinavica*, **1**, 944–950.

Holmgren, A. (1981). Regulation of ribonucleotide reductase. *Current Topics in Cellular Regulation*, **19**, 47–76.

Hopner, T., and Troutwein, A. (1972). Some properties of formate dehydrogenase. *Zeitschrift fur Naturforschung*, **27b**, 1075–1076.

Hurlberg, R.E., and Jacoby, W.B. (1965). Tartaric acid metabolism. *Journal of Biological Chemistry*, **240**, 2772–2777.

Iancu, T.C., and Neustein, H.B. (1977). Ferritin in human liver cells of homozygous beta-thalassaemia: ultrastructural observations. *British Journal of Haematology*, **37**, 527–535.

Jackson, S., and Burrows, T.W. (1956). The virulence-enhancing effect of iron on non-pigmented mutants of virulent strains of *Pasteurella pestis*. *British Journal of Experimental Pathology*, **37**, 577–583.

Jacobs, A. (1980). The pathology of iron overload. In *Iron in Biochemistry and Medicine* (Eds. A. Jacobs and M. Worwood) Vol. II, pp.427–459. Academic Press, London.

Jacobs, A., and Worwood, M. (Eds.) (1974). *Iron in Biochemistry and Medicine*, Vol I. Academic Press, London.

Jacobs, A., and Worwood, M. (Eds.) (1980). *Iron in Biochemistry and Medicine*, Vol. II. Academic Press, London.

Kaye, D., Merselis, Jr., J.G., and Hook, E.W. (1965). *Proceedings of the Society of Experimental Biology and Medicine*, **120**, 810–813.

Kloepper, J.W. Leong, J., Teintze, M., and Schroth, M.N. (1980). Enhanced plant growth by siderophores produced by plant growth-promoting rhizobacteria. *Nature*, **286**, 885–886.

Lankford, C.E. (1973). Bacterial assimilation of iron. *CRC Critical Reviews in Microbiology*, **2**, 273–331.

Lascelles, J. (1964). *Tetrapyrrole Biosynthesis and Its Regulation*. Benjamin, New York.

Leong, J. (1986) Siderophores: their biochemistry and possible role in the biocontrol of plant pathogens. *Annual Review of Phytopathology*, **24**, 187–209.

Light, P.A., and Clegg, R.A. (1974). Metabolism in iron-limited growth. In *Microbial Iron Metabolism: A Comprehensive Treatise* (Ed. J.B. Neilands), pp.35–64. Academic Press, New York.

Lovenberg, W. (1974). Ferredoxin and rubredoxin. In *Microbial Iron Metabolism: A Comprehensive Treatise* (Ed. J.B. Neilands) pp.161–185. Academic Press, New York.

McCandliss, R.J., and Herrmann,K.M. (1978). Iron, an essential element for biosynthesis of aromatic compounds. *Proceedings of the National Academy of Sciences (USA)*, **75**, 4810–4813.

McCord, J.M. (1974). Free radicals and inflammation: protection of synovial fluid by superoxide dismutase. *Science*, **185**, 529–531.

Markert, M., Glass, G.A., and Babior, B.M. (1985). Respiratory burst oxidase from human neutrophils: purification and some properties. *Proceedings of the National Academy of Sciences (USA)*, **82**, 3144–3148.

May, P.M., and Williams, D.R. (1980). The inorganic chemistry of iron metabolism. In *Iron in Biochemistry and Medicine* (Eds. A. Jacobs and M. Worwood), Vol. II, pp.1–28. Academic Press, London.

Miles, A.A., Khimji, P.L., and Maskell, J. (1979). The variable response of bacteria to excess ferric iron in host tissues. *Journal of Medical Microbiology*, **12**, 17–28.

Miller, R.E. (1974). Glutamase synthase. In *Microbial Iron Metabolism: A Comprehensive Treatise* (Ed. J.B. Neilands), pp.283–302. Academic Press, New York.
Morgan, E.H. (1981). Transferrin, biochemistry, physiology and clinical significance. *Molecular Aspects of Medicine*, **4**, 1–123.
Mortensen, L.E., and Chen, J.S. (1974). Hydrogenase. In *Microbial Iron Metabolism: A Comprehensive Treatise* (Ed. J.B. Neilands), pp.231–282. Academic Press, New York.
Murphy, M.J., and Siegel, L.M. (1973). Siroheme and sirohydrochlorin: the basis for a new type of prophyrin-related prosthetic group common to both assimilatory and dissimilatory sulfite reductases. *Journal of Biological Chemistry*, **248**, 6911–6919.
Neilands, J.B. (Ed.) (1974). *Microbial Iron Metabolism: A Comprehensive Treatise*. Academic Press, New York.
Neilands, J.B. (1981). Microbial iron compounds. *Annual Review of Biochemistry*, **50**, 715–731.
Neilands, J.B. (1984) Siderophores of bacteria and fungi. *Microbiological Sciences*, **1**, 9–14.
Nozaki, M., and Ishimura, Y. (1974). Oxygenases. In *Microbial Iron Metabolism: A Comprehensive Treatise* (Ed. J.B. Neilands), pp.417–444. Academic Press, New York.
Ohnishi, T., Schleyer, H., and Chance, B. (1969). Studies on non-heme iron proteins and the piercidin A binding site of submitochondrial particles from *Candida utilis* cells grown in media of varying iron concentrations. *Biochemical Biophysical Research Communications*, **36**, 487–493.
Orme-Johnson, W.H., Beinert, H., and Blakley, R.L. (1974). Cobamides and ribonucleotide reduction. *Journal of Biological Chemistry*, **249**, 2338–2343.
Osborne, T.B., and Campbell, G.F. (1900). The protein constituents of egg white. *Journal of the American Chemical Society*, **22**, 422–450.
Palmour, R.M., and Sutton, H.E. (1971). Vertebrate transferrins: molecular weights, chemical compositions and iron binding studies. *Biochemistry*, **10**, 4026–4032.
Payne, S.M., and Finkelstein, R.A. (1975). Pathogenesis and immunology of experimental gonococcal infection: role of iron in virulence. *Infection and Immunity*, **12**, 1313–1318.
Powell, L.W., and Halliday, J.W. (1980). Idiopathic haemochromatosis. In *Iron in Biochemistry and Medicine* (Eds. A. Jacobs and M. Worwood), Vol. II, pp.462–498. Academic Press, London.
Propper, R.D., and Marino, S.K. (1978). The relationship of ascorbic acid (C) and deferoxamine (DF) to non-transferrin bound iron (free Fe) in patients with thalassemia major. *Blood*, **52**, No. 5, Supplement 1, 37.
Quinn, P.J., and Williams, W.P. (1978). Plant lipids and their role in membrane function. *Progress in Biophysics and Molecular Biology*, **34**, 109–173.
Reichard, P., and Ehrenberg, A. (1983). Ribonucleotide reductase—a radical enzyme. *Science*, **221**, 514–519.
Robins-Browne, R.M., and Prpic, J.K. (1985). Effects of iron and desferrioxamine on infections with *Yersinia enterocolitica*. *Infection and Immunity*, **47**, 774–779.
Rosen, H., and Klebanoff, S.J. (1985). Oxidation of iron-sulfur centers by the myeloperoxidase–H_2O_2–halide antimicrobial system. *Infection and Immunity*, **47**, 613–618.
Sagers, R.D. (1974). Other iron-containing or iron-activated enzymes: enzymes acting on certain amino acids, amines and acetyl phosphate. In *Microbial Iron Metabolism: A Comprehensive Treatise* (Ed. J.B. Neilands), pp.445–453. Academic Press, New York.

Schade, A.L. (1963). Significance of serum iron for growth, biological characteristics and metabolism of *Staphylococcus aureus*. *Biochemische Zeitschrift*, **338**, 140–148.
Schade, A.L., and Caroline, L. (1944). Raw hen egg white and the role of iron in growth inhibition of *Shigella dysenteriae, Staphylococcus aureus, Escherichia coli* and *Saccharomyces cerevisiae*. *Science*, **100**, 14–15.
Schade, A.L., and Caroline, L. (1946). An iron binding component in human blood plasma. *Science*, **104**, 340–341.
Schroth, M.N., and Hancock, J.G. (1982). Disease-suppressive soil and root-colonizing bacteria. *Science*, **216**, 1376–1381.
Segal, A.W. (1984). How do phagocytic cells kill bacteria? *Medical Biology*, **62**, 81–84.
Siegel, L.M., Faeder, E.J., and Kamin, H. (1972). Flavin interaction in NADPH-sulfite reductase. *Zeitschrift fur Naturforschung*, **27b**, 1087–1089.
Smith, S.T., Rajagopalan, K.V., and Handler, P. (1967). Purification and properties of xanthine dehydrogenase from *Micrococcus lactilyticus*. *Journal of Biological Chemistry*, **242**, 4108–4117.
Spiro, T.G., and Saltman, P. (1969). Polynuclear complexes of iron and their biological implications. *Structure and Bonding*, **6**, 116–156.
Spiro, T.G., and Saltman, P. (1974). Inorganic chemistry. In *Iron in Biochemistry and Medicine* (Eds. A. Jacobs and M. Worwood), Vol.I, pp.1–28. Academic Press, London.
Spitznagel, J.K. (1983). Microbial interactions with neutrophils. *Reviews of Infectious Diseases*, **5**, Supplement 4, S806–S822.
Streicher, S.L., and Valentine, R.C. (1974). The nitrogen fixation (Nif) operon(s) of *Klebsiella pneumoniae*. In *Microbial Iron Metabolism: A Comprehensive Treatise* (Ed. J.B. Neilands), pp.211–229. Academic Press, New York.
Sword, C.P. (1966). Mechanism of pathogenesis in *Listeria monocytogenes* infection: I, influence of iron. *Journal of Bacteriology*, **92**, 536–542.
Takeshize, K., and Minakami, S. (1979). NADH and NADPH-dependent formation of superoxide anions by bovine heart submitochondial particles and NADH-ubiquinone reductase preparation. *Biochemical Journal*, **180**, 129–135.
Thelander, L., and Reichard, P. (1979). Reduction of ribonucleotides. *Annual Review of Biochemistry*, **48**, 133–158.
Theodore, T.S., and Schade, A.L. (1965). Carbohydrate metabolism of iron-rich and iron-poor *Staphylococcus aureus*. *Journal of General Microbiology*, **40**, 385–395.
Tiffin, L.O. (1970). Translocation of iron citrate and phosphorus in xylem exudate of soybean. *Plant Physiology*, **45**, 280–283.
Veeger, C., Dervartanian, D.V., and Zeylemaker, W.P. (1969). In *Methods in Enzymology*, (Ed. J.M. Lowenstein), Vol. 8, p.81. Academic Press, New York.
Walker, A.R.P., and Arvidsson, U.B. (1953), Iron 'overload' in South African Bantu. *Transactions of the Royal Society for Tropical Medicine and Hygiene*, **47**, 536.
Waring, W.S., and Werkman, C.H. (1944). Iron deficiency in bacterial metabolism. *Archives of Biochemistry*, **4**, 75–87.
Weinberg, E.D. (1984). Iron withholding; a defense against infection and neoplasia. *Physiological Reviews*, **64**, 65–102.
Williams, J. (1982). The evolution of transferrin. *Trends in Biochemical Sciences*, **7**, 394–397.
Williams, M.D., and Chance, B. (1983). Spontaneous chemiluminescence of human breath: spectrum, lifetime, temporal distribution and correlation with peroxide. *Journal of Biological Chemistry*, **258**. 3628–3631.
Wong, S.F., Halliwell, B., Richmond, R., and Skowroneck, W.R. (1981). The role of superoxide and hydroxyl radicals in the degradation of hyaluronic acid induced by metal ions and by ascorbic acid. *Journal of Inorganic Biochemistry*, **14**, 127–134.

Wrigglesworth, J.M., and Baum, H. (1980). The biochemical functions of iron. In *Iron in Biochemistry and Medicine* (Eds. A. Jacobs and M. Worwood). Vol. II. pp.29–86. Academic Press, London.

Wright, A.C., Simpson, L.M., and Oliver, J.D. (1981). Role of iron in the pathogenesis of *Vibrio vulnificus*. *Infection and Immunity*, **34**, 503–507.

Yamanaka, T., and Okunuki, K. (1974). Cytochromes. In *Microbial Iron Metabolism, A Comprehensive Treatise* (Ed. J.B. Neilands), pp.349–400. Academic Press, New York.

Yariv, J., Kalb, A.J., Sperling, R., Bauminger, E.R., Cohen, S.G., and Ofer, S. (1981). The composition and structure of bacterioferritin of *Escherichia coli*. *Biochemical Journal*, **197**, 171–175.

Iron and Infection
Edited by J.J. Bullen and E. Griffiths

Chapter 2

Iron proteins

A. BEZKOROVAINY

Department of Biochemistry,
Rush-Presbyterian-St. Luke's Medical Center,
1753 West Congress Parkway,
Chicago, Illinois 60612, USA

1. INTRODUCTION

Proteins containing iron are widely distributed in nature and perform a variety of functions. In an attempt to develop a classification scheme for such proteins, I have used a scheme developed by the Nomenclature Committee of the International Union of Biochemistry (1979), which provided a rational way of looking at the iron–sulphur proteins. A classification, based on both the structural and functional aspects of iron proteins, is presented in Fig. 1.

The haem proteins are perhaps the most abundant iron proteins found in nature. The haemoglobins and myoglobins are oxygen carriers, and much chemical pathology has been associated with various mutations in haemoglobin structures. The cytochrome-type proteins are concerned with electron transport, while other haem proteins may function as oxygenase-type enzymes, or serve to detoxify peroxides and the superoxide anion. Iron in haem proteins is

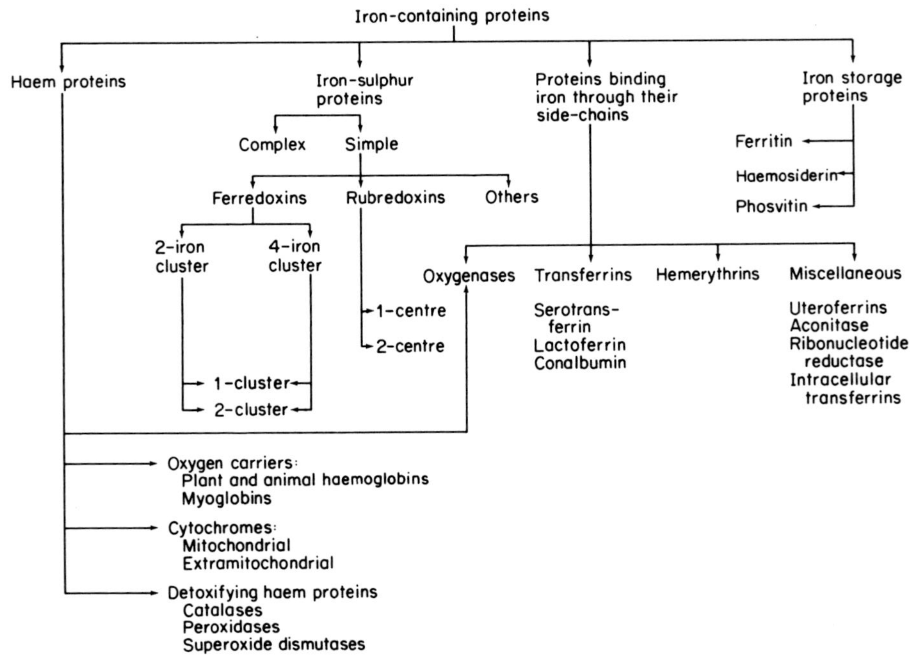

Figure 1 Proposed classification of iron proteins

associated with the protophorphyrin ring structure. In myoglobin and the haemoglobins, the iron is normally in the ferrous state, whereas in other haem proteins its oxidation state may vary under physiological conditions from the ferrous to the ferric state (Reed, 1981).

The iron–sulphur proteins are found in both the plant and animal kingdoms and their function is largely to act as electron carriers. The simpler iron–sulphur proteins are termed ferredoxins and rubredoxins. The former contain inorganic sulphur, which along with sulphydryl groups of cysteine is bonded with iron. The inorganic sulphur can be released from ferredoxins as H_2S by acid. Rubredoxins, present only in microorganisms, do not contain inorganic sulphur. In mammalian systems, ferredoxins appear as components of the oxidative phosphorylation pathway and as cofactors in cytochrome P-450 mediated reactions such as hydroxylation of steroids and vitamin D biosynthesis (Orme-Johnson and Orme-Johnson, 1978; Sweeney and Rabinowitz, 1980; Beinert and Albracht, 1982).

Ferritin and phosvitin are iron-storage proteins. Phosvitin occurs in the egg yolks of numerous species including birds, fish, reptiles and amphibians. It contains iron clusters associated with phosphoserine and threonine residues of the polypeptide chain. The iron is presumably utilized for the development of the embryo (Taborsky, 1974). Ferritin is a mammalian tissue protein (though it occurs in some plants as well) which has been well characterized. Iron in ferritin occurs in the form of iron hydroxide–phosphate micelles, and the iron is in the ferric state. The apoferritin consists of some 24 subunits with a molecular weight of near 20,000 each, there being two types of subunits. Circulating ferritin has been used in the clinical biochemistry laboratory to estimate total iron stores in the organism. Haemosiderin is considered to be a denatured and partially degraded form of ferritin (Bezkorovainy, 1980, pp. 207–269).

There are several classes of iron proteins that sequester iron through their amino acid side-chains. Haemerythrins are oxygen carriers in the haemolymph of animals that lack haemoglobin. The iron oxygenases are enzymes that catalyse the introduction of molecular oxygen into organic substances (Bezkorovainy, 1980, pp. 399–413). A recently discovered group of proteins are the purple acid phosphatases (uteroferrins), whose iron status has yet to be settled (Antanaitis, Aisen and Lilienthal, 1983). The transferrins are iron carriers found in the bloodstream of vertebrates, in egg white and in mammalian cellular secretions. They are respectively termed serotransferins (hereafter referred to as transferrins), conalbumins or ovotransferrins, and lactoferrins or lactotransferrins. They function as antimicrobial agents and, in the case of transferrin, as the means of delivering iron to various tissues (Bezkorovainy, 1980, pp. 127–206 and 271–304).

This chapter will deal only with those iron proteins which play the greatest role in the development of infection or protection against it in vertebrate species. These are the transferrins, lactoferrins, ferritins and the haemoglobins.

2. THE TRANSFERRINS

2.1 General

The discovery of the transferrins is generally associated with the observation of Schade and Caroline (1944) that raw egg white was inhibitory to bacterial growth and that such inhibition could be abolished by the addition of iron. The active component was shown to be conalbumin by Alderton, Ward and Fevold (1946), which previously had been isolated from egg white by Osborne and Campbell (1900). Schade and Caroline (1946) also obtained the first transferrin preparation from a human plasma fraction and showed that it, too, was a microbial growth inhibitor. The subsequent forty years have witnessed a remarkable development in the area of transferrin biochemistry and physiology.

The transferrins are present in numerous vertebrate biological fluids. In blood plasma, the presence of transferrin is reflected by total iron (TI) and total iron-binding capacity (TIBC) measurements, which are common clinical biochemistry tools in the assessment of human iron metabolic status (International Committee for Standardization in Haematology, 1978). Thus, the transferrins bind two gram-atoms of iron per mole of protein (molecular weight near 80,000), but in the human bloodstream, only about one-third of the transferrin iron-binding sites are occupied by iron. TI therefore is usually equal to $\frac{1}{3}$TIBC. In cases of iron overload, which may be either induced (e.g. repeated blood transfusions) or endogenous (e.g. idiopathic haemochromatosis), TI$\geqslant$TIBC, and in well-developed iron deficiency anaemia, TI$\ll\frac{1}{3}$TIBC. Lactoferrin in mammals occurs both intracellularly and in various secretions. Its main source in the laboratory has been milk, since it is present only in very

Table 1 Levels of transferrins in blood serum/plasma and other biological fluids

Protein	Animal species	Biological fluid	Concentration (mg/ml)
Transferrin	Human	Serum	2.6
	Rabbit	Serum	2.8
	Cattle	Serum	3.4
	Dog	Serum	3.0
Lactoferrin	Human	Colostrum	4.9
	Human	Milk	1.0
Conalbumin	Hen	Egg white	125

From Bezkorovainy (1980).

small amounts in plasma (Brown, Rickard and Kronenberg 1983; Estevenon and Figarella, 1983). Table 1 presents the approximate levels of transferrins in various biological fluids.

Of special interest is the presence of lactoferrin in animal white blood cells. Neutrophils contain the highest quantities of lactoferrin: an average of 17.8 μg/10^6 in human males, 10 μg/10^6 in premenopausal females and 20.8 μg/10^6 in females over the age of 50. However, other authors give rather lower figures (See Chapter 6, p.222). Some lactoferrin is also found in monocytes but none in lymphocytes (Bennett and Kokocinski, 1978).

2.2 Isolation of the transferrins

Transferrins can be isolated without undue difficulty. The properties of which advantage can be taken in the various isolation procedures available are their solubility in water (except lactoferrin in some instances) and their electric properties. The isoelectric point of human transferrin is near 5.5. and that of conalbumin is near 6 in the iron-free state. These proteins move with the beta globulins at pH 8.6. Thus, various preparative electrophoretic and ion-exchange chromatography procedures are useful, especially in combination with an initial ammonium sulphate precipitation step (Gordon and Louis, 1963; Azari and Baugh, 1967; Frenoy, Goussault and Burrillon, 1971). Another series of methods involves the use of Rivanol® (2-ethoxy-6,9-diaminoacridine lactate), which precipitates most proteins from human serum with the exception of the immunoglobulins and transferrin. The latter are then easily separated on the basis of their solubility properties or ion-exchange chromatography (Sutton and Karp, 1965; Roop and Putnam, 1967).

Procedures for the isolation of lactoferrin have utilized combinations of salting-out and ion-exchange chromatography methods (Johansson, 1969; Querinjean, Masson and Heremans, 1971). A 'single chromatographic step' method has also been reported (Blackberg and Hernell, 1980). Lactoferrin in bovine milk is much less plentiful than in human milk and it is usually associated with other fractions during isolation procedures. It may be extracted from either commercial casein preparations (Groves, 1960) or alpha lact-albumin (Castellino, Fish and Mann, 1970). Lactoferrin is less soluble in aqueous solutions than is transferrin and its isoelectric point is higher than that of transferrin.

2.3 Physical properties

The physical properties of transferrins most thoroughly studied are summarized in Table 2. The transferrins are rather compact molecules with molecular weights in the range of 75,000–80,000. Older reports have generally listed molecular weights in the 90,000 range, which was in part due to the use of

Table 2 Physical properties of the transferrins

Protein	Form	$S^{o}_{20,w}$ (s units)	$D_{20,w}$ (cm^2/s)	[η] (dl/g)	V (ml/g)	$E^{1\%}_{465}$	pI[a]	Molecular weight[b]	Shape[d]	Molecular volume ($Å^3 \times 10^4$)	Molecular dimensions	Reference
Human serum transferrin	Fe_2	5.4	5.8	0.040	0.722	0.595	—	86,000[c]	P	15.5	—	Bezkorovainy (1966)
	Fe_2	—	—	0.037	—	—	—	—	P	16.9	55 × 27.6	Rosseneu-Motreff *et al*. (1971)
	Fe_2	4.92	5.85	—	—	—	—	73,800[c]	P[e]	—	97.8 × 62.1	Roberts, Makey and Seal (1966), Wright and Baxter (1976)
	Apo	5.25	—	0.040	0.725	—	—	76,600[c]	—	—	—	Mann *et al*. (1970)
	Apo	—	—	—	—	—	—	75,000[f]	O	14.4	46.6 × 46.6 × 15.8[k]	Martel, Kim and Powell (1980)
	Fe_2	5.54	—	—	0.765	—	—	83.000[g]	—	—	—	Lundh (1973)
	Fe_2	5.0	—	—	—	0.570	5.80[h]	90,000[c]	—	—	—	Keller and Pennell (1959)
	Fe_2	5.5	5.4	—	0.725	0.57	5.60[i]	89,600[c]	—	—	—	Bearn and Parker (1966)

Hen's egg conalbumin	Apo	4.47	—	—	—	—	—	—	P	—	68 × 21	Yeh, Iwai and Feeney (1979)
	Apo	5.4	5.66	—	0.731	—	6.0	87,000[c]	—	—	—	Bain and Deutsch (1948)
Human lactoferrin	Apo	4.94	5.6	—	0.716	—	—	76,800[j]	—	—	—	Querinjean, Masson and Heremans (1971)
	Fe_2	5.02	—	—	0.726	—	—	82,600[c]	—	—	—	Haupt and Baudner (1973)
Bovine lactoferrin	Fe_2	5.55	5.75	—	0.725	0.47	7.8	86,100[c]	—	—	—	Groves (1960)

[a] Isoelectric points of diferric- and apo-conalbumins have been reported at 5.78 and 6.73 respectively (Wenn and Williams, 1968), and 5.2 and 5.6 for human diferric- and apo-transferrins respectively (Hovanessian and Awdeh, 1976).

[b] Amino acid sequence studies gave molecular weights of 79,550 for human transferrin (MacGillivray *et al.*, 1982) and 77,770 for hen's egg conalbumin (Williams *et al.*, 1982); and 84,884 for human transferrin (DeLucas *et al.*, 1978) and 81,500 for swine transferrin (Magdoff-Fairchild and Low, 1970) by the method of X-ray diffraction.

[c] Sedimentation velocity or equilibrium methods.

[d] Abbreviations: P = prolate; O = oblate.

[e] Calculated by Wright and Baxter (1976).

[f] Small angle neutron scattering.

[g] Density gradient equilibrium centrifugation.

[h] p*I* reported at 5.45 for the apo form.

[i] p*I* reported at 5.4 for the apo form.

[j] Polyacrylamide gel electrophoresis; the sedementation method gave a molecular weight of 75,000.

[k] X-ray diffraction analysis at 6 Å resolution showed molecular dimensions of 95 × 60 × 50 Å for rabbit transferrin (Gorinsky *et al.*, 1979).

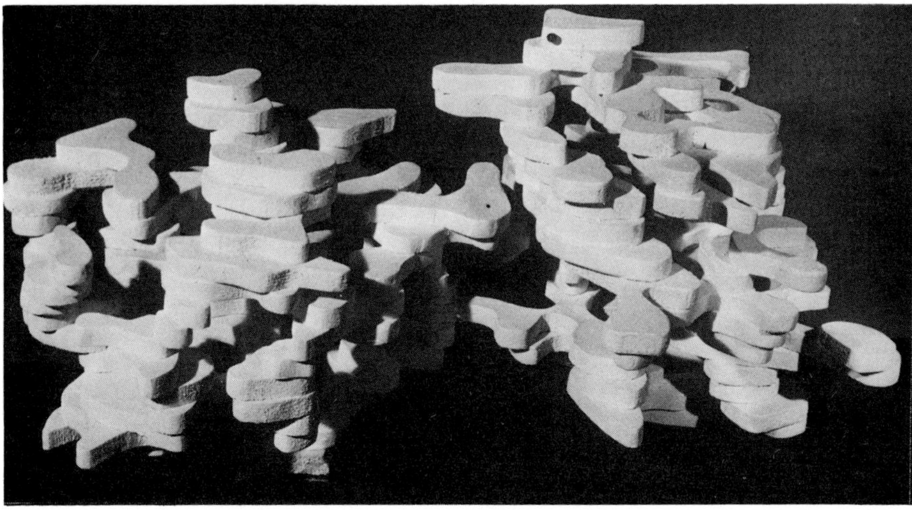

Figure 2 Three-dimensional appearance of rabbit transferrin. *From Gorinsky* et al. *(1979). Reprinted by permission of Macmillan Journals Limited*

incorrect partial specific volumes in the sedimentation–molecular weight calculations (Mann *et al.*, 1970). The exact amino acid and carbohydrate moiety sequences for human transferrin and hen's egg conalbumin are known, and these give molecular weights of 79,550 and 77,770 respectively. Thorough X-ray diffraction studies on transferrin crystals have not yet been performed. The best resolution (to 6 Å) was obtained by Gorinsky *et al.* (1979), which shows that rabbit transferrin consists of two lobes joined by a narrow polypeptide bridge (Fig. 2). Such a bilobal structure has previously been suggested by work involving proteolytic cleavage of the transferrin into half-molecules, each possessing iron-binding properties. The fact that the transferrins are not simple ellipsoids of revolution has also been shown by neutron-scattering experiments, which showed that whereas the molecular volume is 144×10^3 Å^3, the shape-independent volume is only 98×10^3 Å^3 Such differences in volumes generally indicate grooves or clefts in a protein molecule (Martel, Kim and Powell, 1980).

The fact that the transferrins contain two iron-binding sites suggested that the molecule consists of two subunits, and in fact a report appeared to that effect (Jeppsson, 1967). However, extensive work by others failed to substantiate this finding and it is now well established that transferrins are single-chain proteins (Bezkorovainy and Grohlich, 1967; Greene and Feeney, 1968; Mann *et al.*, 1970).

2.4 Primary structures

The transferrins are glycoproteins. The amino acid and carbohydrate contents of some representative transferrins are given in Table 3. The amino acid sequences of human transferrin and hen's egg conalbumin are now established (MacGillivray *et al.*, 1982, 1983; Williams *et al.*, 1982) and the messenger RNA sequence of the conalbumin is also known (Jeltsch and Chambon, 1982). Structure analysis of the human lactoferrin polypeptide chain is well under way (Metz-Boutigue *et al.*, 1981a; Mazurier *et al.*, 1983). The amino acid sequence of human transferrin is presented in Fig. 3.

Amino acid sequences of the three transferrins indicate internal homology, and, in fact, the entire transferrin molecule can be separated on this basis into two 'domains'. These are termed the 'N-terminal domain' and the 'C-terminal domain'. In human transferrin, 151 of some 362 amino acids in the two domains occupy the same position (41.7 per cent homology). This fact is believed to have been the result of a gene-duplication process, which occurred some 500 million years ago, the ancestral protein having had a molecular weight of near 40,000 (Williams, 1982b). In human transferrin, the carbohydrate is present in the form of two oligosaccharide chains linked to asparagine residues at positions 413 and 611. In hen's egg conalbumin, the single oligosaccharide chain is linked to an asparagine residue in position 473. In lactoferrin, the two oligosaccharide residues are each located in the N-terminal and the C-terminal domains. The bridge linking the two domains in the transferrins is apparently quite short: seven residues in transferrin and nine residues in conalbumin. The N-terminal domain of transferrin is thus composed of residues 1–336, residues 337–678 comprising the C-terminal domain. The corresponding domains in conalbumin comprise residues 1–332 and 342–686, with residues 333–341 accounting for the bridge. In transferrin, the bridge linking the two domains may be cleaved by thermolysin. The cleavage occurs between residues 341 and 342 (Pro–Val bond), and the N-terminal fragment with a molecular weight of about 35,600 can be isolated intact. The preparation is as expected, free of carbohydrate, which is located entirely in the C-terminal domain (Lineback-Zins and Brew, 1980).

The three types of transferrins are homologous proteins. If the amino acid sequences of human transferrin and hen's egg conalbumin are compared, some 348 out of 699 residues are found to occupy identical positions (49.8 per cent homology). The same relationship exists between human transferrin and lactoferrin. On the other hand, a 44 per cent homology exists between human lactoferrin and hen's egg conalbumin. These facts suggest that the gene-duplication process referred to above took place first, followed by the divergence of the transferrins and conalbumins and then by the divergence of transferrin and lactoferrin. The latter is thus the youngest transferrin species

Table 3 Amino acid and carbohydrate content of the transferrins (in moles/mole protein). Footnotes *a* to *g* indicate sources, molecular weights, and other comments

Component	Hen's egg conalbumin			Human lactoferrin	Human transferrin	
	a	*b*	*c*	*d*	*e*	*f*
Lys	56	58	59	47±5	58	52
His	12	12	12	11±1	18	17
Arg	28	29	31	49±5	26	23
Asp	72	46	72	65±6	45	75
Asn		32			33	
Thr	33	37	33	29±3	30	28
Ser	40	47	39	46±5	41	37
Glu	67	45	66	64±6	41	54
Gln		22			18	
Pro	26	28	27	33±3	32	37
Gly	52	52	51	48±5	50	46
Ala	55	53	54	58±6	57	56
Val	52	49	47	49±5	45	39
Met	8	11	10	6	9	8
Ile	24	27	24	15±2	16	13
Leu	49	50	47	57±6	59	55
Tyr	20	21	20	19±2	26	27
Phe	26	26	26	27±3	28	30
Cys	31	30	28	30±3	38	35
Trp	—	11	15	11±1	8	—
NAcGlu[g]	4.8	—	5.6	8.96±0.62	—	8
Gal	3.6	—	—	4.87±0.60	—	4
Man		—	3.0	—	—	6
NAcNeu	—	—	—	2.60±0.30	—	4
Fuc	—	—	—	2.86±0.64	—	—

[a] Keung, Azani and Phillips (1982); molecular weight assumed was 76,000.
[b] Williams *et al.* (1982); calculated from conalbumin DNA sequence (Jeltsch and Chambon, 1982).
[c] Same as *b* by direct analysis; carbohydrate analysis from Dorland *et al.* (1979).
[d] Metz-Boutigue *et al.* (1981a); the polypeptide chain only has a molecular weight of 73,900±7,400. Carbohydrate analysis from Spik *et al.* (1982), which assumes an overall molecular weight of 80,000.
[e] Calculated from amino acid sequence (MacGillivray *et al.*, 1983); overall molecular weight used was 79,550.
[f] Montreuil and Spik (1975); molecular weight used was 75,200.
[g] Abbreviations: NAcGlu = *N*-acetylglucosamine; Man = mannose; Gal = galactose; Fuc = fucose; NAcNeu = acetylneuraminic acid.

Figure 3 Primary structure of human serum transferrin showing internal homology between the N-terminal domain (residues 1–336) and the C-terminal domain (residues 337–678). Predicted secondary structures are designated as - - - for alpha helix, ∼∼ for pleated sheets and — for bends. *From MacGillivray* et al *(1982)*

10 20 30
VAL PRO ASP LYS THR VAL ARG TRP CYS ALA VAL SER GLU HIS GLU ALA THR LYS CYS GLN SER PHE ARG ASP HIS MET LYS SER VAL ILE
ASN GLU CYS LYS PRO VAL LYS TRP CYS ALA LEU SER HIS HIS GLU ARG LEU LYS CYS ASN GLU TRP SER VAL SER ASP VAL GLY LYS ILE
337 340 350 360

40 50 60
PRO SER ASP GLY PRO SER VAL ALA CYS VAL LYS LYS ALA SER TYR LEU ASP CYS ILE ARG ALA ILE ALA ALA ASN GLU ALA ASP ALA VAL
GLU ———— CYS VAL SER ALA GLU THR THR GLU ASP CYS ILE ALA LYS ILE MET ASN GLY GLU ALA ASP ALA MET
370 380

70 80 90
THR LEU ASP ALA GLY LEU VAL TYR ASP ALA TYR LEU ALA PRO ASN ASN LEU LYS PRO VAL VAL ALA GLU PHE TYR GLY SER LYS GLU ASP
SER LEU ASP GLY GLY PHE VAL TYR ILE ALA ——— GLY LYS CYS GLY LEU VAL PRO VAL LEU ALA GLU ASN TYR ASN LYS SER ASP ASP
390 400 410

100 110
——— PRO GLU THR PHE TYR TYR ALA VAL ALA VAL VAL LYS LYS — ASP SER GLY PHE GLN MET ASN GLN LEU ARG GLY LYS
CYS GLU GLN THR PRO ALA ASP GLY TYR PHE ALA VAL ALA VAL VAL LYS LYS SER ALA SER ASP LEU THR TRP ASP ASN LEU LYS GLY LYS
420 430 440

120 130 140
LYS SER CYS HIS THR GLY LEU GLY ARG SER ALA GLY TRP ASN ILE PRO ILE GLY LEU LEU TYR CYS ASP LEU PRO GLU PRO ARG LYS PRO
LYS SER CYS HIS THR ALA VAL GLY ARG THR ALA GLY TRP ASN ILE PRO MET GLY LEU LEU TYR ASN LYS ILE ASN HIS CYS ARG PHE ASP
450 460 470

150 160 170
LEU GLU LYS ALA VAL ALA ASN PHE PHE SER GLY SER CYS ALA PRO CYS ALA ASP GLY THR ASP PHE PRO GLN LEU CYS GLN LEU CYS PRO
——— GLU PHE PHE SER GLU GLY CYS ALA PRO ——— GLY SER LYS LYS ASP SER SER LEU CYS LYS LEU CYS MET
480 490

180 190 200
GLY CYS GLY ——— CYS SER THR LEU ASP ——— GLU TYR PHE GLY TYR SER GLY ALA PHE LYS CYS LEU LYS ASP GLY ALA GLY
GLY SER GLY LEU ASN LEU CYS GLU PRO ASN ASN LYS GLU GLY TYR TYR GLY TYR THR GLY ALA PHE ARG CYS LEU — VAL GLU LYS GLY
500 510 520

210 220
ASP VAL ALA PHE VAL LYS HIS SER THR ILE PHE GLU ASN LEU ALA ASN LYS ——— ALA ASP ARG ASP GLN TYR
ASP VAL ALA PHE VAL LYS HIS GLN THR VAL THR GLN ASN PRO GLY GLY LYS ASN PRO ASP TRP PRO ALA LYS ASP LEU ASN GLU LYS TYR
530 540 550

230 240 250
GLU LEU LEU CYS LEU ASP ASN THR ARG LYS PRO VAL GLN ASP TYR LYS ASP CYS HIS LEU ALA GLU VAL PRO SER HIS THR VAL VAL ALA
ASN GLU LEU CYS LEU ASP GLY THR ARG LYS PRO VAL GLN GLU TYR ALA ASN CYS HIS LEU ALA ARG ALA PRO ASN HIS ALA VAL VAL THR
560 570 580

260 270 280
ARG SER MET GLY GLY LYS GLU ASP LEU ILE TRP GLU LEU LEU ASN GLN ALA GLN GLU HIS PHE GLY LYS ASP LYS SER LYS GLU PHE GLN
ARG LYS ASP ——— LYS GLU ALA CYS VAL HIS LYS ILE LEU ARG GLN GLN GLN HIS LEU PHE GLY SER ASN VAL THR ASP CYS SER GLY
590 600 610

290 300 310
LEU PHE ——— SER SER PRO HIS GLY LYS ASN LEU LEU PHE LYS ASP SER ALA HIS GLY PHE LEU LYS VAL PRO PRO ARG MET ASN ALA
ASN PHE CYS LEU PHE ARG SER GLU THR LYS ASP LEU LEU PHE ARG ASP ASP THR VAL CYS LEU ALA LYS LEU HIS ASP ARG ASN THR TYR
620 630 640

320 330 336
LYS MET TYR LEU GLY TYR GLU TYR VAL THR ALA ILE ARG ASN LEU ARG GLU GLY THR CYS ——— PRO GLU ALA PRO THR ———
GLU LYS TYR LEU GLY GLN GLU TYR VAL LYS ALA VAL GLY ASN LEU ARG LYS CYS SER THR SER SER LEU LEU GLU ALA CYS THR PHE ARG
650 660 670

ARG PRO
678

from the evolutionary point of view. It has also recently been shown that an homology exists between caeruloplasmin and the transferrins. This is especially clear when copper-containing fragments of caeruloplasmin and certain lactoferrin fragments are compared (Metz-Boutigue *et al.*, 1981b).

Disulphide linkages in the transferrins have been located by the isolation and sequencing of cystine-containing fragments. Though differences among the transferrins do exist, for the most part the number and positions of these linkages are the same for all transferrins. Figure 4 indicates a rope model of hen's egg conalbumin constructed on the basis of such cystine-containing peptide sequences. The shapes of transferrin and lactoferrin are believed to be quite similar to that shown in Fig. 4 (Mazurier *et al.*, 1983). Thus, the overall structure of the transferrin group of proteins deduced from amino acid sequencing and positioning of disulphide bonds is remarkably similar to that synthesized from X-ray diffraction data (Gorinsky *et al.*, 1979).

The transferrins are glycoproteins containing hexoses, *N*-acetylglucosamine,

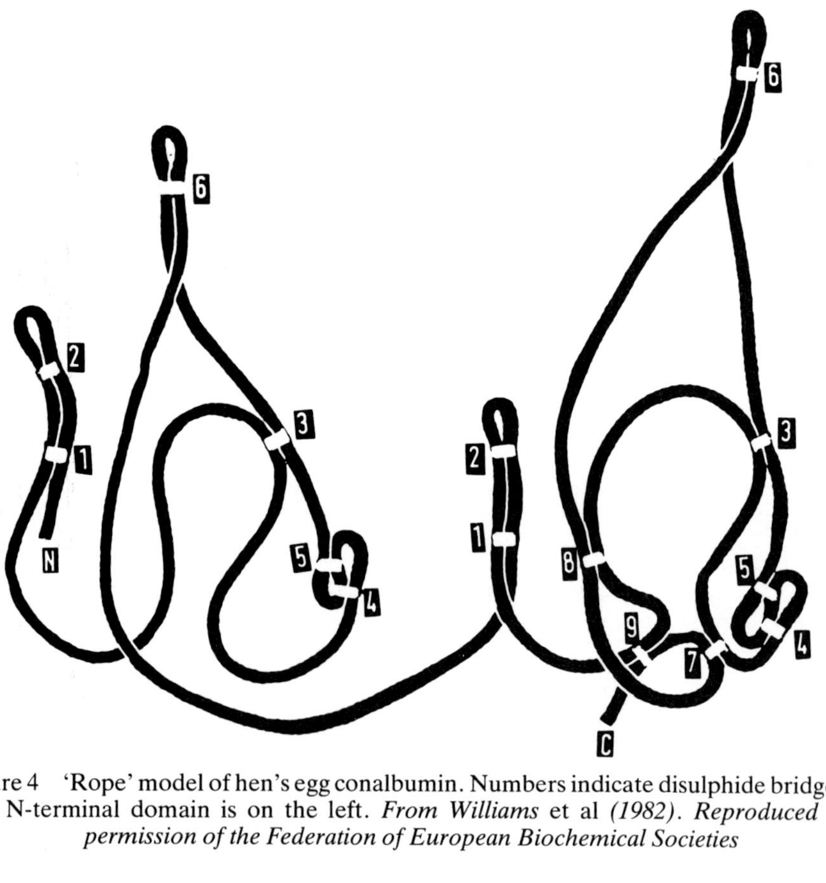

Figure 4 'Rope' model of hen's egg conalbumin. Numbers indicate disulphide bridges. The N-terminal domain is on the left. *From Williams* et al *(1982). Reproduced by permission of the Federation of European Biochemical Societies*

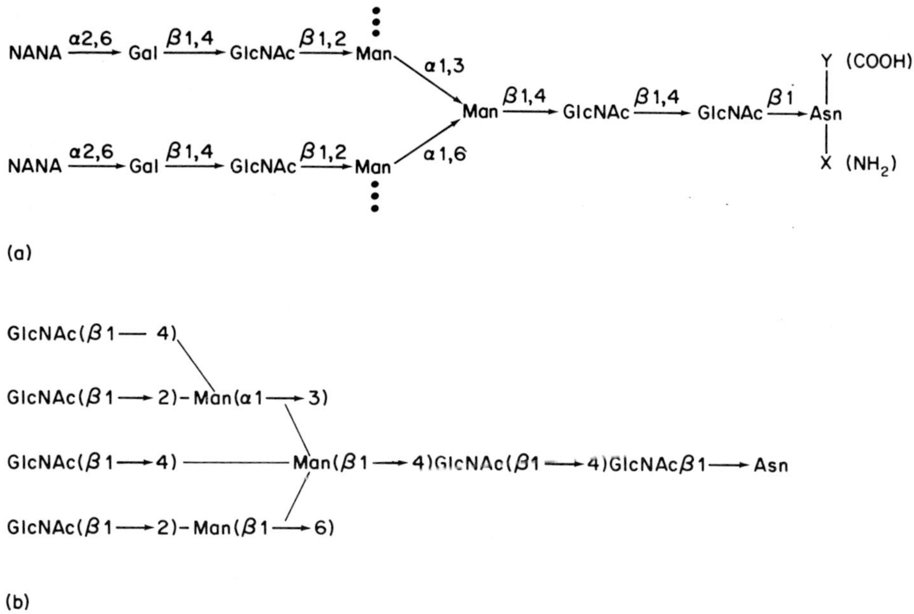

Figure 5 Structures of the carbohydrate moieties of (a) human serum transferrin and (b) hen's egg conalbumin. Dotted line in (a) indicates possible locations of additional sialic acid–Gal–GlcNAc units (*Wong* et al., *1978*). (a) *From Spik* et al *(1975)*. (b) *From Dorland* et al (1979). Reproduced by permission of the Federation of European Biochemical Societies

fucose and sialic acid (see Table 3). As has been stated previously, the carbohydrate moiety in the form of oligosaccharide chains is attached to specific asparagine residues in the C-terminal domains of transferrin and conalbumin: two such chains in transferrin and one in conalbumin. The two oligosaccharide chains in lactoferrin are each present in the N- and C-terminal domains.

The structures of the two oligosaccharide chains of transferrin (Spik *et al.*, 1975) and that of hen's egg conalbumin (Dorland *et al.*, 1979) are given in Fig. 5. The two oligosaccharide units of lactoferrin are similar to that of transferrin; however, there exists a polydisperity from one molecule to another (Matsumoto *et al.*, 1982; Spik *et al.*, 1982) based on the position of fucose as well as the presence or absence of sialic acid on one or both antennae of the oligosaccharide chain. The specific function of the carbohydrate units in transferrin physiology is unknown.

The two-domain structure of the transferrins had been anticipated more than a decade before the evidence was unambiguously established by primary structure studies. Thus Greene and Feeney (1968) proposed that the transferrins had arisen through a gene-duplication process and that the two halves of the transferrin molecule should be very similar, if not identical. Shortly thereafter reports on the partial fragmentation of the transferrins using limited proteolysis began to appear. All transferrins thus tested were susceptible to limited proteolysis yielding either the C-terminal or the N-terminal half-molecule, or both, under various sets of conditions. Such work to the end of 1979 has been summarized by Bezkorovainy (1980, p. 185). One recent application of the limited cleavage technique has been the testing of the hypothesis that the modern transferrins are the descendants of a primitive transferrin with a molecular weight of 40,000. The N- and C-terminal half-molecules of hen's egg conalbumin were injected into mice, but were rapidly cleared by the kidneys in contrast to the intact conalbumin. It is argued on the basis of these experiments that the ancestral protein could not have been a serum protein, and was most probably a plasma membrane metal ion receptor (Williams, Grace and Williams, 1982). It has also been speculated that the need for a gene-duplication process was dictated by a need to have an iron-carrying plasma protein that would not be cleared by the kidneys (Zak, Leibman and Aisen, 1983).

2.5 Secondary structure

The secondary structure of transferrins has been studied by analysing their circular dichroic and optical rotatory dispersion spectra. In hen's egg conalbumin, some 11 per cent of the amino acid residues are in the alpha helical conformation, 32 per cent in the form of pleated sheets and the rest as random coil (Yeh, Iwai and Feeney, 1979). Human ferro- and apotransferrins and lactoferrins have approximately 20 per cent alpha helix, 65 per cent pleated sheet and 15 per cent random coil conformations (Mazurier *et al.*, 1976). MacGillivray *et al.* (1982) have attempted to predict the secondary structure of human transferrin from its amino acid sequence. They found that some 14 per cent of the amino acid residues have a high probability of being in the alpha helical conformation, some 10 per cent in the random coil state and the rest presumably in the pleated sheet conformation or in the form of bends. There are more than a dozen alpha helical regions predicted. Direct determination of the secondary structures of the two domains of hen's egg conalbumin was carried out by Keung, Azari and Phillips (1982). These workers were able to cleave iron-saturated conalbumin into the C- and the N-terminal domains with immobilized subtilisin. Each fragment had a molecular weight of near 39,000. Circular dichroic analysis of the intact protein and both halves revealed, 7, 4 and 8 per cent alpha helix in intact conalbumin, the N-terminal domain and the C-terminal domain respectively. The corresponding pleated sheet components were 46, 46 and 45 per cent, the rest of the amino acid residues being in the random coil state. These values are somewhat off the mark in regard to the theoretical predictions mentioned above. The secondary structural characterization of the transferrins must thus await a detailed X-ray diffraction study of suitably crystallized proteins. In view of the availability of their primary structures, such work should now receive a much needed impetus.

2.6 Metal-binding characteristics

The transferrins bind two atoms of ferric iron per molecule of protein. When iron is bound, the protein acquires the typical salmon-pink colour, the intensity of which is proportional to the degree of saturation with iron. The absorbance of the fully saturated protein is close to 0.5 at the absorption maximum of 460 nm. It is important to check the maximum, since partially denatured transferrins, or transferrins that bind iron non-specifically (e.g. in the form of ferric hydroxide micelles), give absorption maxima at lower wavelengths. Absorbance at 280 nm increases upon the binding of iron from 10–11 to approximately 14. A typical titration curve of human apotransferrin with iron is shown in Fig. 6.

Ferric iron cannot be presented to transferrin for binding in the 'free' state for two reasons: first, binding takes place at pH values around neutrality, at which point the ferric iron exists in the form of the insoluble ferric hydroxide;

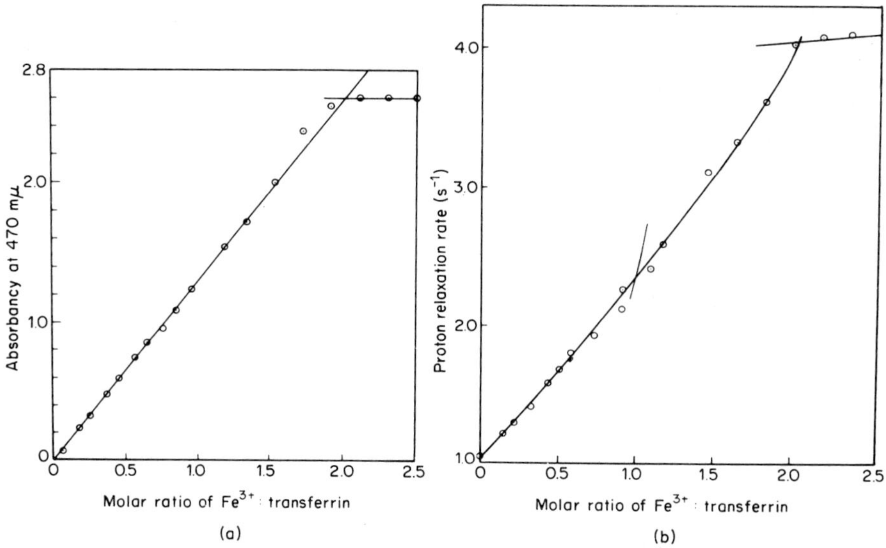

Figure 6 Titration of human serum transferrin with iron, where the iron–protein stoichiometry is indicated by (a) absorbancy or (b) proton relaxation. *From Aisen, Leibman and Reich (1966). Reproduced by permission of The American Society of Biological Chemistry, Inc.*

second, non-specific binding of such ferric hydroxide by the transferrins is possible. Ferric iron must therefore be presented in combination with a small molecular weight chelator such as citrate or nitrilotriacetate. The latter has been routinely used in most laboratories. The reaction between apotransferrin and iron chelate is apparently biphasic and involves a transient intermediate complex. This was shown spectrophotometrically using apotransferrin and iron–acetohydroxamic acid complex (Cowart, Kojima and Bates, 1982). The reactions may be summarized as follows, where TRF is transferrin and $Fe^{3+}(AHA)_3$ is the iron–acetohydroxamic acid complex:

$$TRF + HCO_3^- \rightleftharpoons TRF - CO_3^{2-} + H^+$$

$$Fe^{3+}(AHA)_3 \rightleftharpoons Fe^{3+}(AHA)_2 + AHA$$

$$Fe^{3+}(AHA)_2 + TRF - CO_3^{2-} \rightleftharpoons AHA\text{–}Fe^{3+}\text{–}TRF\text{–}CO_3^{2-} + AHA$$

$$AHA\text{–}Fe^{3+} - TRF - CO_3^{2-} \rightleftharpoons [Fe^{3+}\text{–}TRF\text{–}CO_3^{2-}]\ \text{open} + AHA$$

$$[Fe^{3+} - TRF - CO_3^{2-}]\ \text{open} \rightleftharpoons [Fe^{3+} - TRF - CO_3^{2-}]\ \text{closed}$$

This reaction series proposes that the conformation of apotransferrin is maintained until the penultimate step, at which time, following the loss of the last AHA molecule, the conformation changes to that of the iron-laden transferrin (see below).

When iron is bound by the transferrins, three protons are released per iron atom bound. The iron-laden proteins thus become more acidic than the iron-free proteins. The isoelectric point difference is depicted in Table 2 and its footnotes. Note, however, that the binding of other metals by the transferrins

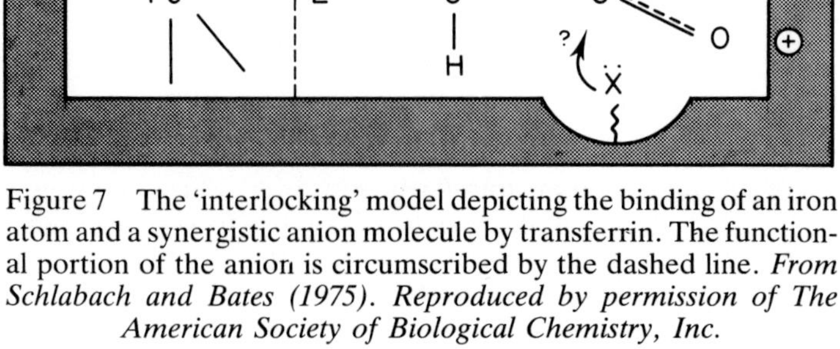

Figure 7 The 'interlocking' model depicting the binding of an iron atom and a synergistic anion molecule by transferrin. The functional portion of the anion is circumscribed by the dashed line. *From Schlabach and Bates (1975). Reproduced by permission of The American Society of Biological Chemistry, Inc.*

may be accompanied by the release of only two protons per atom bound (Gelb and Harris, 1980).

The binding of iron by the transferrins is accompanied by the binding of an anion on a 1:1 molar basis. Presumably this precedes the binding of iron, as shown by the above equations. Physiologically, this anion, termed the 'synergistic' anion, is carbonate. However, under laboratory conditions, other anions can be utilized (Schlabach and Bates, 1975). Iron is not bound in the absence of carbonate or another anion. An 'interlocking' model for the binding of the synergistic anion and iron has been proposed, where one of the iron ligands becomes the carbonate molecule. This model is depicted in Fig. 7.

The transferrins may be saturated with iron by using ferrous iron salts. The ferrous form must of course be oxidized in order to yield the typical iron-transferrin complex. It has been proposed that this oxidation is carried out through the action of the transferrin molecule itself, and it is said to possess ferroxidase activity. Ferrous iron is first loosely bound to transferrin, following which it is oxidized with O_2 or another oxidant, after which it is bound specifically to the appropriate binding sites (Bates, Workmann and Schlabach, 1973).

2.7 The iron-binding ligands

Since the transferrins do not contain protoporphyrin-type prosthetic groups, iron binding must be achieved via their amino acid side-chains. Spectrophotometric titration experiments and the fact that protons are released when iron interacts with transferrins pointed to tyrosine side-chains as being one ligand type involved in iron binding. Eventually electron spin resonance methodology was applied to the transferrins, identifying the phenolic residues as well as nitrogen-containing residues as being involved in the chelation of iron. A model was proposed by Windle *et al* (1963) to account for these findings. It presented the iron-binding centre as an octahedral structure with iron being coordinated to three phenolic and two nitrogen-containing side-chains, with the sixth ligand being the synergistic anion. Copper was visualized as forming a planar structure with four rather than six ligands. Its binding by the transferrins is known to release only two protons. This model has served well as a working hypothesis for a number of years, though evidence now exists that only two rather than three phenolic residues are coordinated with iron. Periodate, which has a peculiar affinity for phenolic residues at the transferrin iron-binding sites, oxidizes only four or five tyrosyl residues per apoprotein molecule. These are largely protected in metal-saturated transferrins (Geoghegan, Dallas and Feeney 1980; Penner *et al.*, 1983). Moreover, using ethylenebis ((*O*-hydroxyphenyl) glycine), a model compound in spectrophotometric studies of transferrins, Pecoraro *et al.* (1981) have shown that only two phenolic side-chains are coordinated with iron. They propose that each iron atom is coordinated with two tyrosine and two histidine side-chains, one synergistic anion, and either a water molecule or a hydroxide anion.

The iron-binding ligands of the transferrins have also been identified by chemical modification methods. Though it is extremely important to distinguish iron-binding alterations brought about by the modification of specific iron-binding sites from those caused by non-specific denaturation, chemical modification techniques under carefully controlled conditions may yield valuable information on the chemical properties of proteins. Early attempts at chemical modification were carried out by various groups (e.g. Komatsu and Feeney, 1967; Line, Grohlich and Bezkorovainy, 1967; Phillips and Azari, 1972), and these were able to confirm the idea that iron is bound via phenolic and imidazole residues in the transferrins. These have also consistently demonstrated that a certain number of tyrosine and histidine side-chains are protected against chemical modification in the iron-laden but not the iron-free states. More recent chemical modification studies have focused on the differences between the two iron-binding sites.

As was stated above, the exact number of each amino acid side-chain involved in the binding of iron is not certain; nor do we know exactly which amino acids in the transferrin sequences are at the iron-binding site, though some educated guesses have been made. Thus Williams (1982a) has determined that the tyrosine side-chains that are protected against nitration by tetranitromethane in the iron-laden conalbumin are located in positions 42, 82, 92, 188, 191, 319, 415, 431, 521 and 524. Eight of these lie in the 'conserved' regions: positions 82, 92, 188, and 191 in the N-terminal domain and 415, 431, 521 and 524 in the C-terminal domain. Arguing from a strictly theoretical point of view, assuming that the iron-binding ligands are the same in all three types of transferrins (i.e. they have been conserved during the course of evolution), Chasteen (1983) has proposed that at least in the N-terminal domain of the human transferrin molecule, a 'pocket' exists where His 207, His 249, His 219, Arg 124, Tyr 185 and Tyr 188 are close together in space. In this pocket, the synergistic anion is possibly bound to Arg 124, and two of the histidines and both tyrosines are coordinated with iron. The pocket is stabilized by a disulphide linkage between Cys 117 and Cys 194. A similar conclusion was reached by Mazurier *et al.* (1983), who proposed as iron-binding sites the so-called ND2 region (approximately residues 110–230) and the CD2 region (approximately residues 448–570) in human transferrin. More direct evidence for the involvement of specific imidazole residues was provided by Shewale and Brew (1982), who looked for decreases in reactivities of lysyl residues towards acetic anhydride as iron was bound by transferrin. Most significant changes occurred with Lys 206 and 534, which are located near His 207 and 535 respectively and which may therefore be implicated in the binding of iron. The two metal-binding sites of human trasferrin are some 42 Å apart (Zweier, 1983).

2.8 Nature of the iron-binding sites

It was believed for many years that the two iron-binding sites of the transferrins were independent and equivalent (e.g. Aisen, Leibman and Reich, 1966). However, it is now well established that the two iron-binding sites are not chemically and physically equivalent. The first indication that this was the case came from chemical modification studies (Line, Grohlich and Bezkorovainy, 1967). Later spectroscopic evidence using electron spin resonance techniques and transferrins carrying such metals as chromium, gallium and iron, or combinations of these, supported this view. More convincing spectroscopic evidence in favour of the inequality of the two sites was obtained using iron-carrying half-molecules of the transferrins. Thus, Zak, Leibman and Aisen (1983) described the preparation of the N-terminal domain of transferrin by thermolysin digestion of the iron-saturated protein. This fragment was subjected to electron spin resonance analysis, and when the spectrum was subtracted from that of the intact molecule, a spectrum differing from that of the N-terminal domain was obtained. In another investigation, Keung, Azari and Phillips (1982) measured the electron spin resonance spectra of the two domains of hen's egg conalbumin. These were decidedly different (Fig. 8), the spectrum of the N-terminal domain being very similar to that of the N-terminal domain of human transferrin. When the spectra of the two domains were added digitally, the spectrum of the intact molecule was regenerated.

The absorption spectra of the two metal-binding sites of hen's egg conalbumin have also proved to be different: the copper complexes of the N- and C-terminal domains had A_{max} of 450 and 430 nm respectively, the fully saturated molecule having A_{max} of 440 nm (Yamamura *et al.*, 1984).

A great impetus towards the preparation of transferrins labelled at one site or another was provided by the finding that the two iron-binding sites responded differently to pH changes (Princiotto and Zapolski, 1975; Lestas, 1976). Thus, iron is lost from one site at a relatively high pH of 6–7, whereas the other site is relatively pH-stable, losing its iron at pH 5–6 (Fig. 9). The acid-labile site (formerly termed site B) is located in the N-terminal domain, whereas the acid-stable site (formerly designated as site A) is located in the C-terminal domain of the transferrin (Frieden and Aisen, 1980). Another technical innovation that has fostered further work in this area has been the finding that the four forms of the transferrins, i.e. the apotransferrin, transferrin carrying iron in either the N-terminal or the C-terminal domain and the diferric transferrin, can be separated by electrophoresis in polyacrylamide gels in the presence of 6 *M* urea (Makey and Seal, 1976; Evans and Williams, 1980). A typical pattern is shown in Fig. 10. We thus have both the means for preparing transferrins labelled at only one iron-binding site and the means to determine which species of the transferrin is present in solution.

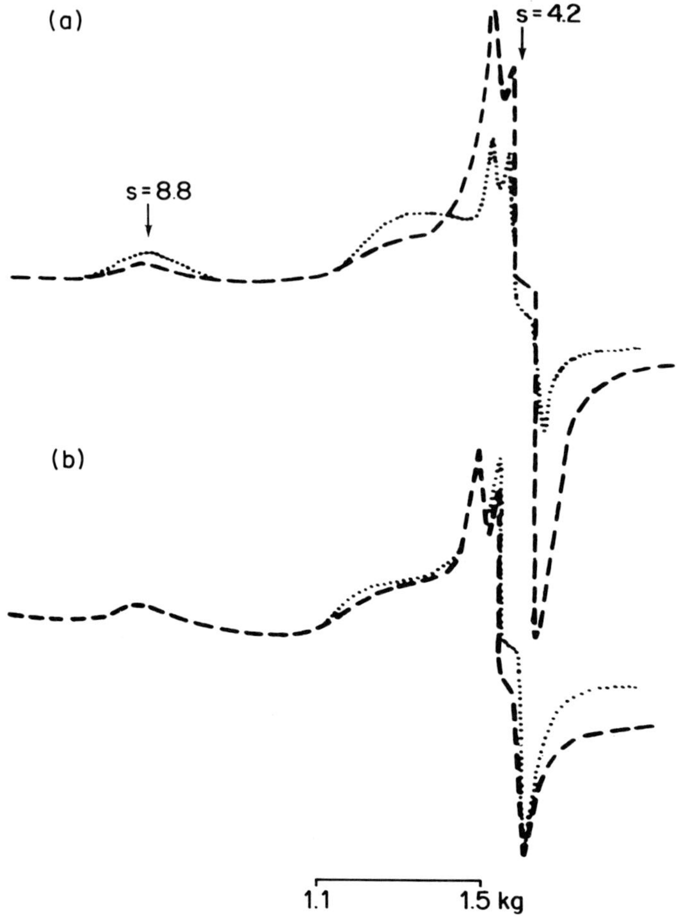

Figure 8 Electron-spin resonance spectra of hen's egg conalbumin and its N- and C-terminal fragments in the iron-saturated state. Curve A: dotted line is the N-terminal and the dashed line is the C-terminal fragment spectra. Curve B: dotted line is the intact conalbumin and the dashed line is a mixture of the two fragments. *From Keung, Azari and Phillips (1982). Reproduced by permission of The American Society of Biological Chemists, Inc.*

One of the first practical applications of the above analytical technique involved the determination of the forms of transferrin present in normal human serum (Leibman and Aisen, 1979; Williams and Moreton, 1980). The most abundant transferrin species is the apo form, followed by monoferric transfer-

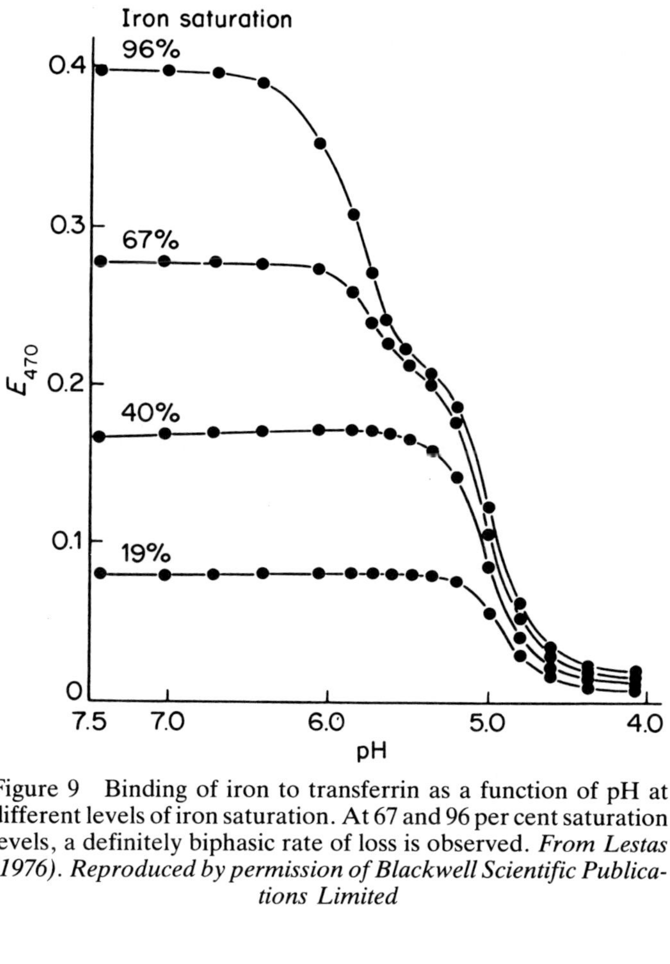

Figure 9 Binding of iron to transferrin as a function of pH at different levels of iron saturation. At 67 and 96 per cent saturation levels, a definitely biphasic rate of loss is observed. *From Lestas (1976). Reproduced by permission of Blackwell Scientific Publications Limited*

rin with the N-terminal site occupied; the diferric form is next in quantity and the monoferric form with the C-terminal site occupied is the least abundant. The predominance of the N forms is apparently maintained by a dialysable iron chelator with a special affinity for that specific iron-binding site. The physiological significance of this curious iron distribution is unknown.

The affinity of the two iron-binding sites for iron and other metals is not identical if the pH is maintained constant. Using intact transferrin in equilibrium dialysis experiments in combination with the Makey and Seal (1976) procedure, Aisen, Leibman and Zweier (1978) were able to measure the intrinsic association constants of the C- and the N-terminal domains for iron, assuming the following model:

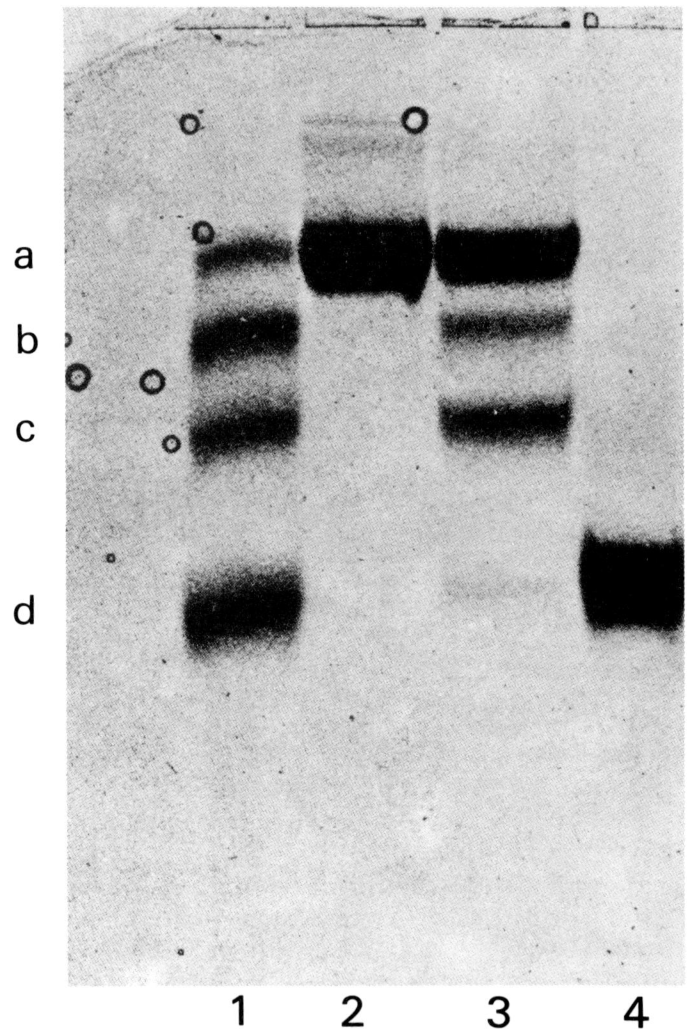

Figure 10 Electrophoresis in polyacrylamide gels and in the presence of 6 *M* urea of various forms of human serum transferrin. Band a is apotransferrin, bands b and c are monoferric transferrins with the C- and N-terminal sites occupied respectively, and band d is diferric transferrin. Tracks 1, 2, 3 and 4 are 60, 0, 30 and 100 per cent iron-saturated transferrins. *From Makey and Seal (1976). Reproduced by permission of J.D. de Vries, Excerpta Medica*

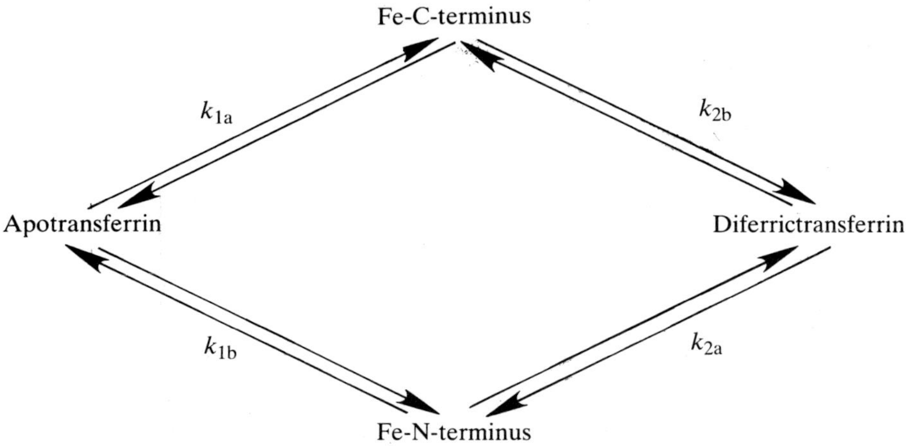

The association constants, k_{1a}, k_{1b}, k_{2a} and k_{2b}, were 4×10^{20}, 6.8×10^{19}, 1.6×10^{20} and 2.8×10^{19} respectively in the presence of nitrilotriacetate. This was confirmed by Zak, Leibman and Aisen (1983), who determined the association constant of the isolated N-terminal domain for iron to be near 1×10^{20} The affinity of the two binding sites for zinc is also different. Using the intact human transferrin, the constants were determined to be $10^{7.8}$ and $10^{6.4}$ for the C- and the N-terminal domains respectively (Harris, 1983). Thus, the affinity for iron and zinc is greater at the C-terminal domain than it is at the N-terminal domain. On the other hand, the affinity of the N site for copper and aluminium is greater than that of the C site (Yamamura *et al.*, 1984).

Finally, we may take a look at the functional characteristics of the two iron-binding sites. Human transferrin is known to transport iron into immature red cells for haemoglobin synthesis and into the liver parenchymal cells for storage. Some years ago, Fletcher and Huehns (1967) proposed that certain cell types would prefer to abstract iron from one iron-binding site of transferrin, whereas others would prefer the other site. Since then numerous publications have appeared, some confirming this, but most disproving it. Current thinking is that functionally the two iron-binding sites of transferrin are equivalent. Thus, human transferrin, labelled either in the C-terminal or the N-terminal domains donated iron equally well to human immature red cells (Van der Heul *et al.*, 1981). In fact, immature red cells prefer the diferric form and remove iron atoms in pairs from the transferrin molecule, whereas hepatocytes prefer to remove the iron from either site, one iron atom at a time (Young, 1982).

We are thus faced with the fact that the two iron-binding sites of the transferrins are not identical chemically and physically, but are identical functionally. What then is the basis for such chemical difference? Are the iron-binding ligands qualitatively or quantitatively different, or are we concerned simply with a difference in neighbouring group effects and/or the physical location of the binding site in the protein molecule? These questions remain largely unanswered, though the scanty evidence that is available points to the latter possibility. It has been shown that a histidyl residue of only one iron-binding site is susceptible to chemical modification by low concentrations of diethyl pyrocarbonate, whereas those of the other site are inaccessible (Mazurier *et al.*, 1981). It was proposed on this basis that the first binding site is fairly close to the surface, whereas the other lies buried in the protein interior. Yeh and Meares (1980) determined that the iron-binding sites of human transferrin may be located as much as 1.7 nm below the protein surface. Furthermore, a size difference in the two sites was also observed: the N-terminal site is smaller than the C-terminal one, so that it will not admit metals greater than europium to be chelated by its ligands (Harris *et al.*, 1981). Electron–nuclear double resonance spectroscopy, on the other hand, was unable to distinguish the nitrogen ligands of the two metal-binding sites of human transferrin (Roberts *et al.*, 1983). This issue might be resolved by further X-ray diffraction data.

2.9 Conformational changes in the transferrins upon binding iron

When apotransferrin reacts with iron, its overall conformation is altered. It is believed that the differences in conformation are responsible for the binding of iron-laden but not iron-depleted transferrin by the specific receptors of the immature red cell plasma membranes. The conformational change results apparently in a redistribution of charges on the surface of the protein molecule; this in turn results in the iron-saturated transferrin being eluted before apotransferrin from DEAE–cellulose columns, contrary to what would be expected on the basis of the pI's of the proteins (Lane, 1971).

Remarkably, little work has been done to determine the shapes of the transferrin molecules in their iron-free and iron-saturated forms. One of the first efforts in this direction was reported by Bezkorovainy (1966), who determined an axial ratio of 2.0 for apotransferrin and 3.0 for the iron-saturated transferrin. He assumed a prolate shape for the molecule. Rosseneu-Motreff *et. al.* (1971) reported axial ratios of 2.5 and 2.0 respectively. They, too, came to the conclusion that the molecules were prolate in shape. Further, Hendrickx *et. al.* (1968), using dielectric dispersion methods, found that the axial ratio of the iron-saturated material was near 4.9, whereas that of the apoform was 4.6. The shape was determined to be prolate. As pointed out in Table 2, work involving small angle neutron scattering (Martel, Kim and Powell, 1980) indicates that the shape of the transferrins may be that of an oblate rather than prolate ellipsoid of revolution, in which case the earlier work must be reevaluated. At any rate, we can only be certain that the loss or gain of iron by the transferrins is accompanied by a change of shape which, though not of exceptional magnitude, is sufficient to alter recognition by the plasma membrane iron–transferrin receptors of immature red cells and perhaps even hepatocytes.

3. THE FERRITINS

Ferritins are intracellular iron-storage proteins present in most animal tissues and in some plants. Their chemistry and physiology has been the subject of a number of recent reviews (Aisen and Listowsky, 1980; Bezkorovainy, 1980, Chap. 5; Jacobs and Worwood, 1980, Chap. 4; Ford *et al.*, 1984). Ferritin is water soluble, of large molecular weight and present in the extra-mitochondrial spaces of the cell. It is responsible for giving the typical diffuse blue colouration that is observed when tissues are stained with Prussian blue. Its main function is to store (or detoxify) iron, but other functions have been ascribed to ferritin as well. Thus it is held by some investigators that ferritin is the cytosolic iron carrier that delivers iron to the mitochondria of the immature red cells where iron is inserted into the protoporphyrin IX ring structure through the action of ferrochelatase to give haem. Ferritin receptors have been detected on mitochondrial membranes (Ulvik, 1982). Others have disputed this function of ferritin (Grasso, Hillis and Mooney-Frank, 1984).

The ferritin molecule can be viewed as consisting of a polypeptidic apoferritin portion and an iron hydroxide–phosphate micelle. The latter may be represented by $(FeOOH)_8(FeOOPO_3H_2)$, where iron accounts for about 57 per cent of the micellar weight. The apoferritin portion is a hollow sphere about 124–130 Å in diameter, and an inside diameter of 70–80 Å wherein the iron hydroxide–phosphate micelle may reside. The shell has a thickness of about 25 Å. The apoferritin portion of the molecule is composed of some twenty-four subunits, the average molecular weight of each being close to 20,000. Thus the molecular weight of horse spleen apoferritin molecule is close to 450,000. The apoferritin molecule can accommodate approximately 4,500 iron atoms, the inorganic micelle thus being capable of contributing some 442,000 daltons to the maximum molecular weight of ferritin.

The subunits of horse spleen apoferritin are nearly cylindrical, with a height of 55 Å and a diameter of 27 Å. Each subunit has a high alpha helical content with five distinct alpha helical segments connected by unordered polypeptide chains. The alpha helical arrays account for about two-thirds of the 163 amino acid residues present in each subunit (Banyard, Stammers and Harrison, 1978). The subunits of apoferritin are held together by physical interactions of which polar bonds play a major role. Each molecule has a number of channels that are 3–4 Å in diameter at their narrowest point connecting the apoferritin interior with the outside. There are two types of channels: six hydrophobic ones lined with leucine residues and eight hydrophilic channels lined with aspartate and glutamate residues (Ford *et al.*, 1984). It is not clear if either

Table 4 Amino acid content of the H and L subunits of human apoferritin/ferritin in residues per molecule, assuming molecular weights of 21,000 for the H species and 19,500 for the L species

Amino acid	H subunit	L subunit
Asx	28	22
Thr	8	7
Ser	11	9
Glx	30	25
Pro	4	4
Gly	12	13
Ala	17	16
Cys	2	1–2
Val	7	7
Met	4	4
Ile	6	4
Leu	23	27
Tyr	7	6
Phe	6	8
Lys	13	12
His	7	6
Arg	9	11

From Otsuka, Maruyama and Listowsky, (1981).

channel type is selective for iron or other small molecules that enter the ferritin interior.

The subunits of mammalian ferritins or apoferritins are not necessarily identical. It has been proposed that two types of subunits exist, termed the H and the L-subunits, with molecular weights of 21,000 and 19,500 respectively. They differ immunochemically, and have different amino acid compositions (Table 4). Circular dichroic spectra have shown that the L subunit has some 50 per cent alpha helical structure, whereas the H subunit has only 30 per cent alpha helix in the human material (Otsuka, Maruyama and Listowsky, 1981). The existence of the two types of subunits then provides an opportunity for the formation of both homo- and heteropolymers. Indeed, it has been proposed that the resolution of various tissue ferritins into the characteristic isoferritin patterns is due to the presence of different proportions of homo- and heteropolymers in each specific tissue. This is illustrated in Fig. 11 (Drysdale, 1977).

Iron loading of animals or cell systems causes an increase in the amount of the L type of subunit. This is consistent with the idea that those organs which have a high iron content (e.g. liver, spleen) have a predominance of the L subunits, whereas those with less iron (heart, intestine, pancreas, placenta) have predominantly the H-type subunits (Kohgo, Yokota and Drysdale, 1980;

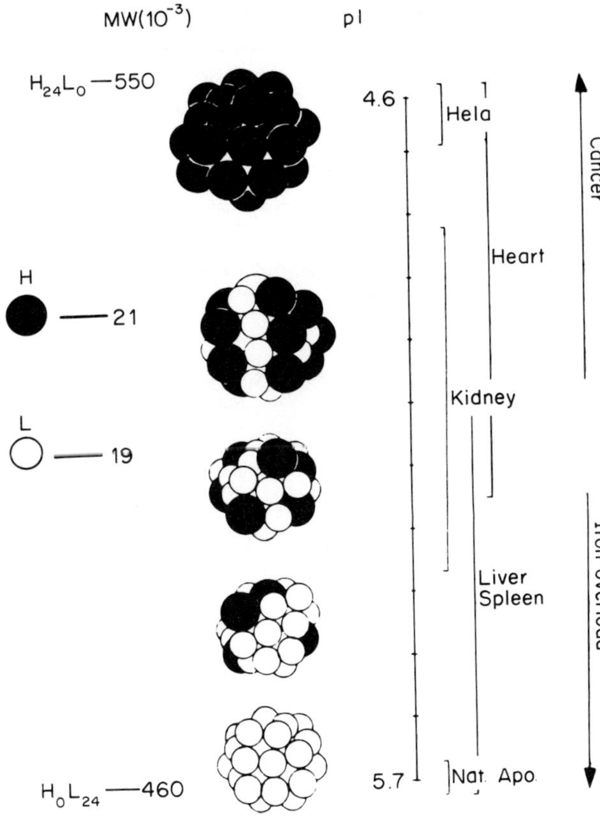

Figure 11 Composition of different types of ferritins that accounts for the isoferritin phenomenon. The two types of subunits shown differ in terms of molecular weights and isoelectric points. *From Drysdale (1977). Reproduced by permission of J.D. de Vries, Excerpta Medica*

Otsuka, Maruyama and Listowsky, 1981). Since the H-homopolymers exchange iron faster with the medium than do the L-homopolymers *in vitro*, it has been argued that the L-type ferritin is concerned primarily with long-term iron storage, whereas the H-type ferritin is concerned primarily with preventing iron-overload intoxication (Drysdale, 1982). There is evidence indicating that there may be additional types of ferritin subunits both of the H (acidic) and the L (basic) types (Asakawa and Mori, 1983; Watanabe and Drysdale, 1983).

The biosynthesis of the apoferritin/ferritin subunits is closely regulated by iron. It is well established that when an animal or even a cell culture is exposed to iron, apoferritin increases. The source is most likely both a *de-novo*

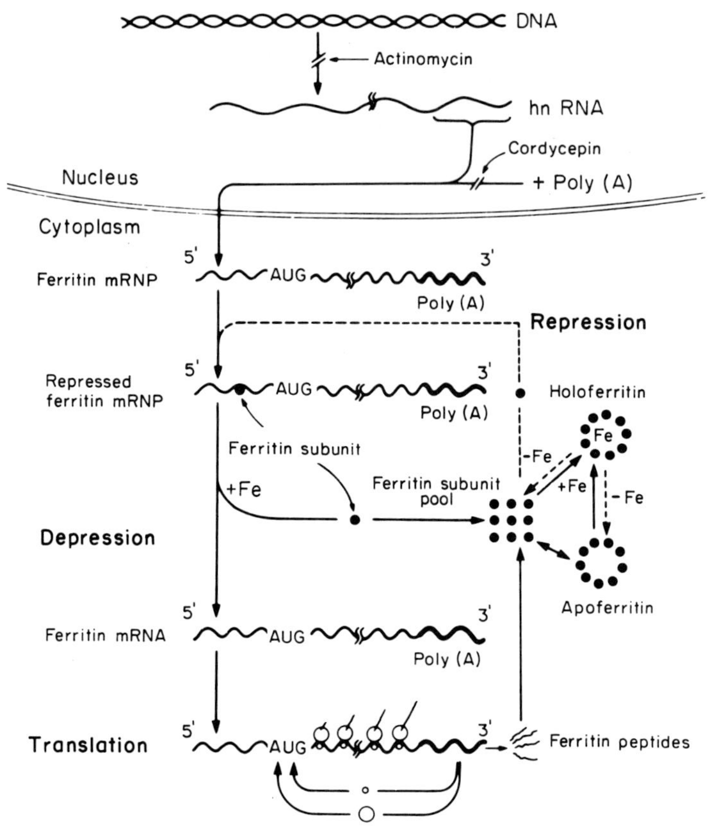

Figure 12 A hypothesis accounting for the post-transcriptional control of apoferritin biosynthesis by iron. mRNP is mRNA of ferritin repressed by ferritin subunits. *From Zähringer, Baliga and Munro (1976)*

biosynthesis and a post-translational release of apoferritin/ferritin subunits. The mechanism originally proposed by Zähringer, Baliga and Munro (1976) and which has so far withstood the test of time is presented in Fig. 12. Repressed apoferritin subunit messenger RNA is stored by the cell in combination with the subunits (the complex is termed mRNP). Under the influence of iron, the subunits are released from mRNP generating free subunits that proceed to aggregate into apoferritin, and the now depressed mRNA induces the *de-novo* biosynthesis of more subunits in the usual manner.

The uptake of iron by apoferritin is believed to involve a two-stage process (Treffry, Sowerby and Harrison, 1979), though other mechanisms have been proposed. In this model, ferrous iron enters the apoferritin molecule through one of the above-mentioned channels, and oxidation to the ferric state is initiated at specific sites on the inside surface of the apoferritin shell using molecular oxygen as the oxidizing agent. As the iron oxide–phosphate micelle continues to grow, oxidation then begins to take place on the surface of the growing micelle, and O_2 no longer becomes essential for the process. Stoichiometric measurements involving oxygen and iron incorporation into apoferritin are consistent with this model (Mayer *et al.*, 1983). The removal of iron from ferritin *in vitro* may be achieved via a reductive process with $FMNH_2$. Reducing factors must be able to travel down the rather narrow channels to the ferritin molecule interior. In view of the small size of the channels, the ability of $FMNH_2$ to do this is somewhat puzzling (Ford *et al.*, 1984).

Certain iron-chelating agents are capable of abstracting ferric iron directly from ferritin. These include certain siderophores (Tidmarsh, Klebba and Rosenberg, 1983) and compounds derived from pyridoxal isonicotinoyl hydrazone (Vitalo, Webb and Saltman, 1984). The former finding has implications in host defence mechanisms (see Chapter 3).

Small amounts of ferritin are found in the circulation, and its levels have been used in clinical biochemistry to assess the iron status of the patient. Serum ferritin levels decrease in iron-deficiency syndromes and increase in tissue iron overload (Kimber, Rudzki and Blunden, 1983).

4. HAEM-CONTAINING PROTEINS

Proteins containing haem or related ring structures are quite common in most forms of life. The haem-containing proteins include the oxygen carriers haemoglobin and myoglobin, enzymes such as catalases, peroxidases and some oxygenases, and electron carriers such as the various cytochromes. Haem proteins, especially the haemoglobins, have been the subject of extensive investigations over a number of years, and excellent reviews and monographs are available on the subject (e.g. Gould, 1971, Chaps. 12, 13 and 19; Jacobs and Worwood, 1980, Chaps. 2 and 8; Dunford *et al.*, 1981, Secs. C, F and G; Dickerson and Geis, 1983). In addition, most standard biochemistry texts have good chapters on the chemistry and physiology of haemoglobin. For this reason, no attempt will be made to present an exhaustive account of the haem proteins. Instead, a brief review of the basic properties of the haemoglobin series will be given, which should be sufficient to refresh the readers' memories on the subject and enable them to understand the role of haemoglobin or myoglobin in certain infections and in host defence mechanisms.

Myoglobin is the simplest haemoglobin-type protein. It is a tissue protein concerned with storage at O_2 for later use by the tissue. It consists of a single polypeptide chain plus the haem prosthetic group. It is believed that myoglobin is the oldest haemoglobin from the evolutionary point of view. Its shape is that of an oblate ellipsoid of revolution with dimensions of 44 × 44 × 25 Å. The molecular weight is close to 18,000 and the sperm whale variety contains 153 amino acids. The haemoglobins are oxygen-binding proteins of red blood cells. They consist of two pairs of polypeptide chains, which are termed the alpha and the beta chains. The alpha chains of human haemoglobin consist of 141 amino acid residues and have a molecular weight of 15,126, whereas the corresponding figures for the beta chains are 146 and 15,867. Each polypeptide chain is associated with a haem residue, molecular weight 616, so that the complete haemoglobin molecule has a molecular weight of 64,450. The protein portion of haemoglobin is sometimes referred to as globin. Normal adult haemoglobin described above is termed HbA_1, or if one wishes to designate its quarternary structure, $\alpha_2{}^A\ \beta_2{}^A$.

The haem residue of the haemoglobins, which is planar in three dimensions, is located in a cleft or pocket of each globin chain. It is anchored to the amino acid residues of globin largely through hydrophobic interactions involving its methyl and vinyl side-chains. Iron present in the haemglobins is of the ferrous type, and it is coordinated with the four nitrogen atoms of the protoporphyrin moiety, as well as with an imidazole residue of the globin chain. This imidazole residue is termed 'proximal' and is located in position 92 of the beta and position 87 of the alpha chains. The sixth ligand of iron is oxygen in oxyhemoglobin, which is also in contact with another imidazole residue of globin termed 'distal'. This is located in position 63 of the beta and position 58 of the alpha chains. Oxyhaemoglobin may be oxidized to methaemoblobin. The ferric iron of methaemoglobin is also coordinated with six ligands, but, rather than binding oxygen, its sixth ligand is either a water molecule or the hydroxide ion. These are also in contact with the 'distal' imidazole residue. Iron in both haemoglobin and methaemoglobin thus has an octahedral geometry. Iron in both deoxy- and methaemoglobin is in the high spin state, whereas in oxyhaemoglobin it is diamagnetic. When ferrous iron interacts with protoporphyrin IX, two protons from the pyrrhole nitrogen atoms are lost. Since the two negative charges thus generated exactly neutralize the two positive charges carried by the ferrous iron, the haem molecule carries no net charge. It thus reacts with neutral substances such as O_2 and CO. Haemin (oxidised haem), on the other hand, has a single net positive charge and therefore prefers to combine with negatively charged particles such as cyanide, formate or chloride. The structure of haem is shown in Fig. 13.

The function of the haemglobins is to bind oxygen. This association may be represented by

$$Hb + nO_2 \leftrightharpoons Hb\,(O_2)_n$$

where the term Hb is used in the generic sense to indicate either haemoglobin or myoglobin. The association constant A may be expressed by

$$A = y/(1-y)\,(pO_2)^n$$

where y is the fraction of Hb saturated with O_2, and n may (but does not

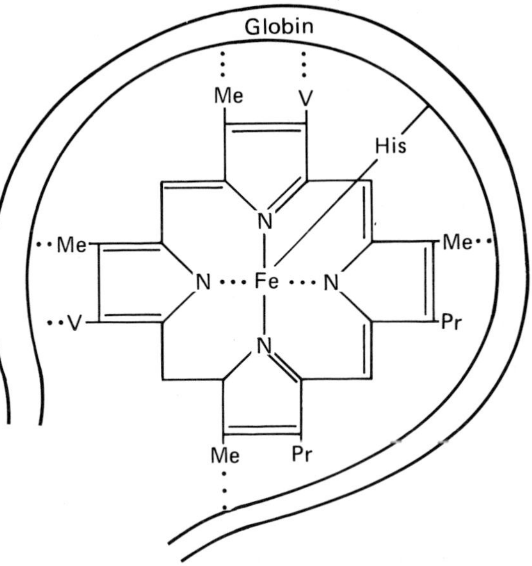

Figure 13 Haem residue of haemoglobin located in a hydrophobic pocket of the globin polypeptide chain. *From Rafelson, Hayashi and Bezkorovainy (1980). Reproduced by permission of Macmillan Publishing Co., Inc.*

necessarily) represent the stoichiometry of the Hb–O_2 interaction. It is termed the Hill coefficient. For myoglobin $n = 1$, whereas for haemoglobin $n = 2.8$. The latter figure indicates cooperation among the different subunits of haemoglobin. If plots are constructed of y (y axis) versus pO_2 (x axis), the typical O_2 saturation curves obtained are as shown in Fig. 14.

A number of factors cause the loss of oxygen by oxyhaemoglobin. Increasing concentrations of CO_2 will result in loss of O_2 if pO_2 is maintained constant. This effect is in large part due to the generation of protons as CO_2 interacts with water to give bicarbonate. Decreasing pH (increasing proton concentration) will also result in a loss of O_2. Thus, the environment that oxyhaemoglobin encounters in the peripheral tissue will favour oxygen loss. Increasing proton concentrations will in fact result in the change of a number of physical properties of haemoglobin. The protons are bound by the side-chains of His β146, Hisα122 and Valα1, resulting in an increase of the pI of the haemoglobin from 7.4 to 7.7. This proton binding is called the Bohr effect. The protonation of the above groups induces the formation of certain salt linkages, which in turn results in a conformational change in the haemoglobin molecule. The deoxyhaemoglobin conformation is termed the tight or T form, whereas that of oxyhaemoglobin is termed the relaxed or R form. The T structure is further

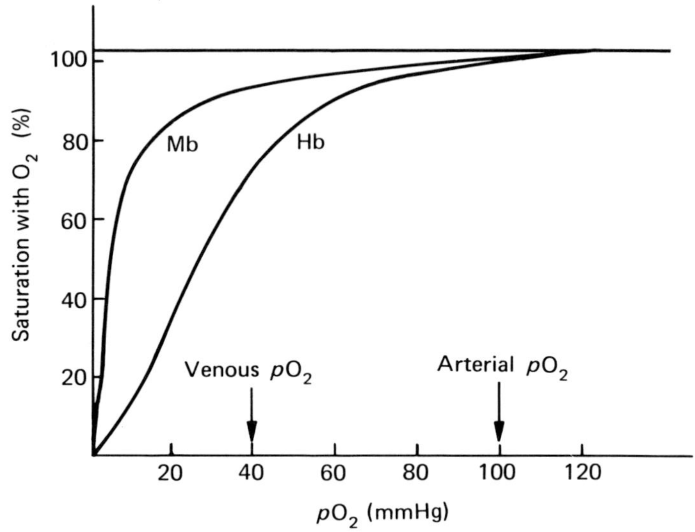

Figure 14 Oxygen saturation curves of myoglobin (Mb) and hemoglobin (Hb). *From Rafelson, Hayashi and Bezkorovainy (1980). Reproduced by permission of Macmillan Publishing Co., Inc.*

stabilized by the binding of 2,3–diphosphoglycerate. The T forms thus have low O_2-binding affinity, whereas the R forms have a high affinity for O_2.

A number of haemoglobin variants exist in human populations, which may be either physiological or the result of disease. Abnormal haemoglobins with point mutations can be classified into the following:

1. Altered solubility.
2. Increased oxygen affinity. These generally have destablized T structures, which may be due to a low affinity for 2,3–diphosphoglycerate, or altered subunit contact possibilities. Their Hill coefficients are near 1.
3. Decreased O_2 affinity, where the R structures are generally destabilized.
4. Unstable haemoglobins, which denature or precipitate easily. The reason for this latter tendency to precipitate may be a lowered affinity for haem by the globin's hydrophobic pocket or the substitution of a Pro residue for an alpha helix forming amino acid in the globin chain.
5. Methaemoglobinaemias, which are due to a propensity of the ferrous iron to be oxidized to ferric iron. This may be due to an increase in size of the haem-containing hydrophobic pocket, resulting in the entry of water which catalyses the oxidation process.

Most abnormal haemoglobins are the result of point mutations in the beta chain, which is more recent than the alpha chain from the evolutionary point of view.

Table 5 Some common deviations from HbA_1[a]

Haemoglobin	Designation	Oxygen-binding affinity	Notes
HbA_2	$\alpha_2{}^A \delta_2$	Normal	Present in normal red cells
HbF	$\alpha_2{}^A \gamma_2{}^F$	High	Foetal haemoglobin
HbH	$\beta_4{}^A$	High	Present in α-thalassaemia (HbH disease)
Hb-Barts	$\gamma_4{}^F$	High	Present in α-thalassaemia
Glycosylated Hb (HbA_{ic})	—	Normal	N-terminal Val of the beta chains carries glucose; increased in diabetics
HbS	$\alpha_2{}^A \beta_2{}^S$	Low	Present in sickle cell disease and trait; precipitates at low O_2 tension; Glu in position 6 of the beta chain replaced by Val
Hb-Gowers 1	$\xi_2 \epsilon_2$	—	Embryonic Hb, replaced by HbF after about 6 weeks of gestation
Hb-Gowers 2	$\alpha_2 \epsilon_2$	—	Same as Hb-Gowers 1
Hb-Portland	$\xi_2 \gamma_2$	—	Same as Hb-Gowers 1

[a] Hb is haemoglobin.

A number of physiologically important non-mutant haemoglobin variants are in existence. These and the sickle cell haemoglobin, the most common haemoglobin mutant, are presented in Table 5.

For host defence purposes, iron conservation and possible prevention of injury to certain tissues, the body has developed the means of sequestering haemoglobin and free haem by specific plasma proteins. The best known of such systems is the formation of a complex between haptoglobin and plasma haemoglobin. Haptoglobin is a plasma glycoprotein which exists in the form of genetically determined phenotypes controlled by two allelic genes. A great majority of individuals fall into one of three phenotypic categories termed the 1–1 (molecular weight of 100,000), 2–1, and 2–2. The 1–1 and 2–2 are homozygotes, whereas the 2–1 is a heterozygote (Javid, 1978).

Work on the stoichiometry of haemoglobin binding of haptoglobin has been largely restricted to haptoglobin 1–1. Binding is associated with a dramatic increase in the peroxidase activity of haemoglobin, which in fact serves as a basis for the assay of haptoglobin. Best evidence to-date indicates that the binding occurs as follows:

$$Hp + (\alpha\beta)^{Hb} \rightarrow \alpha\beta\text{–}Hp \text{ (intermediate complex)}$$

$$\alpha\beta\text{–}Hp + (\alpha\beta)^{Hb} \rightarrow \alpha\beta\text{–}Hp\text{–}\alpha\beta \text{ (saturated complex)}$$

Thus, haptoglobin reacts first with an αβ dimer that comes from the dissociation of haemoglobin and then completes the reaction by binding the other dimer. Final stoichiometry involves one molecule of haemoglobin bound by one molecule of haptoglobin (Nagel and Gibson, 1967; Kawamura *et al.*, 1972). The haemoglobin–haptoglobin complex is rapidly cleared by the hepatocytes, where the haem iron then enters the hepatocyte iron pool. The fractional catabolic rate for haptoglobin is 0.198 per day, whereas that of the haemoglobin–haptoglobin complex is 0.069 per minute. It has been proposed that one of the main reasons for the existence of the haemoglobin sequestering machinery in plasma and its rapid clearance is to make haem (or haem iron) unavailable for potential microbial invaders (Eaton *et al.*, 1982) (See Chapter 7).

Free haem can be bound by a specific haem-binding protein called haemopexin and by serum albumin (Müller-Eberhard and Liem, 1974). Free haem in circulation apparently originates from the breakdown of methaemoglobin, the oxidized form of haemoglobin. Haemopexin is a glycoprotein with a molecular weight of 57,000, and it binds one haem molecule per molecule of protein using two imidazole residues.Iron in the haem–haemopexincomplex is Fe(III) in a low spin state (Aisen *et al.*, 1974). Haemopexin-bound haem is delivered to hepatocytes where the haem may be degraded to bilirubin or incorporated into cytochrome P-450 The maximum amount of haem that can be bound by circulating haemopexin is about 25 mg, so that albumin serves as a backup system for binding of free haem. Not much is known about the fate of albumin-bound haem, though there is evidence, albeit indirect, indicating that such haem is transferred to haemopexin for disposal. The affinity of haemopexin for haem is much greater than that of albumin.

REFERENCES

Aisen, P., Leibman, A., Harris, D.C., and Moss, T. (1974). Human hemopexin. Preparation and magnetic properties. *Journal of Biological Chemistry*, **249**, 6824–6827.

Aisen, P., Leibman, A., and Reich, H.A. (1966). Studies on the binding of iron by transferrin and conalbumin. *Journal of Biological Chemistry*, **241**, 1666–1671.

Aisen, P., Leibman, A., and Zweier, J. (1978). Stoichiometric and site characteristics, of the binding of iron to human transferrin. *Journal of Biological Chemistry*, **253**, 1930–1937.

Aisen, P., and Listowsky, I. (1980). Iron transport and storage proteins. *Annual Review of Biochemistry*, **49**, 357–393.

Alderton, G., Ward, W.H., and Fevold, H.L. (1946). Identification of the bacteria-inhibiting iron-binding protein of egg white as conalbumin. *Archives of Biochemistry and Biophysics*, **11**, 9–13.

Antanaitis, B.C., Aisen, P., and Lilienthal, H.R. (1983). Physical chararcterization of two-iron uteroferrin. *Journal of Biological Chemistry*, **258**, 3166–3172.

Asakawa, H., and Mori, W. (1983). Possibly unique subunit(s) of human ferritins responsible for tissue specificity. *Hoppe-Seyler's Zeitschrift fur Physiologische Chemie (Berlin)*, **364**, 859–862.

Azari, P., and Baugh, R.F. (1967). A simple and rapid procedure for the preparation of large quantities of pure ovotransferrin. *Archives of Biochemistry and Biophysics*, **118**, 138–144.

Bain, J.A., and Deutsch, H.F. (1948). Separation and characterization of conalbumin. *Journal of Biological Chemistry*, **172**, 547–555.

Banyard, S.H., Stammers, D.K., and Harrison, P.M. (1978). Electron density map of apoferritin at 2.8 Å resolution. *Nature*, **271**, 282–284.

Bates, G.W., Workman, E.F., and Schlabach, M.R. (1973). Does transferrin exhibit ferroxidase activity? *Biochemical and Biophysical Research Communications*, **50**, 84–90.

Bearn, A.G., and Parker, W.C. (1966). Transferrin. In *Glycoproteins* (Ed. A. Gottschalk), p. 415. Elsevier, Amsterdam.

Beinert, H., and Albracht, S.P.J. (1982). New insights, ideas, and unanswered questions concerning iron-sulfur clusters in mitochondria. *Biochimica et Biophysica Acta*, **683**, 245–277.

Bennett, R.M., and Kokocinski, T. (1978). Lactoferrin content of peripheral blood cells. *British Journal of Haemotology*, **39**, 509–521.

Bezkorovainy, A. (1966). Comparative study of metal-free, iron-saturated, and sialic acid-free transferrins. *Biochimica et Biophysica Acta*, **127**, 535–537.

Bezkorovainy, A. (1980). *Biochemistry of Nonheme Iron*. Plenum Press, New York.

Bezkorovainy, A., and Grohlich, D. (1967). The behaviour of native and reduced-alkylated human transferrin in urea and guanidine-HCI solutions. *Biochimica et Biophysica Acta*, **147**, 497–510.

Blackberg, L., and Hernell, O. (1980). Isolation of lactoferrin from human whey by a single chromatographic step. *FEBS Letters*, **109**, 180–184.

Brown, R.D., Rickard, K.A., and Kronenberg, H. (1983). Immunoradiometric assay of plasma lactoferrin. *Pathology*, **15**, 27–31.

Castellino, F.J., Fish, W.W., and Mann, K.G. (1970). Strucutral studies on bovine lactoferrin. *Journal of Biological Chemistry*, **245**, 4269–4275.

Chasteen, N.D. (1983). The identification of the probable locus of iron and anion binding in the transferrin. *Trends in Biochemical Sciences*, **8**, 272–275.

Cowart, R.E., Kojima, N., and Bates, G. (1982). The exchange of Fe^{3+} between acetohydroxamic acid and transferrin. *Journal of Biological Chemistry*, **257**, 7560–7565.

DeLucas, L.J., Suddath, F.L., Gams, R.A., and Bugg, C.E. (1978). Preliminary X-ray study of crystals of human transferrin. *Journal of Molecular Biology*, **123**, 285–286.

Dickerson, R.E., and Geis, I. (1983). *Hemoglobin Structure, Function, Evolution, and Pathology*. The Benjamin/Cummings Publishers Company, Menlo Park, California.

Dorland, L., Haverkamp, J., Vliegenthart, J.F.G., Spik, G., Fournet, B., and Montreuil, J. (1979). Investigation by 360 MHz ^{1}H-nuclear magnetic-resonance spectroscopy and methylation analysis of the single glycan chain of chicken ovotransferrin. *European Journal of Biochemistry*, **100**, 569–574.

Drysdale, J.W. (1977). Ferritin phenotypes: structure and metabolism. In *Ciba Foundation Symposium 51, Iron Metabolism*, pp. 41–67. Elsevier–North Holland, Amsterdam.

Drysdale, J.W. (1982). Regulation of ferritin phenotypes. In *Advances in Red Cell Biology* (Ed. D.J. Weatherall), pp. 35–47. Raven Press, New York.

Dunford, H.B., Dolphin, D., Raymond, K.N., and Sieker, L. (1981). *The Biological Chemistry of Iron*, D. Reidel Publishing Company, Dordrecht, Holland.

Eaton, J., Brandt, P., Mahoney, J.R., and Lee, J.T. (1982). Haptoglobin: a natural bacteriostat. *Science*, **215**, 691–692.

Estevenon, J.P., and Figarella, C. (1983). A non competitive enzyme immunoassay of human lactoferrin in biological fluids. *Clinical Chimica Acta (Amsterdam)*, **129**, 311–318.

Evans, R.W., and Williams, J. (1980). The electrophoresis of transferrins in urea/polyacrylamide gels. *Biochemical Journal*, **189**, 541–546.

Fletcher, J., and Huehns, E.R. (1967). Significance of the binding of iron by transferrin. *Nature*, **215**, 584–586.

Ford, G.C., Harrison, P.M., Rice, D.W., Smith, M.A., Trefry, A., White, J.L., and Yariv, J. (1984). Ferritin: design and formation of an iron-storage molecule. *Philosophical Transactions of the Royal Society of London, Series B*, **304**, 551–565.

Frenoy, N., Goussault, Y., and Burrillon, R. (1971). Preparation de la transferrine du serum humain. *Clinica Chimica Acta (Amsterdam)*, **32**, 243–249.

Frieden, E., and Aisen, P. (1980). Forms of iron transferrin. *Trends in Biochemical Sciences*, **5**, xi.

Gelb, M.H., and Harris, D.C. (1980). Correlation of proton release and ultraviolet difference spectra associated with metal binding by transferrin. *Archives of Biochemistry and Biophysics*, **200**, 93–98.

Geoghegan, K.F., Dallas, J.L., and Feeney, R.E. (1980). Periodate inactivation of ovotransferrin and human serum transferrin. *Journal of Biological Chemistry*, **255**, 11429–11434.

Gordon, A.H., and Louis, L.N. (1963). Preparation and properties of rat transferrin. *Biochemical Journal*, **88**, 409–414.

Gorinsky, B., Horsburgh, C., Lindley, P.F., Moss, D.S., Parkar, M., and Watson, J.L. (1979). Evidence for the bilobal nature of differic rabbit plasma transferrin. *Nature*, **281**, 157–158.

Gould, R.F. (1971). *Bioinorganic Chemistry*, American Chemical Society, Washington, DC.

Grasso, J.A., Hillis, T.J., and Mooney-Frank, J.A. (1984). Ferritin is not a required intermediate for iron utilization in heme synthesis. *Biochimica et Biophysica Acta*, **797**, 247–255.

Greene, F.C., and Feeney, R.E. (1968). Physical evidence for transferrins as single polypeptide chains. *Biochemistry*, **7**, 1366–1371.

Groves, M.L. (1960). The isolation of a red protein from milk. *Journal of the American Chemical Society*, **82**, 3345–3350.

Harris, W. (1983). Thermodynamic binding constants of the zinc–human serum transferrin complex. *Biochemistry*, **22**, 3920–3926.

Harris, W.R., Carano, C.J., Pecoraro, V.L., and Raymond, K.N. (1981). Siderophillin metal coordination. I. Complexation of thorium by transferrin: structure-function implications. *Journal of the American Chemical Society*, **103**, 2231–2237.

Haupt, H., and Baudner, S. (1973). Isolierung und Kristallisation von Lactoferrin aus Human-Kolostrum. *Hoppe-Seyler's Zeitschrift fur Physiologische Chemie (Berlin)*, **354**, 944–948.

Hendrickx, H., Verbruggen, R., Rosseneu-Motreff, M.Y., Blaton, V., and Peeters, H. (1968). The dipolar origin of protein relaxation. *Biochemical Journal*, **110**, 419–424.

Hovanessian, A.G., and Awdeh, Z.L. (1976). Gel isoelectric focusing of human serum transferrin. *European Journal of Biochemistry*, **68**, 333–338.

International Committee for Standardization in Haematology (1978). The measurement of total and unsaturated iron-binding capacity in serum. *British Journal of Haematology*, **38**, 281–294.

Jacobs, A., and Worwood, M. (1980). *Iron in Biochemistry and Medicine*, Vol. II. Academic Press, New York.

Javid, J. (1978). Human haptoglobins. *Current Topics in Hematology*, **1**, 151–192.

Jeltsch, J.M., and Chambon, P. (1982). The complete nucleotide sequence of the chicken ovotransferrin mRNA. *European Journal of Biochemistry*, **122**, 291–295.

Jeppsson, J.O. (1967) Subunits of human transferrin. *Acta Chemica Scandinavica*, **21**, 1686–1694.

Johansson, B.G. (1969). Isolation of crystalline lactoferrin from human milk. *Acta Chemica Scandinavica*, **23**, 683–684.

Kawamura, K., Kagiyama, S., Ogawa, A., and Yanase, T. (1972). The reactive unit of hemoglobin in hemoglobin–haptoglobin complex formation. *Biochimica et Biophysica Acta*, **285**, 15–21.

Keller, W., and Pennell, R.B. (1959). Sterilization of plasma components by heat. 1. β_1 -metal combining protein. *Journal of Laboratory and Clinical Medicine*, **53**, 638 645.

Keung, W.M., Azari, P., and Phillips, J.L. (1982). Structure and function of ovotransferrin. I. Production of iron-binding fragments from iron-ovotransferrin by the action of immobilized subtilisin. *Journal of Biological Chemistry*, **257**, 1177–1183.

Kimber, R.J., Rudzki, Z., and Blunden, R.W. (1983). Clinching the diagnosis: 1. Iron deficiency and iron overload: serum ferritin and serum iron in clinical medicine. *Pathology*, **15**, 497–503.

Kohgo, Y., Yokota, M., and Drysdale, J.W. (1980). Differential turnover of rat liver isoferritins. *Journal of Biological Chemistry*, **255**, 5195–5200.

Komatsu, S.K., and Feeney, R.E. (1967). Role of tyrosyl groups in metal binding properties of transferrins. *Biochemistry*, **6**, 1136–1141.

Lane, R.S. (1971). DEAE-cellulose chromatography of human transferrin. The effect of increasing iron saturation and copper (II) binding. *Biochimica et Biophysica Acta*. **243**, 193–202.

Leibman, A., and Aisen, P. (1979). Distribution of iron between the binding sites of transferrin in serum: methods and results in normal human subjects. *Blood*, **53**, 1058–1065.

Lestas, A.N. (1976). The effect of pH on human transferrin: selective labelling of the two iron-binding sites. *British Journal of Haematology*, **32**, 341–350.

Line, W.F., Grohlich, D., and Bezkorovainy, A. (1967). The effect of chemical modification on the iron-binding properties of human transferrin. *Biochemistry*, **6**, 3393–3402.

Lineback-Zins, J., and Brew, K. (1980). Preparation and characterization of an NH_2-terminal fragment of human serum transferrin containing a single iron-binding site. *Journal of Biological Chemistry*, **255**, 708–713.

Lundh, S. (1973). Determination of the molecular weight and partial specific volume of human transferrin by means of a new two-stage density gradient equilibrium method. *International Journal of Peptide Protein Research*, **5**, 309–325.

MacGillivray, R.T.A., Mendez, E., Sinha, S.K., Sutton, M.R., Lineback-Zins, J., and Brew, K. (1982). The complete amino acid sequence of human serum transferrin. *Proceedings of the National Academy of Sciences (USA)*, **79**, 2504–2508.

MacGillivray, R.T.A., Mendez, E., Sinha, S.K., Sutton, M.R., Lineback-Zins, J., and Brew, K. (1983). The primary structure of human serum transferrin. *Journal of Biological Chemistry*, **258**, 3543–3553.

Magdoff-Fairchild, B., and Low, B.W. (1970). Preliminary X-ray crystallographic study of porcine transferrin. *Archives of Biochemistry and Biophysics*, **138**, 703–705.

Makey, D.G., and Seal, U.S. (1976). The detection of four molecular forms of human transferrin during the iron binding process. *Biochimica et Biophysica Acta*, **453**, 250–256.

Mann, K.G., Fish, W.W., Cox, A.C., and Tanford, C. (1970). Single-chain nature of human serum transferrin. *Biochemistry*, **9**, 1348–1354.

Martel, P., Kim, S.M., and Powell, B.M. (1980). Physical characteristics of human transferrin from small angle neutron scattering. *Biophysical Journal*, **31**, 371–380.

Matsumoto, A., Yoshima, H., Takasaki, S., and Kobata, A. (1982). Structural study of the sugar chains of human lactoferrin: finding of four novel complex-type asparagine-linked sugar chains. *Journal of Biochemistry*, **91**, 143–155.

Mayer, D.E., Rohrer, J.S., Schoeller, D.A., and Harris, D.C. (1983). Fate of oxygen during ferritin iron incorporation. *Biochemistry*, **22**, 876–880.

Mazurier, J., Aubert, J. -P., Loucheux-Lefevre, M. -H., and Spik, G. (1976). Comparative circular dichroism studies of iron-free and iron-saturated forms of human serotransferrin and lactotransferrin. *FEBS Letters*, **66**, 238–242.

Mazurier, J., Leger, D., Tordera, V., Montreuil, J., and Spik, G. (1981). Comparative study of the iron-binding properties of transferrins. Differences in the involvement of histidine residues as revealed by carboxyethylation. *European Journal of Biochemistry*, **119**, 537–543.

Mazurier, J., Metz-Boutigue, M. -H., Jolles, J., Spik, G., Montreuil, J., and Jolles, P. (1983). Human lactotransferrin: molecular, functional, and evolutionary comparisons with human transferrin and ovotransferrin. *Experientia*, **39**, 135–141.

Metz-Boutigue, M.-H., Mazurier, J., Jolles, J., Spik, G., Montreuil, J., and Jolles, P. (1981a). The present state of the human lactotransferrin sequence. Study and alignment of the cyanogen bromide fragments and characterization of N- and C-terminal domains. *Biochimica et Biophysica Acta*, **670**, 243–254.

Metz-Boutigue, M. -H., Jolles, J., Mazurier, J., Spik, G., Montreuil J. and Jolles, P. (1981b). Structural relatedness between human lactotransferrin and human ceruloplasmin. *FEBS Letters*, **132**, 239–242.

Montreuil, J., and Spik, G. (1975). Comparative studies of carbohydrate and protein moieties of human serotransferrin and lactotransferrin. In *Proteins of Iron Storage and Transport in Biochemistry and Medicine* (Ed. R.R. Crichton), pp. 27–38. North Holland, Amsterdam.

Müller-Eberhard, U., and Liem, H.H., (1974). Hemopexin, the heme-binding serum β-glycoprotein. In *Structure and Function of Plasma Proteins* (Ed. A.C. Allison), pp. 35–53. Plenum Press, London.

Nagel, R.L., and Gibson, Q.H. (1967). Kinetics and mechanism of complex formation between hemoglobin and haptoglobin. *Journal of Biological Chemistry*, **242**, 3428–3434.

Nomenclature Committee of the International Union of Biochemistry (1979). Nomenclature of iron–sulfur proteins. Recommendations. *European Journal of Biochemistry*, **93**, 427–430.

Orme-Johnson, W.H., and Orme-Johnson, N.R. (1978). Overview of iron-sulfur proteins. *Methods in Enzymology*, **58**, 259–268.

Osborne, T.B., and Campbell, G.F. (1900). The protein constituents of egg white. *Journal of the American Chemical Society*, **22**, 422–450.

Otsuka, S., Maruyama, H., and Listowsky, I. (1981). Structure, assembly, conformation, and immunological properties of the two subunit classes of ferritin. *Biochemistry*, **20**, 5226–5232.

Pecoraro, V.L., Harris, W.R., Carrano, C.J., and Raymond, K.N. (1981). Siderophilin metal coordination. Different ultraviolet spectroscopy of di-, tri-, and tetravalent

metal ions with ethylenebis (*O*-hydroxyphenyl) glycine. *Biochemistry*, **20**, 7033–7039.
Penner, M.H., Yamasaki, R.B., Osuga, D.T., Babin, D.R., Meares, C.F., and Feeney, R.E. (1983). Comparative oxidations of tyrosines and methionines in transferrins: human serum transferrin, human lactotransferrin, and chicken ovotransferrin. *Archives of Biochemistry and Biophysics*, **225**, 740–747.
Phillips, J.L., and Azari, P. (1972). Iodination of ovotransferrin and its iron complex. Extent of involvement of tyrosine phenolic groups in the iron binding. *Archives of Biochemistry and Biophysics*, **151**, 445–452.
Princiotto, J.V., and Zapolski, E.J. (1975). Difference between the two iron-binding sites of transferrin. *Nature*, **255**, 87–88.
Querinjean, P., Masson, P.L., and Heremans, J.F. (1971). Molecular weight, single-chain structure, and amino acid composition of human lactoferrin. *European Journal of Biochemistry*, **20**, 420–425.
Rafelson, M.E., Hayashi, J.A., and Bezkorovainy, A. (1980). *Basic Biochemistry* Macmillan Press, New York.
Reed, C.A. (1981). Oxidation states, redox potentials, and spin states. In *The Biological Chemistry of Iron* (Eds. H.B. Dunford, D. Dolphin, K.N. Raymond and L. Sieker), pp. 25–42. D. Riedel Publishing Company, Boston, Massachusetts.
Roberts, J.E., Brown, T.G., Hoffman, B.M., and Aisen, P. (1983). Electron-nuclear double resonance of copper complexes of human transferrin. *Biochimica et Biophysica Acta*, **747**, 49–54.
Roberts, R.C., Makey, D.G., and Seal, U.S. (1966). Human transferrin. Molecular weight and sedimentation properties. *Journal of Biological Chemistry*, **241**, 4907–4913.
Roop, W.E., and Putnam, F.W. (1967). Purification and properties of human transferrin C and a slow moving genetic variant. *Journal of Biological Chemistry*, **242**, 2507–2513.
Rosseneu-Motreff, M.Y., Soetewey, F., Lamote, R., and Peeters, H. (1971). Size and shape determination of apotransferrin and transferrin monomers. *Biopolymers*, **10**, 1039–1048.
Schade, A.L., and Caroline, L. (1944). Raw hen egg white and the role of iron in growth inhibition of *Shigella dysenteriae, Staphylococcus aureus, Escherichia coli*, and *Saccharomyces cerevisiae*. *Science*, **100**, 14–15.
Schade, A.L., and Caroline, L. (1946). An iron-binding component of human blood plasma. *Science*, **104**, 340–341.
Schlabach, M.R., and Bates, G. (1975). The synergistic binding of anions and Fe^{3+} by transferrin. *Journal of Biological Chemistry*, **250**, 2182–2188.
Shewale, J.G., and Brew, K. (1982). Effects of Fe^{3+} binding on the microenvironments of individual amino groups in human serum transferrin as determined by differential kinetic labelling. *Journal of Biological Chemistry*, **257**, 9406–9415.
Spik, G., Baynard, B., Fournet, B., Strecker, G., Bouquelet, S., and Montreuil, J. (1975). Studies on glycoconjugates. LXIV. Complete structure of two carbohydrate units of human serotransferrin. *FEBS Letters*, **50**, 296–299.
Spik, G., Strecker, G., Fournet, B., Bouquelet, S., Montreuil, J., Dorland, L., Van Halbeek, H., and Vliegenthart, J.F.G. (1982). Primary structure of the glycans from human lactotransferrin. *European Journal of Biochemistry*, **121**, 413–419.
Sutton, H.E., and Karp, Jr., G.W. (1965). Adsorption of rivanol by potato starch in the isolation of transferrins. *Biochimica et Biophysica Acta*, **107**, 153–154.
Sweeney, W.V., and Rabinowitz, J.C. (1980). Proteins containing 4Fe–4S clusters: an overview. *Annual Review of Biochemistry*, **49**, 139–161.
Taborsky, G. (1974). Phosphoproteins. *Advances in Protein Chemistry*, **29**, 1–210.
Tidmarsh, G.F., Klebba, P.E., and Rosenberg, L.T. (1983). Rapid release of iron from

ferritin by siderophores. *Journal of Inorganic Biochemistry*, **18**, 161–168.
Treffry, A., Sowerby, J.M., and Harrison, P.M. (1979). Oxidant specificity in ferritin formation. *FEBS Letters*, **100**, 33–36.
Ulvik, R.J. (1982). Relevance of ferritin-binding sites on isolated mitochondria to the mobilization of iron from ferritin. *Biochimica et Biophysica Acta*, **715**, 42–45.
Van der Heul, C., Kroos, M.J., van Noort, W.L., and van Eijk, H.G. (1981). No functional difference of the two iron-binding sites of human transferrin *in vitro*. *Clinical Science*, **60**, 185–190.
Vitalo, M.L., Webb, J., and Saltman, P. (1984). Release of iron from ferritin by pyridoxal isonicotinoyl hydrazone and related compounds. *Journal of Inorganic Biochemistry*, **20**, 255–262.
Watanabe, N., and Drysdale, J. (1983). Studies on the heterogeneity in ferritin subunits. *Biochimica Biophysica Acta*, **743**, 98–105.
Wenn, R.V., and Williams, J. (1968). The isoelectric fractionation of hen's egg ovotransferrin. *Biochemical Journal*, **108**, 69–74.
Williams, J. (1982a). The identification of protected tyrosine residues in iron-ovotransferrin. *Biochemical Journal*, **201**, 647–651.
Williams, J. (1982b). The evolution of transferrin. *Trends in Biochemical Science*, **7**, 394–397.
Williams, J., Elleman, T.C., Kingston, I.B., Wilkins, A.G., and Kuhn, K.A. (1982). The primary structure of hen ovotransferrin. *European Journal of Biochemistry*, **122**, 297–303.
Williams, J., Grace, S.A., and Williams, J.M. (1982). Evolutionary significance of the renal excretion of transferrin half-molecule fragments. *Biochemical Journal*, **201**, 417–419.
Williams, J., and Moreton, K. (1980). The distribution of iron between the metal-binding sites of transferrin in human serum. *Biochemical Journal*, **185**, 483–488.
Windle, J.J., Wiersema, A.K., Clark, J.R., and Feeney, R.E. (1963). Investigation of the iron and copper complexes of avian conalbumins and human transferrins by electron paragmagnetic resonance. *Biochemistry*, **2**, 1341–1345.
Wong, K.L., Debaune, M.T., Hatton, M.W.C., and Regoeczi, E. (1978). Human transferrin, asialotransferrin, and the intermediate forms. *International Journal of Protein Research*, **12**, 27–37.
Wright, K.A., and Baxter, J.E. (1976). A numerical inversion of the Perrin equation for rotational and translational diffusion constants by iterative techniques. *Biophysical Journal*, **16**, 931–938.
Yamamura, T., Hagiwara, S., Nakazato, K., and Satake, K. (1984). Copper complexes at N- and C- site of ovotransferrin: quantitative determination and visible absorption spectrum of each complex. *Biochemical and Biophysical Research Communications*, **119**, 298–304.
Yeh, S.M., and Meares, C.F. (1980). Characterization of transferrin-metal-binding sites by diffusion-enhanced energy transfer. *Biochemistry*, **19**, 5057–5062.
Yeh, Y., Iwai, S., and Feeney, R.E. (1979). Conformations of denatured and renatured ovotransferrin. *Biochemistry*, **18**, 882–889.
Young, S.P. (1982). Evidence for the functional equivalence of the iron-binding sites of rat transferrin. *Biochimica et Biophysica Acta*, **718**, 35–41.
Zähringer, J., Baliga, B.S. and Munro, H.N. (1976). Novel mechanism for translational control in regulation of ferritin synthesis by iron. *Proceedings of the National Academy of Sciences (USA)*, **73**, 857–861.
Zak, O., Leibman, A., and Aisen, P. (1983). Metal-binding properties of a single-sited transferrin fragment. *Biochimica et Biophysica Acta*, **742**, 490–495.

Zweier, J.L. (1983). Electron paramagnetic resonance measurement of the distance between the metal binding sites of transferrin. *Journal of Biological Chemistry*, **258**, 13759–13760.

Iron and Infection
Edited by J.J. Bullen and E. Griffiths

Chapter 3

The iron-uptake systems of pathogenic bacteria

E. GRIFFITHS
*National Institute for Biological Standards and Control,
Holly Hill,
Hampstead,
London, NW3 6RB, England*

1. INTRODUCTION

One common and essential factor in all infections is the ability of the invading pathogen to multiply successfully in the tissues of the host. Here bacteria must produce the full complement of virulence determinants required for pathogenicity. Most investigations into bacterial virulence have been carried out with organisms grown *in vitro* under conditions that do not necessarily reflect microbial behaviour *in vivo*. It is well known that bacteria can alter their metabolism rapidly in response to environmental changes and that they are

Table 1 Distribution of host iron-binding glycoproteins

Lactoferrin	Saliva Tears Nasal secretions Intraocular fluids Intestinal fluids Seminal fluids Cervical mucus Colostrum Milk (human) Polymorphonuclear leucocytes
Transferrin	Serum Lymph
Ovotransferrin	Avian egg white

capable of existing in a variety of physiological states that can be quite different from one another. In general, little is known about the alterations that occur in pathogenic bacteria as they adapt to and multiply in the environment found in host tissues under bacterial attack. These are not only poorly defined but also likely to change as an infection proceeds.

Perhaps one of the best understood aspects of the host environment at present, and of the effects it has on bacterial growth, concerns the availability of iron. As has been discussed in Chapters 1 and 2, most of the body's iron is found intracellularly, in ferritin, haemosiderin or haem, and that which is extracellular in body fluids is attached to the high affinity iron-binding glycoproteins transferrin and lactoferrin (Table 1; see also Chapter 2). A related protein, called ovotransferrin, occurs in avian egg white. Since these iron-binding proteins are usually only partially saturated with iron and have association constants of approximately 10^{36}, the amount of free iron in equilibrium with the proteins is about $10^{-18}M$. Thus, although there is normally an abundance of iron present in body fluids, the amount of free iron is far too small to sustain bacterial growth (Bullen, Rogers and Griffiths, 1978; Bullen, 1981). In addition, during infection the host reduces the total amount of iron bound to serum transferrin (Cartwright *et al.*, 1946). This decrease, called the hypoferraemia of infection, can be reproduced experimentally by injecting small amounts of endotoxin (Baker and Wilson, 1965) which acts by stimulating the release from polymorphonuclear leukocytes of a factor which seems identical to leukocytic pyrogen (Merriman, Pulliam and Kampschmidt, 1977). Leukocyte pyrogen (interleukin I; see Chapter 7) induces fever, leukocytosis and the release of the contents of specific granules from polymorphs (Leffell and Spitznagel, 1974; Klempner, Dinarello and Gallin, 1978; see also Chapter 7). Although the triggering signal appears to be due to leukocyte pyrogen, the subsequent processes which lead to the reduction of serum iron levels are not fully understood. Van Snick, Masson and Heremans (1974) have reported evidence for an accelerated removal of iron from the serum transferrin pool during inflammation. They suggest that lactoferrin released from polymorphs removes iron from transferrin and that the Fe^{3+}- loaded lactoferrin is taken up by the macrophages and removed rapidly from the circulation by the reticuloendothelial system. It has been shown that lactoferrin does accumulate at sites of inflammation and that, unlike transferrin, whose iron-binding ability is dimished below pH 6, it retains its iron-binding properties in the more acidic conditions which often prevail at such sites (McClelland and van Furth, 1976; Ainscough *et al.*, 1980; Aisen, 1980; Morgan, 1981). However, others have evidence that, in mice at least, hypoferraemia is due not to an accelerated removal of iron from the serum transferrin pool but to an altered processing of iron within the reticuloendothelial system which limits the supply of the metal to the extracellular pool (Letendre and Holbein, 1983; 1984; Beaumier, Caldwell and Holbein, 1984; Brock, Esparza and Logie, 1984). Hypoferraemia of infection is discussed in more detail in Chapter 7.

2. ACQUISITION OF IRON

In spite of the virtual absence of freely available iron in normal body fluids, and of the hypoferraemia of infection, pathogenic bacteria can multiply successfully *in vivo* to establish an infection. Since all known bacterial pathogens need iron to multiply, they must, initially, be able to adapt to the iron-restricted environment usually found *in vivo* and develop mechanisms for assimilating protein-bound iron or for acquiring it from liberated haem. Under normal physiological conditions bacteria might be expected to assimilate the iron bound by the high affinity iron-binding glycoproteins of the host in one of four ways:

1. Through proteolytic cleavage of the iron-binding glycoprotein, disrupting the iron-binding site and releasing iron
2. By reduction of Fe^{3+} complex to Fe^{2+} complex and the consequent release of Fe^{2+} from the glycoprotein
3. Through direct interaction between receptors on the bacterial cell surface and the Fe^{3+}–glycoprotein complex in a manner analogous to the reaction occurring between transferrin and the reticulocyte
4. By producing low molecular mass iron-chelating compounds, known as siderophores, that are able to remove iron from the Fe^{3+}–glycoprotein complex and to deliver the iron to the bacterial cell

So far there is little evidence that bacterial pathogens in general are able to degrade either transferrin or lactoferrin, although recent data indicate that some strains of *Bacteroides* species are able to do so (Carlsson, Hofling and Sundqvist, 1984). It is suggested that the ability of these organisms to degrade not only transferrin but also haemopexin and haptoglobin may contribute to their virulence. Similarly, to date, there is only one instance where it has been suggested that a pathogen uses a soluble reductant to remove iron from an iron-binding protein. Cowart and Foster (1985) have shown that, *in vitro*, *Listeria monocytogenes* secretes a soluble reductant that effectively removes iron from the Fe^{3+}–transferrin complex in a manner analogous to the chemical reductive mechanism described by Kojima and Bates (1979). Whether such a reductive process can actually operate *in vivo* remains to be seen. However, it is worth noting that the growth of *Clostridium perfringens in vivo* leads to a progressive generalized decrease in the Eh of the infected tissues, with the Eh finally reaching -400 mV at pH 6.5 (Rogers, Bullen and Cushnie, 1970; Bullen, 1981). These highly reduced conditions, as well as the acid pH, will facilitate the release of iron from transferrin and promote the growth of this pathogen (see also Chapter 7).

An iron-uptake mechanism involving the direct interaction of the pathogen with an iron-binding protein is thought to operate in *Neisseria gonorrhoeae* and in *N. meningitidis*, and this is discussed in detail in Section 2.2. The best understood systems used by pathogens to assimilate iron from host iron-binding proteins are those which depend on the production of siderophores, and these will be considered in some detail below. Of course, the fact that such systems are the best understood at present does not necessarily mean that they are the most common, nor indeed the most efficient mechanisms for assimilating iron. It may merely reflect the relative ease with which such mechanisms can be studied.

2.1 Iron-uptake systems which depend on siderophores

Many microorganisms combat the biological unavailability of iron in aerobic environments (see Chapter 1) by producing siderophores (Raymond and Carrano 1979; Neilands, 1981). These low molecular weight chelators are part of what is termed the 'high affinity' iron transport system. A 'low affinity' iron transport system is thought to operate when iron is freely available, but little is known about the mechanisms involved.

Escherichia, Klebsiella, Salmonella, Shigella: the siderophores

Perhaps the best studied 'high affinity' iron transport systems are those produced by bacteria of the genera *Salmonella, Escherichia, Klebsiella* and *Shigella*. *Escherichia coli, K.pneumoniae, S.typhimurium* and some species of *Shigella* secrete the iron-chelator enterobactin (also called enterochelin) under conditions of iron restriction *in vitro* (O'Brien and Gibson, 1970; Pollack and Neilands, 1970; Rogers, 1973; Rogers *et al.*, 1977; Perry and San Clemente, 1979; Lawlor and Payne, 1984). This compound, which is the cyclic triester of

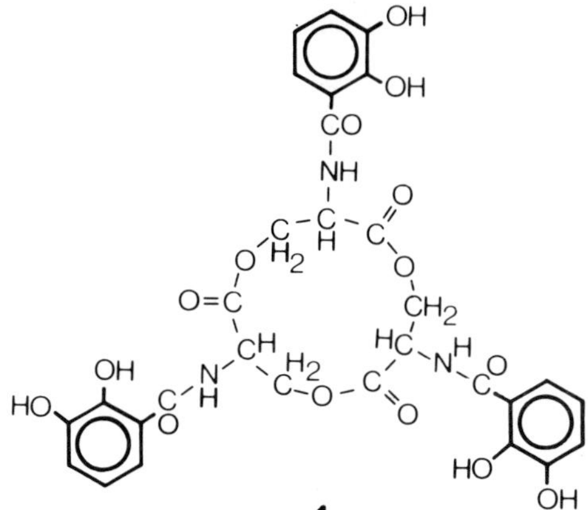

1

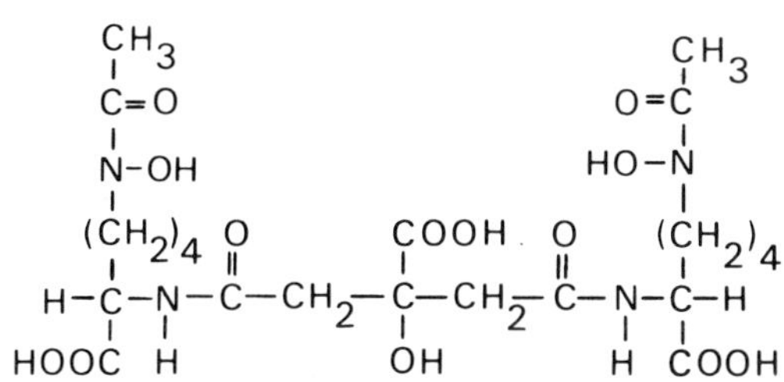

2

Figure 1 Structural formula of (**1**) enterobactin; (**2**) aerobactin

2,3-dihydroxy-*N*-benzoyl serine (Fig. 1), is made only under conditions of iron restriction, and it both removes iron from iron-binding proteins efficiently and promotes bacterial growth (Rogers, 1973; Miles and Khimji, 1975; Rogers *et al.*, 1977; Carrano and Raymond, 1979). The fact that an enterobactin-producing strain of *Salmonella paratyphi* B obtained iron from transferrin when the protein was inside a dialysis bag shows that contact between the transferrin and the bacterial cell surface is not required for siderophore-mediated removal of iron (Tidmarsh and Rosenberg, 1981). The single most outstanding feature of siderophores is their extremely high affinity for ferric iron. The formation constant for ferric enterobactin is the highest ever recorded for a ferric iron chelator, being near 10^{52} at neutral pH (Harris, Carrano

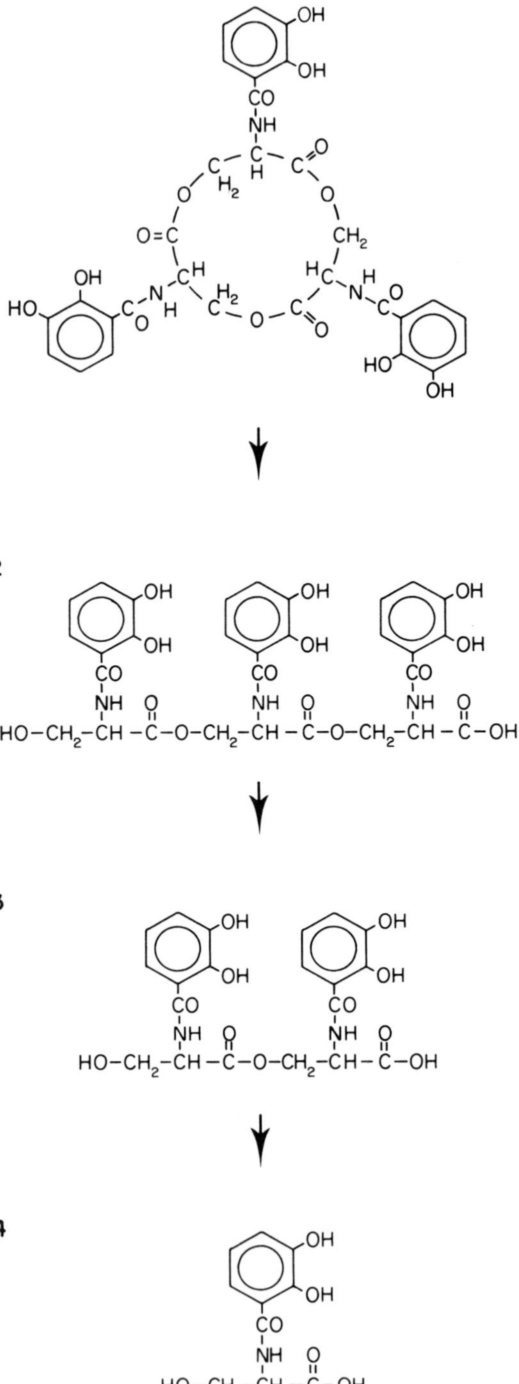

1

2

3

4

and Raymond, 1979a; Harris *et al.*, 1979). Organisms using enterobactin-mediated iron transport are, therefore, able to compete effectively for complexed iron. However, the chelator is used only once for transporting iron into the bacterial cell. This is because the cyclic triester linkages of the Fe^{3+}–enterobactin are cleaved by a specific esterase when the molecule enters the cell, ultimately producing 2,3–dihydroxybenzoylserine which is then discarded (Rosenberg and Young 1974; Greenwood and Luke 1978) (Fig. 2). It has been proposed that hydrolysis of the bonds is necessary to release the iron because the ferric–ester has too low a reduction potential to enable enterobactin reduction to release the metal (Cooper, McArdle and Raymond, 1978; Harris *et al.*, 1979; Raymond and Carrano, 1979). The fact that a carbocyclic analogue of enterobactin, which lacks ester bonds, effectively supplies iron to an enterobactin-deficient strain of *E. coli* has, however, raised questions about the exact role of the esterase, and these questions have not yet been satisfactorily answered (Hollifield and Neilands, 1978). A ferrous–enterobactin complex has been identified and it has been suggested that this might play a part in translocating iron across the cytoplasmic membrane (Hider *et al.*, 1979). In this complex the metal is held much less tightly than in the ferric–enterobactin form and it might be expected that it could donate the iron readily to other coordinating ligands within the cell. Nevertheless, whatever the exact function of the esterase, *E.coli fes* mutants, which lack esterase activity, are unable to use the ferric complex; such cells accumulate Fe^{3+}–enterobactin with the result that a sedimented pellet of these cells is distinctly pink (Langman *et al.*, 1972; Rosenberg and Young, 1974).

The enterobactin-dependent 'high affinity' iron-uptake system has been studied mainly *in vitro* with the laboratory strain *E.coli* K12, but it is known that pathogenic strains of *E.coli* also synthesize the siderophore (Rogers, 1973; Rogers *et al.*, 1977). Indeed, nearly all wild-type and clinical isolates of *E.coli* seem to produce enterobactin. Furthermore, it is known to be produced *in vivo* during infection (Griffiths and Humphreys, 1980); enterobactin and its degradation products were detected in the peritoneal washings from guinea-pigs infected with *E.coli* 0111, a finding which supports the notion that the presence of iron-binding proteins in body fluids maintains an iron-restricted environment *in vivo*. In 1979 Yancey, Breeding and Lankford reported that the loss by mutation of the ability to synthesize enterobactin inhibited the ability of *S.typhimurium* to grow in human serum and also reduced greatly its virulence for mice. This work suggested that the production of enterobactin was important for the virulence of *S.typhimurium*. Very recently, however, Benjamin *et al.* (1985) have reported results which are at variance with those of Yancey,

Figure 2 Enterobactin and its hydrolytic breakdown products: (**1**) enterobactin; (**2**) linear trimer of 2,3-dihydroxybenzoylserine; (**3**) 2,3-dihydroxybenzoylserine dimer; (**4**) 2,3-dihydroxybenzoylserine

Breeding and Lankford (1979). Benjamin *et al.* (1985) found that although enterobactin-negative mutants of *S.typhimurium* failed to multiply in normal mouse serum, an inability to make enterobactin did not alter the virulence of the organisms for several inbred strains of mice. Since *S.typhimurium* is an intracellular pathogen, it is suggested that the failure of the *ent* mutation to affect the virulence of the organism in mice is because enterobactin may not be required for growth once the pathogen has entered the cells of the reticulo-endothelial system. More work is needed to resolve these apparently contradictory results and to define more clearly the role of siderophores in the pathogenesis of both extra- and intracellular pathogens.

Although enterobactin-mediated iron uptake seems to be the main endogenous system used by *E.coli*, *Salmonella* and *Klebsiella* for accumulating iron in media containing low levels of available iron, these organisms also have the remarkable capability for obtaining iron via a variety of hydroxamate-type siderophores which are not synthesized by the organisms themselves but produced by other microorganisms (Leong and Neilands, 1976; Konisky, 1979; Raymond and Carrano, 1979; Neilands, 1981). Two exogenous chelators studied in some detail are ferrichrome and ferrioxamine B (Fig. 3), which are produced by certain fungi and actinomyces respectively. Although it is not known if such chelators normally operate *in vivo*, exogenously supplied desferrioxamine B can certainly enhance both *Klebsiella* (Khimji and Miles, 1978) and *Salmonella* (Jones *et al.*, 1977) infections. The methane sulphonate salt of desferrioxamine B is available commercially from Ciba–Geigy as Desferal and is widely used in deferration therapy. The possibility that it might increase the susceptibility of treated individuals to bacterial infections should, therefore, not be overlooked (see Chapter 8). Unlike enterobactin, ferrichrome is not destroyed when transporting iron into *E.coli* (Leong and Neilands, 1976), but it does appear to be acetylated on one of the hydroxylamino oxygens after reductive separation of Fe^{3+} (Hartmann and Braun, 1980); this seems to be an essential step in the ferrichrome-mediated iron-transport system.

Citrate is another compound which can supply iron to *E.coli*. Some strains possess a citrate-mediated iron-transport system which is induced when the bacteria are grown in an iron-limited medium containing citrate (Frost and Rosenberg, 1973; Rosenberg and Young, 1974; Hancock, Hantke and Braun, 1976; Woodrow *et al.*, 1978; Hussein, Hantke and Braun, 1981; Zimmerman, Hantke and Braun, 1984). However, it is not known how widely distributed is this system in pathogenic strains of *E.coli*, nor whether it can function *in vivo* during infection. *Salmonella typhimurium* lacks the citrate-dependent iron-transport system although, paradoxically, citrate can be used as a carbon source by *Salmonella* but not normally by *E.coli* (Kay and Cameron, 1978; Neilands, 1981; Wagegg and Braun, 1981). *Escherichia coli* containing H1 plasmids can, however, utilize citrate as the sole energy source (Smith, Parsell and Green, 1978).

1

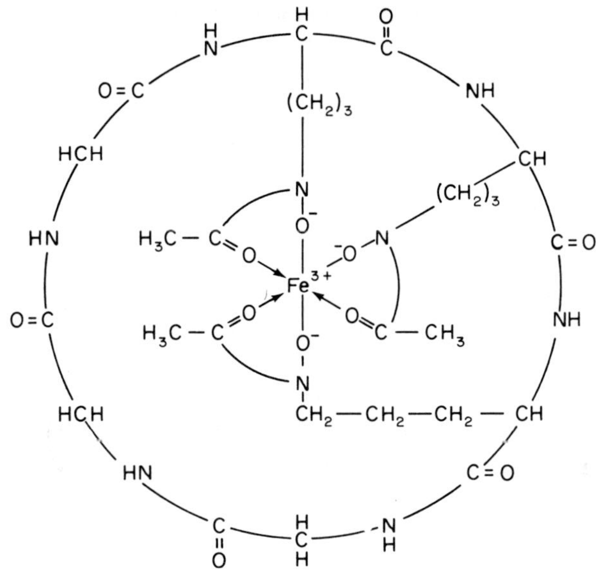

Ferrichrome

2

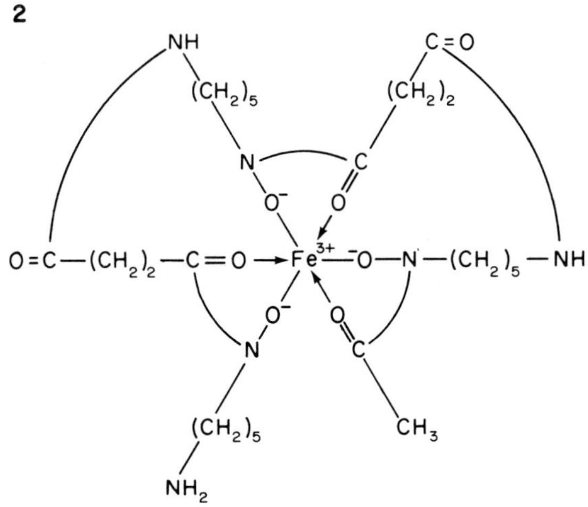

Ferrioxamine B

Figure 3 The structural formula of (**1**) ferrichrome; (**2**) ferrioxamine B

Many strains of *E. coli* that are capable of causing generalized extraintestinal infections in man and animals, and which carry the Colicin V plasmid (pColV), synthesize a plasmid-encoded hydroxamate-type siderophore called aerobactin, in addition to enterobactin (Braun, 1981; Warner *et al.*, 1981; Crosa, 1984). A detailed discussion of plasmid-mediated iron-transport systems can be found in Chapter 4. Aerobactin (Fig. 1) is a member of the hydroxamic acid–citrate family of siderophores and was originally isolated from *Aerobacter aerogenes* (Gibson and Magrath, 1969). It is a conjugate of 6-(*N*-acetyl-*N*-hydroxyamino)-2-aminohexanoic acid and citric acid and it has been shown to form an octahedral complex with ferric iron using the two bidentate hydroxamate groups, the central carboxylate and probably the citrate hydroxyl group (Harris, Carrano and Raymond, 1979b). Although its production is thought to play an important part in the virulence of *E. coli* strains carrying ColV plasmids (Williams, 1979a; Stuart, Greenwood and Luke, 1980; Williams and Warner, 1980; Warner *et al.*, 1981; Crosa, 1984), it is not clear how acquiring the ability to make this siderophore confers a selective advantage on organisms already capable of synthesizing enterobactin. At pH 7.4, enterobactin is by far the most effective siderophore characterizied (Harris *et al.*, 1979). The formation constant for ferric enterobactin (log K_f) is 52, and this is about 29 orders of magnitude larger than that of aerobactin (log K_f=22.9) (Harris, Carrano and Raymond, 1979b). However, by themselves the formation constants say little about the ability of ligands to compete with each other for ferric iron at a given pH. This is because of variations in the ligand protonation constants and of concentration dependencies. In order to obtain a more direct ranking of ligands under specific conditions, Harris and colleagues (Harris, Carrano and Raymond, 1979a; Harris *et al.*, 1979) report what they call p*M* values, which are the negative logarithms of the free ferric ion concentration under different conditions, calculated from the various equilibrium values involved. Even so, as can be seen in Table 2, the p*M* value of enterobactin at pH 7.4 is still more than ten orders of magnitude higher than that of aerobactin; indeed aerobactin is marginally less effective than transferrin. It also seems that, in general, hydroxamate-based chelating agents are kinetically inferior to catecholate-type siderophores in removing iron from transferrin (Carrano and Raymond, 1979). In 1980, Stuart, Greenwood and Luke proposed that ColV plasmid specified aerobactin is bound to the bacterial cell wall and is, therefore, functionally different and somehow more efficient than the secreted enterobactin in acquiring iron from iron-binding proteins. However, this conclusion contrasts with the known relative effectiveness of the two compounds as iron chelators and the cell-free mode of action of aerobactin, as indicated by genetic and other data (Williams and Warner, 1980; Warner *et al.*, 1981; Crosa, 1984). Aerobactin is secreted into culture media of aerobactin-producing bacteria (Gibson and Magrath, 1969; Braun, 1981, Warner *et al.*, 1981; van Tiel-Menkveld *et al.*, 1982) and there is, in addition, a specific

Table 2 Values of p*M* for solutions of ferric complexes of biological ligands

Ligand	pM_1[a]	pM_2[b]
Enterobactin	36.7	35.25
Ferrichrome	27.25	25.2
Transferrin	25.62	23.6
Aerobactin	25.37	23.32

[a] Total metal $10^{-6}M$: total ligand $10^{-3}M$, pH 7.4.
[b] Total metal $10^{-6}M$: total ligand $10^{-5}M$, pH 7.4.

From Griffiths (1985). Data from Harris, Carrano and Raymond (1979b) and Raymond and Carrano (1979). Reproduced by permission of the Society for General Microbiology.

receptor for ferric–aerobactin in the outer membrane of these organisms (see below).

One possible important difference between the mode of action of enterobactin and aerobactin is that the latter appears to be recycled (Braun, Brazel-Faisst and Schneider, 1984). Since enterobactin is used only once for transporting iron into the bacterial cell, it is an energetically expensive way of assimilating iron (Raymond and Carrano, 1979). Harris, Carrano and Raymond (1979b) consider that the high affinity, low capacity and energetically expensive iron-transport system using enterobactin might operate under conditions of extreme iron stress and the low affinity, high capacity system using aerobactin, under conditions of mild iron stress. Others, however, have concluded that enterobactin is produced under conditions of mild iron limitation and that aerobactin production is maximal under iron-deficient conditions (van Tiel-Menkveld *et al.*, 1982). Experimentally it can be shown that both these siderophores are produced simultaneously, although aerobactin is synthesized mainly in the late exponential and stationary phases of growth (Gibson and Magrath, 1969; Stuart, Greenwood and Luke, 1980; van Tiel-Menkveld *et al.*, 1982). However, care must be taken in extrapolating data obtained with bacteria in iron-deficient media, in which the quantity of iron is limiting and the organisms starved of iron, to the situation *in vivo* during infection. A clear distinction must be made between the quantity of iron present in a medium and its availability to bacteria. *In vivo*, there is plenty of iron present, although it is not normally readily available to bacteria because of the presence of the iron-binding glycoproteins. As far as infection is concerned, it is the relative ability of these chelators to remove iron from transferrin or lactoferrin and to transport it back to the bacterial cell that is important. These processes take place in tissue fluids, such as serum or mucosal secretions, not in broth or minimal medium. The presence of other factors in body fluids could well influence the overall effectiveness of different siderophores. Pollack *et al.* (1976) and Konopka, Binderief and Neilands (1982) have shown that the kinetic barrier to efficient hydroxamate-mediated, and in particular aerobactin-mediated, removal of iron from transferrin can be partially overcome by adding other anions to the system; such a phenomenon could operate in serum. Furthermore, the presence in serum of anti-enterobactin antibodies which inhibit enterobactin-mediated iron uptake (Moore *et al.*, 1980; Moore and Earhart, 1981), and anti-'O' polysaccharide antibodies which interfere with enterobactin secretion (Fitzgerald and Rogers, 1980) as well as antibodies directed against the bacterial receptor for ferric–enterobactin (Griffiths *et al.*, 1985a) could reduce the effectiveness of enterobactin-mediated iron-uptake systems in serum and favour aerobactin-mediated iron transport (see Chapter 5). Also, serum albumin has been reported to bind enterobactin, decreasing its effective concentration in serum and impeding enterobactin-mediated mobilization of transferrin iron (Konopka and Neilands, 1984). Since albumin had no detectable binding effect on aerobactin this siderophore could still mediate iron transport from transferrin to *E.coli* unhindered in the presence of serum proteins. All of these mechanisms, as well as the relatively low water solubility (Pollack and Neilands, 1970) and chemical instability of the enterobactin molecule (Neilands, 1981), could well restrict the overall effectiveness of enterobactin-mediated iron-uptake systems in serum and favour aerobactin-mediated iron transport. The growth of *E.coli* strains which rely entirely on enterobactin for supplying iron might then be expected to be restricted, and such organisms would find themselves at a disadvantage compared to aerobactin producers.

Although aerobactin production by *E.coli* was originally correlated with the presence of ColV plasmids, surveys of large numbers of clinical isolates of *E.coli* have shown that the genes for aerobactin synthesis can be located on a plamid or in the chromosome (Montgomerie *et al.*, 1984; Valvano and Crosa, 1984; Bindereif and Neilands, 1985; see also Chapter 4). These surveys have shown that the incidence of aerobactin-positive *E.coli* is highest among isolates from blood (Stuart, Greenwood and Luke, 1982; Montgomerie *et al.*, 1984). In the study carried out by Montgomerie *et al.* (1984), 75 per cent of blood isolates were aerobactin producers, suggesting that the production of aerobactin is associated with the ability to cause septicaemia. Smith and Huggins (1980) showed that although the loss of a ColV plasmid from the pathogenic strain *E.coli* 018 K1 H7 (strain H247) resulted in the loss of virulence, higher doses of the ColV$^-$ bacteria produced a disease which was clinically and bacteriologically similar to that produced by organisms of the ColV$^+$ parent. The fact that the higher levels of ColV$^-$ bacteria, which lack the aerobactin-mediated iron-uptake system (Williams, 1979a; Smith and Huggins, 1980), grew as well as the ColV$^+$ strain in host tissues suggests that the enterobactin-mediated iron-uptake mechanism can function effectively *in vivo* or that some other iron-uptake system is operating. Similar results have been obtained with this strain in guinea-pigs (Griffiths and Stevenson, unpublished data).

These results suggest that the aerobactin iron-uptake system may be particularly important at a low infective dose. What is not clear at present is whether both the enterobactin and aerobactin systems need to be present for full virulence. Stated another way, it could be asked if the ability to make both iron chelators gives *E.coli* an advantage *in vivo*. So far, this question has not been answered, although to date no Ent^-/Aer^+ strains of *E.coli* have been found among clinical isolates. However, recently it has been reported that most clinical isolates of *Shigella flexneri* produce only aerobactin (Payne *et al.*, 1983). A few isolates and laboratory variants of *S.flexneri* did, however, produce enterobactin as well as aerobactin. Interestingly enough, those strains synthesizing enterobactin appeared to have a distinct advantage in the laboratory (Payne *et al.*, 1983). Ent^+ strains grew faster than Ent^- strains and were better able to compete with iron chelators such as ethylene diamine-dihydroxyphenylacetic acid (EDDA); strains producing aerobactin alone were inhibited by such chelators. However, care must be taken when using such data to predict what might happen during an infection. Although most strains of *S. flexneri* failed to synthesize enterobactin, it appears that the necessary genetic information was present in the cells (Payne *et al.*, 1983). The genes involved in synthesizing aerobactin in *S. flexneri* have been located in the chromosome (Lawlor and Payne, 1984; Griffiths *et al.*, 1985b). Indeed, analysis of various *E.coli* K12 transconjugants has shown that these genes are linked to the *mtl* chromosomal marker of *S.flexneri*, one of three chromosomal segments associated with the virulence of this pathogen (Griffiths *et al.*, 1985b). Of course, this does not prove that aerobactin-mediated iron transport is a virulence determinant, but the evidence suggests that this is highly likely. Since *Shigella* species are invasive pathogens and mutliply intracellularly (Formal, Hale and Boedeker, 1983; Formal, Hale and Sansonetti, 1983), it may be that their ability to remove iron from ferritin is more important than their ability to utilize the iron in transferrin or lactoferrin. It is not known if aerobactin can remove iron from ferritin, but enterobactin has been shown to be capable of doing so (Tidmarsh, Klebba and Rosenberg, 1983). However, the rate and extent of iron exchanged was shown to depend critically both on the siderophore concentration and on the degree of loading of the ferritin. When the iron load in ferritin was decreased, the percentage of iron released by enterobactin dropped dramatically (Tidmarsh, Klebba and Rosenberg, 1983).

Salmonella typhimurium is another pathogen which can grow intracellularly during infection (Mackaness, Blanden and Collins, 1966; Lowrie, Aber and Carrol, 1979; O'Brien, 1982) but usually *Salmonella* produce only enterobactin. Recently, however, certain epidemic strains of *Salmonella* have been shown to harbour FI*me* plasmids which carry ISI elements encoding an hydroxamate-mediated iron-uptake system similar to the aerobactin system encoded by ColV plasmids (Colonna *et al.*, 1985). FI*me* plasmids are conjugative or defective conjugative multiple-drug resistance plasmids ranging in size from 100 to 180 kilobase pairs. A particularly interesting fact is the change in the clinical and epidemiological behaviour of strains which carry these plasmids. For example, before 1969 the *S.wien* serotype occurred at very low frequency in human pathology and the isolates tested were susceptible to a variety of antibiotics (LeMinor 1972), which suggests that this strain had not acquired the FI*me* plasmids at that time. On acquiring FI*me* plasmids, *S.wien* strains have become resistant to many antibiotics, express an hydroxamate-mediated iron-uptake mechanism and, moreover, produce epidemics characterized by a high incidence of septicaemia or meningitis. Strains of *S.typhimurium* carrying these FI*me* plasmids also cause a high incidence of septicaemia and meningitis (Anderson *et al.*, 1977; Rangneker, Banker and Jhala, 1983). The data suggest that plasmids encoding an hydroxamate iron-uptake system promote the ability of the pathogen to cause septicaemia and meningitis, in the same way as does the presence of a ColV plasmid encoding the aerobactin system in *E.coli*. However, it must be pointed out that neither *S.flexneri*, nor the enteroinvasive shigella-like *E.coli* usually cause septicaemias, although both produce aerobactin (Griffiths *et al.*, 1985b). Clearly, much more work is needed before we can fully understand the relative importance of the different high affinity iron-uptake mechanisms in promoting the growth of pathogenic bacteria extracellularly in the bloodstream or intracellularly, where in fact little is known about the availability of iron.

Whatever may be the nature of the advantage that the ability to make aerobactin confers on certain of the enterobacteriaceae, it must be noted that there is a large group of enteropathogenic and enterotoxigenic *E.coli* which cause severe diarrhoeal disease but which produce only enterobactin as an iron chelator. It should also be noted that not all species of *Shigella* produce aerobactin. Lawlor and Payne (1984) found that *S.dysenteriae* neither synthesized nor utilized aerobactin but made and used enterobactin. Similarly, *S.sonnei* failed to synthesize aerobactin but it could use it for acquiring iron; *S. sonnei* also made and used enterobactin.

Escherichia, Klebsiella, Salmonella, Shigella: iron-regulated outer membrane proteins

An essential part of high affinity iron-uptake systems based on siderophores is the production of outer membrane protein receptors and enzymes which are involved in the uptake and release of iron from the iron chelator (Neilands, 1982). These proteins are not normally synthesized in significant amounts by the iron-replete bacteria. The need for specific receptors is due, in part, to the fact that the molecular weights of some of the siderophores exceed the diffusion limit (about 600) of the small water-filled pores of the outer membrane (Nikaido, 1979). However, the molecular mass of the iron–citrate complex ($Fe(Cit)_2$) is probably no greater than 443. The fact that there is a specific

Table 3 Functions of well-characterized iron-regulated outer membrane proteins of *Escherichia coli*

Protein	Apparent molecular mass	Receptor for phage/ colicin	Function
Cir protein	74 KDa	Colicin I	Unknown
ColV-aerobactin receptor	74 KDa	Cloacin DF13	Uptake of Fe^{3+} – aerobactin
Fhu protein	78 KDa	Phages T1, T5 and ϕ 80 Colicin M	Uptake of ferrichrome
Fec A protein	80.5 KDa	—	Uptake of Fe^{3+} – citrate
Fep A protein	81 KDa	Colicin B	Uptake of Fe^{3+} – enterobactin
83 KDa protein	83 KDa	—	Unknown

receptor for this iron complex, too, suggests that the iron requirements of the cell can be satisfied only by initial adsorption of the iron-loaded siderophore to the surface receptors where iron can be accumulated relative to the concentration in the growth environment. The strict requirement for receptor proteins in the outer membrane is shown by the fact that mutants lacking such proteins are completely devoid of transport activity (Grewal, Warner and Williams, 1982). Such mutants can be obtained reasonably easily in *E.coli* since most of the siderophore receptors also function as receptors for bacteriophages and/or colicins (Table 3).

The iron-regulated proteins of the enteric bacteria have apparent molecular masses in the range 74–84 kDa. In *E.coli* these proteins are usually designated according to their molecular masses as 83, 81, 78 and 74 kDa proteins (Braun *et al.*, 1976). The 81 kDa protein (Fep A protein) is the receptor for Fe^{3+}-enterobactin and is the product of the *fep* gene, mapping in the *ent, fep, fes* gene cluster at approximately 13 minutes (Hollifield and Neilands, 1978; Konisky, 1979; Braun and Hantke, 1981; Fiss, Stanley-Samuelson and Neilands, 1982; Neilands, 1982). This gene cluster, which has now been cloned, is responsible for the biosynthesis, transport and hydrolysis of enterobactin (Rosenberg and Young, 1974; Laird *et al.*, 1980; Bachmann, 1983; Fleming *et al.*, 1985). The 78 kDa protein (Ton A protein; sometimes also referred to as the Fhu A protein for ferric hydroxamate-uptake protein) is the receptor for ferrichrome and is the product of the *ton* A gene (Konisky, 1979; Braun and Hantke, 1981; Neilands, 1982). Although the 83 kDa protein and the 74 kDa (Cir) protein, which is the product of the *cir* gene (Soucek and Konisky, 1977; Konisky, 1979; Neilands, 1982; Worsham and Konisky, 1985), are both produced by *E.coli* under iron restriction, their function is currently unknown. Some strains of *E.coli* also produce another outer membrane protein with an apparent molecular weight of about 81,000 (Fec A protein) when growing in iron-restricted media containing 1 m*M* citrate (Frost and Rosenberg, 1973; Hancock, Hantke and Braun, 1976; Wagegg and Braun, 1981). This protein is part of the citrate-mediated iron-transport system and is induced by the presence of ferric dicitrate in the medium (Hussein, Hantke and Braun, 1981; Wagegg and Braun, 1981; Zimmermann, Hantke and Braun, 1984).

A specific receptor is also required for the uptake of aerobactin (Williams and Warner, 1980). An outer membrane protein specified by ColV plasmid, regulated by iron and involved in aerobactin-mediated iron transport, has been identified (Bindereif, Braun and Hantke, 1982; Grewal, Warner and Williams, 1982). It has an apparent molecular weight of 74,000 and is revealed only in *cir* mutants, which lack the 74 kDa Cir protein. Like many other siderophore receptors, this protein also functions as a receptor for a bacteriocin, in this particular case for cloacin DF13, which is produced by *Enterobacter cloacae* (Oudega *et al.*, 1979; Bindereif, Braun and Hantke, 1982; Van Tiel-Menkveld *et al.*, 1982). Although the aerobactin receptor specified by the ColV plasmid is a 74 kDa protein, that in *S.flexneri* and in *E.coli* K12–*Shigella* hybrids seems to have an apparent molecular weight of 76,000 (Griffiths *et al.*, 1985b). Enteroinvasive strains of *E.coli* which produce dysentery-like illnesses also produce a 76 kDa outer membrane protein, as well as synthesizing aerobactin. Indeed, the pattern of the iron-regulated proteins expressed by these enteroinvasive *E.coli* strains is virtually identical to that seen in laboratory-constructed *E.coli* K12–*Shigella* hybrids under the same growth conditions (Fig. 4). The 76 kDa protein of *Shigella* also acts as a receptor for cloacin DF13 although the *Shigella* lipopolysaccharide normally intereferes with the reaction; the action of cloacin DF13 can be seen in the *E.coli* K12–*Shigella* hybrids expressing the 76 kDa protein or in rough mutants of *Shigella* (P.Derbyshire, T.Baldwin, P.Stevenson and E.Griffiths, unpublished data; S.Payne, personal communication, 1985).

It is interesting to note that *K.edwardsii* S15 also expresses an iron-regulated 76 kDa protein which again acts as a receptor for both cloacin DF13 and for aerobactin (Krone *et al.*, 1985). In *E.cloacae*, however, these same functions are mediated by an 85 kDa protein (Oudega *et al.*, 1979). Clearly, more work is required to understand the structural relationships between these functionally similar outer membrane proteins.

Although the outer membrane receptors are siderophore specific, inner or cytoplasmic membrane components, also necessary for siderophore-mediated iron transport, are less specific. Hydroxamate siderophores use common transport functions specified by the *fhu* C, D and B genes (Braun *et al.*, 1982, 1983; Fecker and Braun, 1983), and a functional locus called *ton* B is required for the utilization of all high affinity iron carriers, including citrate (Braun *et*

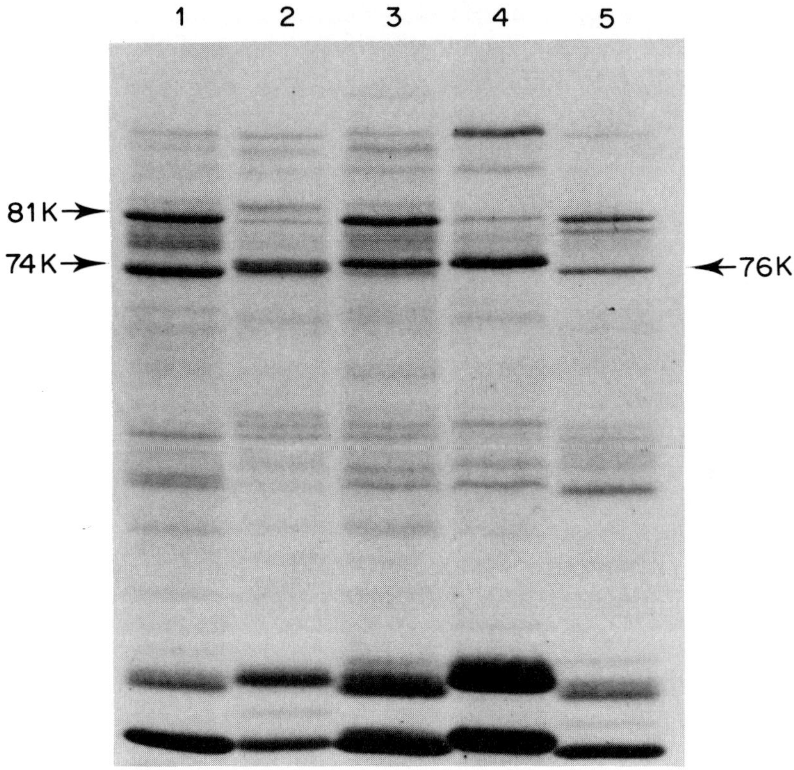

Figure 4 SDS-polyacrylamide gel electrophoresis profiles of outer membrane proteins isolated from bacteria grown in trypticase soy broth containing ovotransferrin: lane (1) *E.coli* K12; (2) enteroinvasive strain *E.coli* 0164; (3) *E.coli* K12–*S.flexneri*, hybrid strain; (4) *S.flexneri*; (5) *E.coli* W3110 carrying ColV-K30 plasmid. The position of the iron-regulated 81kDa enterobactin receptor protein, the 74kDa Cir protein and the 76kDa *Shigella* aerobactin receptor are indicated by arrows. The iron-regulated aerobactin receptor proteins of the ColV-K30 cannot be seen since is has an apparent molecular weight of 74kDa and comigrates with the 74kDa Cir protein. *From Griffiths* et al. *(1985b). Reproduced by permission of the American Society for Microbiology*

al., 1982; Neilands, 1982; Prody and Neilands, 1984). The *ton* B function is not apparently regulated by iron, nor is it specific for iron transport; it is also involved in the utilization of other nutrients such as vitamin B_{12} (Hantke, 1981; Neilands, 1982).

Most of the work on the iron-regulated outer membrane proteins of *E.coli* has been carried out with laboratory strains, such as *E.coli* K12. However, it has now been shown that pathogenic strains produce similar new proteins when grown *in vitro* in the presence of iron-binding proteins (Griffiths, Stevenson

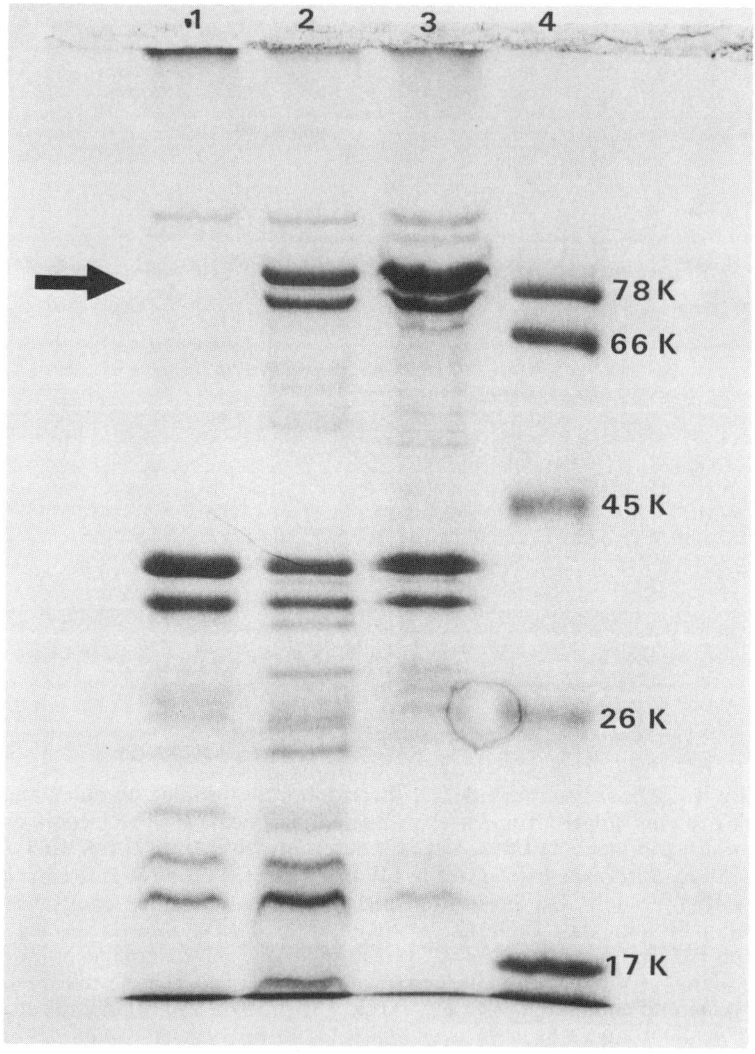

Figure 5 SDS-polyacrylamide gel electrophoresis of outer membrane proteins of *E.coli* 0111 grown in (1) trypticase soy broth; (2) trypticase soy broth containing ovotransferrin; (3) the peritoneal cavities of infected guinea-pigs. The positions of the iron-regulated outer membrane proteins are shown by the arrow. *From Griffiths, Stevenson and Joyce (1983). Reproduced by permission of* FEMS Microbiology Letters

and Joyce, 1983; Griffiths *et al.*, 1985a, 1985b). The relative abundance of the 83, 81, 78 and 74 kDa proteins expressed in different pathogenic *E.coli* strains under the same iron-restricted growth conditions, however, varies consider-

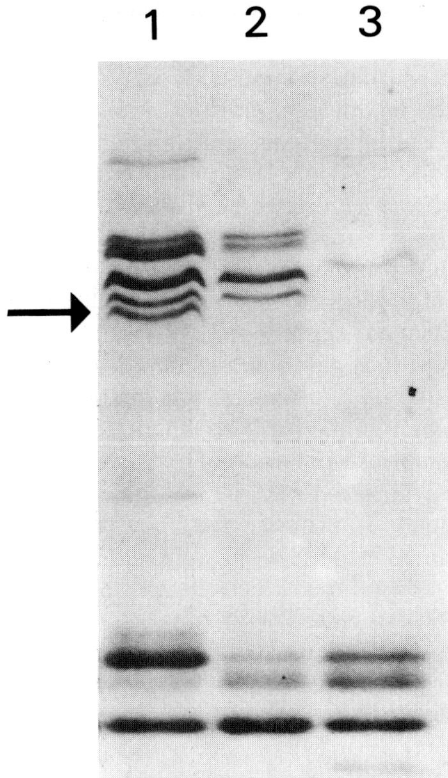

Figure 6 SDS-polyacrylamide gel electrophoresis of the outer membrane proteins of *E.coli* 018 K1 H7, a strain isolated from a child with meningitis; bacteria grown in (1) *in vivo* in experimental infection; (2) in trypticase soy broth containing ovotransferrin; (3) in trypticase soy broth alone. The position of the extra protein band expressed by *in vivo*-grown cells is indicated by the arrow. *From Griffiths* et al. *(1985a). Reproduced by permission of the American Society for Microbilogy*

ably and, in general, the pathogens produce more of the iron-regulated proteins than do *E.coli* K12. Furthermore, some pathogenic strains produce additional iron-regulated outer membrane proteins, ones not usually seen in *E.coli* K12 (Griffiths *et al.*, 1985a, 1985b). Generally, pathogenic *E.coli* isolated from extraintestinal sources express several iron-regulated proteins in their outer membranes, whereas those causing enteric infections mainly synthesize the 81 and 74 kDa proteins (compare Figs. 5 and 6). The enteroinvasive

E.coli strains discussed above are an exception in that they produce a 76 kDa protein under iron restriction (Chart and Griffiths, unpublished data; Griffiths *et al.*, 1985b). Since surface components play such an important part in host–bacteria interactions these alterations, induced in the bacterial cell envelope by host iron-binding proteins, are clearly of interest, especially since it has been shown that the same new outer membrane proteins are expressed by *E.coli* growing *in vivo* during infection (Griffiths, Stevenson and Joyce, 1983). Figure 5 shows that the iron-regulated outer membrane proteins of *E.coli* O111 recovered without subculture from the peritoneal cavities of infected guinea-pigs were major components of the outer membrane and were present in amounts equal to, or even slightly greater than, the so-called major outer membrane proteins with apparent molecular weights in the range 30,000–42,000. Unlike *E.coli* O111, however, which showed the same pattern of iron-regulated outer membrane proteins when grown *in vivo* during infection as when grown *in vitro* in the presence of ovotransferrin, *E.coli* 018 K1 H7, a pathogenic strain carrying a ColV plasmid, produced not only the iron-regulated proteins seen *in vitro* but an extra new protein during growth *in vivo* (Fig. 6) (Griffiths *et al.*, 1985a). This protein had a molecular weight of about 68,000, but it is not known if it is directly related to bacterial iron metabolism; its appearance is not associated with the presence of the ColV plasmid. Interesting differences in the pattern of the major outer membrane proteins of *E.coli* 018 (molecular weights of 30,000–40,000) were also seen when the outer membrane protein profile of the *in vivo* grown bacteria was compared with that obtained from the bacteria grown *in vitro* with ovotransferrin (Fig. 6). These changes may well reflect other environmental changes experienced by the bacteria *in vivo*.

Although it remains to be seen whether *E.coli* express the iron-regulated membrane proteins when colonizing all body sites, it has been shown that

Table 4 Pathogenic bacteria shown to express iron-regulated proteins *in vivo* during infection

Organism	Source	Host
Escherichia coli	Peritoneal cavity	Guinea-pig
Escherichia coli	Urine	Human with urinary tract infection
Klebsiella pneumoniae	Urine	Human with urinary tract infection
Proteus mirabilis	Urine	Human with urinary tract infection
Pseudomonas aeruginosa	Lung	Human with cystic fibrosis
Vibrio cholerae	Intestines	Rabbits

E.coli isolated without subculture from the urine of patients suffering from urinary tract infections, like those recovered from the peritoneal cavities of guinea-pigs, do produce the iron-regulated outer membrane proteins (Lam *et al.*, 1984) (Table 4). *Klebsiella pneumoniae* and *Proteus mirabilis*, isolated directly from the urine of two patients with urinary tract infection, also expressed iron-regulated outer membrane proteins, showing that bacteria in urinary tract infection grow under iron-restricted conditions (Shand *et al.*,1985). Similar results have been obtained by Brown, Anwar and Lambert (1984), who showed that *Pseudomonas aeruginosa* obtained without subculture from the sputum of a patient with cystic fibrosis expressed three iron-regulated proteins in its outer membrane, and by Sciortino and Finkelstein (1983), who found that *Vibrio cholerae* expressed iron-regulated membrane proteins when grown *in vivo* in the intestines of infant rabbits (Table 4).

Understanding the nature of the changes which occur in pathogenic bacteria as they grow *in vivo* is highly germane to the development of new preventive and therapeutic measures against bacterial infections. Since it has been shown that, in several cases (Table 4), the iron-regulated outer membrane proteins are expressed *in vivo* during clinical infection, the possibility that the receptors for ferric siderophores are important protective antigens is worth exploring. The siderophore receptors of some pathogenic strains of *E.coli* have been shown to be exposed on the cell surface and to interact with fairly large proteins in solution (Griffiths, Stevenson and Joyce, 1983; Griffiths *et al.*, 1985a). It is possible, therefore, that they are sufficiently exposed to, and can react with, antibodies. The discovery of naturally occurring antibodies which react with the iron-regulated outer membrane proteins of *E.coli* is discussed in Chapter 5. As part of an investigation into the possible protective role of such antibodies, Chart and Griffiths (1985b) examined the antigenic homology of the ferric–enterobactin receptor protein in different strains of *E.coli*. Their results (Fig. 7) showed that both the molecular weight and at least some of the antigenic properties of the enterobactin receptor are highly conserved within strains of *E.coli*. The antiserum used in the study, which was raised using the purified enterobactin receptor protein of *E.coli* O111, also cross-reacted with an iron-regulated 81K protein in the outer membrane of *S.typhimurium*; this is not surprising since the organism can both synthesize and utilize enterobactin (Neilands, 1982). However, the same antiserum reacted with an 83 kDa iron-regulated outer membrane protein in *K.pneumoniae*. Williams, Brown and Lambert (1984) reported that under iron-restricted conditions, *K.aerogenes* produced an 83 kDa protein in its outer membrane but no 81 kDa protein, although the organism could use ferric–enterobactin as an iron source. From these observations it would seem that in *K.pneumoniae* and *K.aerogenes* the enterobactin receptor has a molecular weight of 83,000, not 81,000.

Not all of the *E.coli* strains examined by Chart and Griffiths (1985b) expressed an iron-regulated 81 kDa protein. Of seventeen strains tested the

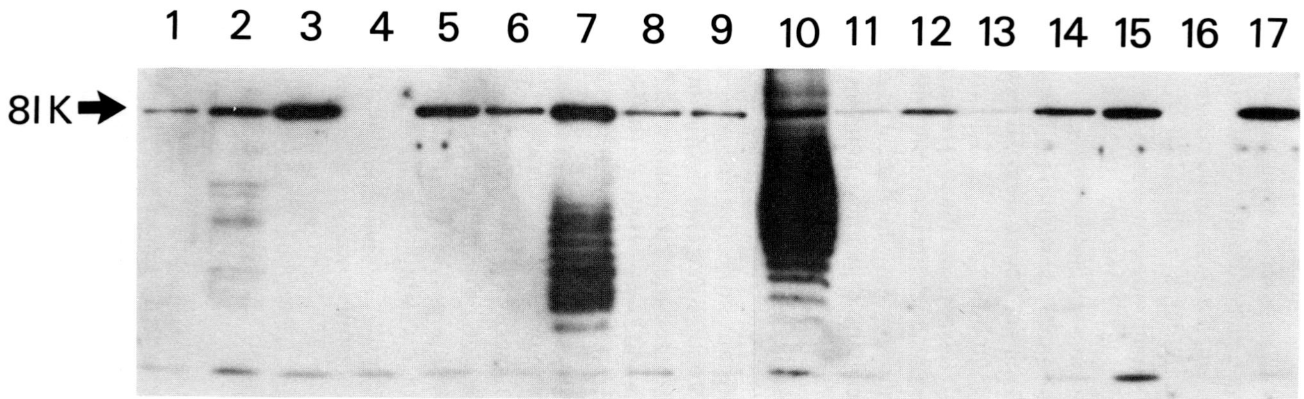

Figure 7 Autoradiograph of an immunoblot showing antibodies raised to purified ferric enterobactin receptor protein of *E.coli* 0111 reacting with an 81K protein (→) in the outer membrane protein profile of all *E.coli* strains tested, except *E.coli* C (lane 4) and *E.coli* 0164 (lane 16). Lane numbers refer to proteins from: *E.coli* strain (1) K12; (2) W3110; (3) W; (4) C; (5) MRE 600; (6) enteropathogenic strain 0128 K67 H2; (7) enteropathogenic strain 0111 K58 H2; (8) enteropathogenic strain 015; (9) 078 K80, and extraintestinal strain; (10) 018 K1 H7, and extraintestinal pathogen; (11) 02 H1, and extraintestinal pathogen; (12) enterotoxigenic strain 0128 H49; (13) enterotoxigenic strain 0159 H20; (14) enterotoxigenic strain 078 K2 H11; (15) enterotoxigenic strain 0149 K91 H10; (16) enteroinvasive strain 0164 H^-. (17) enteroinvasive strain 0124 H30. *(from Chart and Griffiths, 1985b). Reproduced by permission of the Society for General Microbiology.*

laboratory strain, *E.coli* C, and a pathogenic enteronivasive strain, *E.coli* 0164, failed to produce an enterobactin receptor protein during iron-restricted growth (Fig. 7). Subsequent work showed that the same enteroinvasive strain, *E.coli* 0164, was, however, capable of expressing an 81 kDa protein under certain growth conditions (Griffiths *et al.*, 1985b). The difference in the behaviour of this strain was traced to a difference in the way iron restriction had been produced, and the work suggests that some caution should be exercised when interpreting data concerning the nature of iron-regulated proteins expressed by different strains. When *E.coli* 0164 was grown in the presence of the iron chelator αα'-dipyridyl, a chelator which has often been used to induce iron restriction (Stevenson and Griffiths, 1985), the 81 kDa protein was not expressed (Chart and Griffiths, 1985b); in contrast, when the same organism was grown in the presence of the iron-binding protein ovotransferrin, the 81 kDa protein was expressed. *E.coli* C failed to express an 81 kDa protein under both of these growth conditions (Chart *et al.*, 1986).

Vibrio *species*

Iron-sequestering systems based on siderophores, similar to those of the enteric bacteria, have been found in other pathogens although, in general, much less is known about them or their role during infection. A particularly interesting case is that of the pathogen *Vibrio anguillarum* which is responsible for the disease vibriosis in fish. This is a devastating disease which is characterized by terminal haemorrhagic septicaemia (Harbell, Hodgins and Schiewe, 1979; Ransom *et al.*, 1984). Highly virulent strains of *V.anguillarum* isolated in the Pacific Northwest of the United States of America have been shown to carry a 65 kb plasmid designated pJMl (Crosa, 1984). This plasmid encodes an efficient iron-uptake system that allows the organism to grow under iron-restricted conditions. On losing the plasmid, *V.anguillarum* loses its virulence for fish and also its ability to grow under iron-limited conditions (Crosa, 1980; Crosa and Hodges, 1981). Genetic analysis, discussed in detail in Chapter 4, has shown that plasmid pJMI-mediated iron uptake is based on a siderophore, the molecular nature of which has not yet been determined, and an 86 kDa outer membrane receptor protein (Crosa, 1980; Crosa and Hodges, 1981; Crosa, 1984; Tolmasky and Crosa, 1984). Pathogenic strains of *V.anguillarum* isolated from the Atlantic Coast of the United States of America and from European waters have been shown to be similar to those from the Pacific Northwest in that virulence can be correlated with their ability to grow under conditions of iron limitation (Toranzo *et al.*, 1983; Tolmasky *et al.*, 1985). However, strains from the American Atlantic Coast did not contain plasmids and the genes encoding the high affinity iron-uptake system were located on the chromosome (Toranzo *et al.*, 1983; Crosa, 1984). Recent work suggests that the iron-uptake system which was originally described as being encoded by plasmid pJMl may be part of a recombinational unit, possibly a transposition sequence. The discovery of repeated sequences flanking the iron-uptake region of plasmid pJMl is consistent with this idea (Crosa, 1984; and see Chapter 4).

Studies on *Vibrio cholerae*, the causative agent of cholera in man, have shown that this *Vibrio* also expresses a siderophore-mediated high affinity iron-uptake system when grown under iron-restricted conditions. During iron restriction, *V.cholerae* produces the phenolate chelator shown in Fig. 8 (Payne and Finkelstein, 1978a; Sigel and Payne, 1982; Griffiths *et al.*, 1984). This siderophore, called vibriobactin, has a novel structure and belongs to the catecholamide family of iron chelators; it contains three residues of 2,3-dihydroxybenzoic acid, two residues of threonine and the polyamine backbone of the molecule contains the rare norspermidine (*N*-(3-aminopropyl)-1,3-diamino propane) (Griffiths *et al.*, 1984). Like enterobactin, the synthesis of vibriobactin involves a pathway via chorismic acid. Although *V.cholerae* synthesizes and uses vibriobactin as an iron chelator, the organism can also utilize a similar siderophore called agrobactin, which is the siderophore synthesized by iron-deficient cultures of *Agrobacterium tumefascians* (Ong, Peterson and Neilands, 1979; Peterson *et al.*, 1980), as well as ferrichrome and enterobactin or enterobactin breakdown products (Sigel and Payne, 1982; Griffiths *et al.*, 1984). Some strains of *V.cholerae*, like *E.coli*, are able to utilize citrate for acquiring iron (Sigel, Stoebner and Payne, 1985).

In addition to synthesizing vibriobactin, *V.cholerae* has been shown to produce at least six new proteins in its outer membrane during iron starvation (Sigel and Payne, 1982). Five of these proteins have apparent molecular weights in the range 62,000–77,000 and it has been suggested that one or more may be part of the uptake system for iron siderophores. These proteins are not detected when the cells are grown in iron-replete media. Similar iron-regulated outer membrane proteins have been found in *V.cholerae* grown *in vivo* in the intestines of infant rabbits (Sciortino and Finkelstein, 1983).

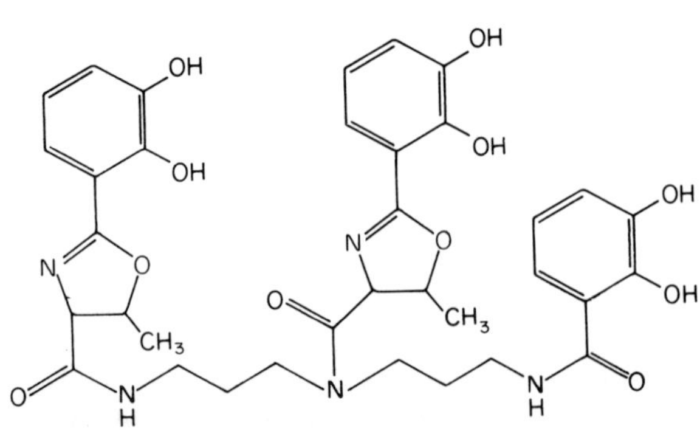

Figure 8 Structural formula of vibriobactin

Sigel, Stoebner and Payne (1985) have claimed that the ferric–vibriobactin transport systems is not required for the virulence of *V.cholerae*. Their view is based on experiments which showed that two mutants of *V.cholerae* which were defective in the iron–vibriobactin transport system retained their ability to multiply and produce disease in an infant mouse infection model. While it has certainly not been shown that the high affinity iron-uptake system based on vibriobactin is necessary for virulence, the data presented by Sigel, Stoebner and Payne (1985) do not permit one to conclude that the system is not necessary. The authors claim that both mutants multiplied normally *in vivo* and indeed the numbers of mutant bacteria recovered from infected animals were similar to those obtained using the wild-type parent strains. However, high inocula of iron-replete cells were used in these experiments (about 10^7 cells) and considerable multiplication of mutant *V.cholerae* might be expected before the organisms become starved of iron and fail to multiply. It is doubtful, therefore, if the experiments carried out by Sigel, Stoebner and Payne would have been able to detect any differences between the rate of multiplication of the two mutants and their parent strains, even if such a difference existed under iron-restricted conditions.

Vibrio vulnificus is a marine *Vibrio* recently recognized as capable of causing lethal septicaemia in humans (Blake *et al.*, 1979; Wright, Simpson and Oliver, 1981; Oliver, Warner and Cleland, 1983). The organism appears to cause disease via skin lesions or after the ingestion of raw shellfish. Putative siderophores of both phenolate and hydroxamate type have been described for *V.vulnificus* (Simpson and Oliver, 1983) and the organism synthesizes two new outer membranes proteins when grown in the presence of an iron-binding protein (Chart and Griffiths, 1985a). Although these proteins have molecular weights of 81,000 and 74,000, they do not appear to be related to the iron-regulated 81 and 74 kDa proteins of *E.coli*; furthermore, *V.vulnificus* cannot use ferric–enterobactin as an iron source (Simpson and Oliver, 1983). Indeed, the involvement of the two apparently iron-regulated membrane proteins described by Chart and Griffiths (1985a) as receptors for *V.vulnificus* siderophores has not been established. The fact that multiplication was inhibited, virtually completely, both in a medium containing ovotransferrin or transferrin and in normal human serum, suggests that the organism does not possess an efficient high affinity iron-uptake system. An ability to use haemoglobin as a source of iron may mean that the availability of haem at the site of infection might be an important factor in pathogenesis (Helms, Oliver and Travis, 1984; Chart and Griffiths, 1985a). However, usually the life-threatening septicaemic infections caused by *V.vulnificus* occur only in patients with underlying diseases which result in elevated serum iron levels, and it appears that the organism is an opportunistic pathogen which relies on the iron which is often freely available in the serum of such individuals (Wright, Simpson and Oliver, 1981; Chart and Griffiths, 1985a; Gutteridge *et al.*, 1985; see also Chapters 5, 7 and 8).

Pseudomonas *species*

Pseudomonas aeruginosa is primarily an opportunistic pathogen involved with diseases of compromised patients, e.g. those with cystic fibrosis, neoplasms or burns. Several extracellular products, such as toxin A, proteases and lipopolysaccharide, are produced by the organism and these may contribute to its pathogenicity (Liu, 1966; Bjorn *et al.*, 1979, Young, 1980; see also Chapter 4). However, the ability of the organism to sequester iron may also be important in cases where host iron metabolism has not been perturbed so as to increase the availability of iron *in vivo* (Hunter *et al.*, 1984). Brown, Anwar and Lambert (1984) showed that mucoid *Ps. aeruginosa* in the cystic fibrosis lung grows under iron-restricted conditions (Table 4). Indeed, their work gave the first direct biochemical evidence of the physiological state of bacteria when infecting humans. The outer membrane protein composition of mucoid *Pseudomonas* recovered without subculture from the sputum of a cystic fibrosis patient was shown to contain three iron-regulated outer membrane proteins with molecular weights in the range 80,000–90,000. These iron-regulated proteins were shown to be antigenic and recognized by antibodies in the patient's serum (Anwar *et al.*, 1984). Similar iron-regulated high molecular weight proteins have been seen in the outer membranes of several *Pseudomonas* species by Meyer, Mock and Abdallah, (1979) and by Sokol and Woods (1983).

Pseudomonas species are known to produce several siderophores during iron restriction: ferribactin, ferrioxamines, pyoverdin, pyochelin and pseudobactin (Liu and Shokrani, 1978; Cox and Graham, 1979; Cox, 1980; Neilands, 1982; Sokol, 1984; Yang and Leong, 1984). Of these, it is pyochelin and pyoverdin which are of most interest as regards infection. Although pyoverdin, which has a binding constant for iron of 10^{32} (Wendenbaum *et al.*, 1983), has been shown to promote the growth of *Pseudomonas* in the presence of transferrin (Cox and Adams, 1985), pyoverdin negative strains have been isolated from human infections. In contrast, no pyochelin negative strains have been found and this siderophore does have dramatic effects on the virulence of *Ps. aeruginosa* (Cox, 1982). Pyochelin (Fig. 9) is a salicylic acid-substituted cysteinyl peptide siderophore (Cox *et al.*, 1981), and it has been shown to promote experimental *Pseudomonas* infections in mice (Cox, 1982). The uptake of ferric–pyochelin by *Pseudomonas* occurs in two stages, an energy-independent step, presumably involving binding to the cell surface, followed by an energy-dependent process (Cox, 1980). The role of the high moleular weight iron-regulated outer membrane proteins of *Pseudomonas* in pyochelin transport, however, is not clear. Sokol and Woods (1983) and Sokol (1984) have shown that ferric–pyochelin binds, *in vitro*, to a protein with a molecular weight of 14,000; this low molecular weight protein is also expressed in greater amounts in cells grown under iron limitation. These workers suggest that the high molecular weight membrane proteins induced by iron limitation are not

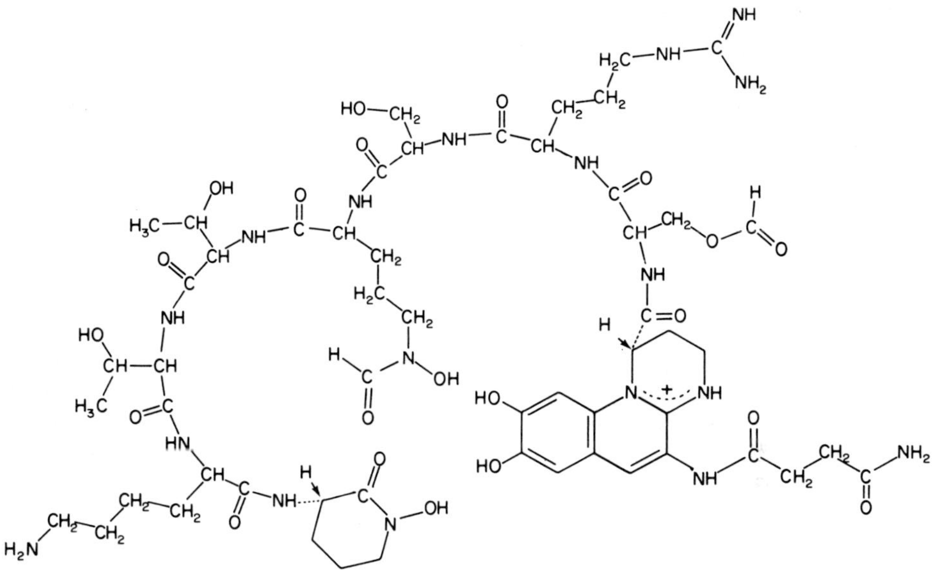

1

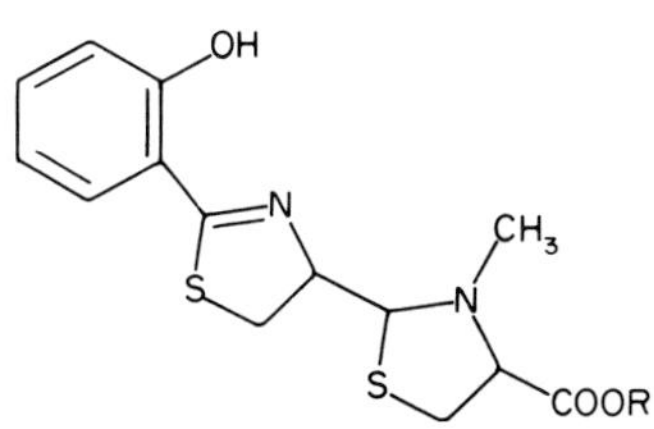

2

Figure 9 Structural formulae of two siderophores from *Pseudomonas aeruginosa*: (1) pyoverdin, (2) pyochelin

involved in the binding of ferric–pyochelin to the bacterial cell. However, so far there is no direct evidence that the 14 kDa protein plays a part in the transport of ferric–pyochelin in intact *Ps.aeruginosa*. Furthermore, although there has been considerable interest in pyochelin as a siderophore, recent work suggests that the synthesis of pyoverdin (Fig. 9) may be more important for the growth of *Ps.aeruginosa* in serum (Ankenbauer, Sriyosachati and Cox, 1985); pyochelin is, apparently, synthesized only very poorly by the bacteria when in serum and offers little benefit to the organism. Detailed genetic analysis of these high affinity iron-transport systems is required to understand more clearly the role they play in infections caused by *Pseudomonas*. Although *Ps.aeruginosa* does not synthesize enterobactin, it can utilize this chelator as well as pyochelin (Liu and Shokrani, 1978) and, like *E.coli*, it can also use ferric citrate as a source of iron (Cox, 1980).

Aeromonas salmonicida

Aeromonas salmonicida is an important pathogen of fish (Herman, 1968). Many strains grow rapidly *in vivo* producing a septicaemia which is often accompanied at the terminal stages by a severe necrosis of the tissues. One of the major virulence determinants of this organism consists of a hydrophobic 49 kDa protein which covers the bacterial cell surface, the so-called A layer (Udey and Fryer, 1978; Kay *et al.*, 1981; Munn *et al.*, 1982). This protein layer appears to play an important part in protecting the pathogen from host defences (Munn *et al.*, 1982; Trust *et al.*, 1982; Phipps *et al.*, 1983). In addition to withstanding host defence mechanisms, it would be expected that this pathogen, like *V.anguillarum*, would have an efficient mechanism for obtaining iron from the fish iron-binding proteins. Chart and Trust (1983) found that highly pathogenic strains of *A.salmonicida* could indeed sequester iron from iron-binding proteins very efficiently and utilized one of two distinct mechanisms for doing so. One mechanism involved a siderophore-mediated iron-uptake system. This system, like other siderophore-mediated iron-uptake mechanisms studied, was inducible although the molecular nature of the siderophore has not been determined. The other mechanism, seen only in one particular strain of *A.salmonicida*, involved a non-inducible iron-uptake system which seemed not to involve the production of soluble siderophores. In this latter case, direct contact between the bacterial cell surface and the iron-binding protein was required for iron uptake and in this respect the mechanism resembled that found in *N.meningitidis* and *N.gonorrhoeae* (see Section 2.2).

Although the *A.salmonicida* strain which was able to use the 'direct-contact' iron-uptake mechanism was unable to produce a soluble iron chelator of its own, it was able to utilize the siderophore or siderophores produced by those strains which depended on the siderophore-mediated iron-uptake system. As in the case of other bacterial species, all *A.salmonicida* strains expressed several new outer membrane proteins during growth under iron-restricted conditions. However, the role of these iron-regulated outer membrane proteins in iron uptake is unknown.

Mycobacteria

A comprehensive review of the chemistry and biology of the mycobactins, a

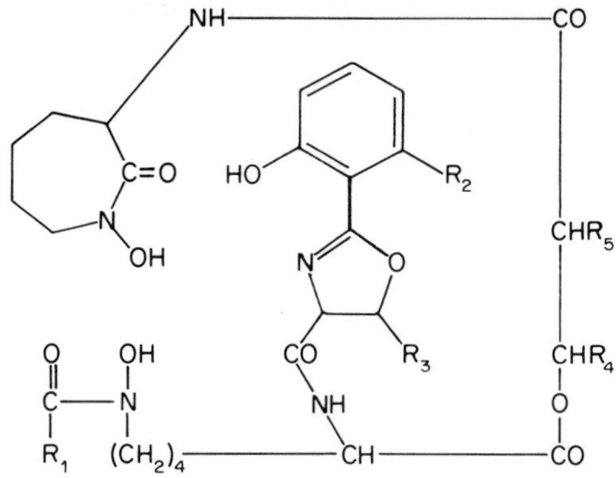

Figure 10 General structure of myobactins: R_1 refers to an acyl side-chain (C_{12}–C_{19}) and R_2–R_5 are usually H or CH_3 moieties

well-characterized group of siderophores produced by the mycobacteria, was made by Snow in 1970. Chemically, the mycobactins consist of two distinct parts: an octahedral iron-binding site, which contains two secondary hydroxamate groups, an oxazoline ring and a phenolic hydroxyl group, and a hydrophobic chain containing up to twenty carbon atoms (Snow, 1970). Figure 10 shows the general structure of the mycobactins. These compounds are virtually insoluble in water but are readily extracted as iron complexes from the bacterial cell into chloroform. The iron complex has an association constant greater than 10^{30} (Snow and White, 1969). Recently, it has been shown that mycobactin is an excellent chemotaxanomic marker for the identification and classification of the mycobacteria (Hall and Ratledge, 1984, 1985).

Since the mycobactins are both essential growth factors for *Mycobacterium paratuberculosis* and also powerful iron chelators, it seems likely that they are involved in mycobacterial iron metabolism (Kochan, 1973). Indeed, the yields of mycobactin from mycobacteria are increased by iron deficiency (Ratledge and Hall, 1971). Also, the addition of mycobactin P or the culture fluids from Bacillus Calmette Guérin (BCG) can abolish the bacteriostatic effect of serum on BCG (Kochan, Pellis and Golden, 1971; Kochan, 1973). More recent data suggests that the assimilation of iron by mycobacteria involves not only mycobactin but also another iron chelator called exochelin (Stephenson and Ratledge, 1979). However, much of the information available is concerned with the mechanisms whereby the avirulent organism *M.smegmatis* obtains iron during growth under iron-restricted conditions (Ratledge, Patel and Mundy, 1982) and the relationship between mycobactin and exochelin and the ability of pathogenic mycobacteria such as *M.tuberculosis* or *M.leprae* to grow *in vivo* is uncertain. Barclay and Ratledge (1983) have shown that some strains of *M.avium*, *M.intracellulare* and *M.scrofulaceum* can produce both mycobactin and exochelin but that *M.paratuberculosis* produced ony exochelin. Ferric citrate also functions as an iron source for *M.smegmatis*, *M.bovis* and BCG *in vitro* (Messenger and Ratledge, 1982), but it remains to be seen if iron chelated to traces of citrate *in vivo* can serve as a source of iron for these organisms. The mycobacteria are, of course, intracellular pathogens and little is known about the capability of microorganisms such as mycobacteria, brucella and listeria to multiply inside polymorphs, macrophages or other host cells. In fact, little is known about intracellular environments although it is known that polymorphs do contain lactoferrin (Moulder, 1979; Bullen, 1981).

Corynebacterium diphtheriae

It is well known that the level of iron in the environment affects the synthesis of diphtheria toxin (see Chapter 4). Maximum levels of diphtheria toxin are produced by *C.diphtheriae* only when cultures are grown in iron-deficient media (Barksdale, 1970; Pappenheimer, 1977). *In vivo*, it would be expected that *C.diphtheriae* would multiply under the iron-restricted conditions imposed by the presence of lactoferrin in mucosal secretions and thus produce the toxin. Recent genetic and biochemical evidence suggests that *C.diphtheriae* obtains iron via a siderophore-dependent iron-transport system (Russell and Holmes, 1983; Russell, Cryz and Holmes, 1984). The molecular nature of the siderophore is not yet known, but it has been shown to stimulate appropriate bacterial indicator strains to transport iron and to multiply under iron-limiting conditions. It is interesting to note that the naturally occurring highly toxinogenic Park Williams Number 8 strain of *C.diphtheriae*, which is used to synthesize toxin for the production of diphtheria toxoid vaccines, grows slowly *in vitro* and is avirulent. Russell and Holmes (1985) have shown that this strain is defective in iron uptake and does not produce the corynebacterium siderophore. Although the genetic and biochemical basis for the phenotype of this strain remains to be determined, it is attractive to postulate that the defect in siderophore production may be an important factor in determining both the poor growth of this organism *in vivo* and its capacity to make large amounts of diphtheria toxin *in vitro* (Russell and Holmes, 1985).

2.2 Iron-uptake mechanisms which do not depend on siderophores

Neisseria *species*

There is no doubt that pathogenic *Neisseria* species can remove iron from iron-binding proteins. However, the means by which this is accomplished is poorly understood and there has been conflicting evidence regarding the role of siderophores in the process. *Neisseria gonorrhoeae* is an obligate human pathogen, causing disease localized primarily on the mucosal surfaces of the genital tract, the oropharynx and the rectum; it occasionally invades the bloodstream and synovial membranes of joints. *Neisseria meningitidis* is normally restricted to the nasopharynx but during systemic infection meningococci grow in a variety of other places in the body, such as the cerebrospinal fluid and blood. In contrast to gonococcal infection, a bacteriaemia occurs in most if not all forms of meningococcal disease. It would be expected that transferrin would be a source of iron for both these organisms in serum and lactoferrin the iron source on mucosal surfaces.

Payne and Finkelstein (1978b) were the first to report the production of a siderophore by certain strains of gonococci; later, Yancey and Finkelstein (1981a) reported finding very small amounts of a hydroxamate-type siderophore in the culture supernatants of both the gonococcus and meningococcus. However, other investigators found no evidence for the existence of either a gonococcal or meningococcal iron chelator (Norrod and Williams, 1978; Archibald and DeVoe, 1979, 1980; Mickelsen and Sparling, 1981; Simonson, Brener and DeVoe, 1982). Recent work by West and Sparling (1985) has shown that certain complex media contain small amounts of siderophore activity as a normal component and it is likely that it was this material that was the source of the iron chelators detected in the culture fluids of *N.gonorrhoeae* and *N.meningitidis* by Yancey and Finkelstein (1981a). Investigators who failed to find siderophores invariably tested culture supernatants of gonococci or meningococci grown in chemically defined iron-deficient media. Although it is now virtually certain that neither the gonococcus nor the meningococcus can synthesize its own siderophore, these organisms can use some exogenous siderophores. For example, *N.meningitidis* and *N.gonorrhoeae* can use ferric citrate as an iron source (Yancey and Finkelstein, 1981b), and the gonococcus has been shown to use aerobactin (West and Sparling, 1985). All of the *Neisseria* isolates examined by Mickelsen and Sparling (1981) were able to use haemin as a sole source of iron and most could also obtain iron from haemoglobin. However, desferrioxime B (Disferal) could not function as an iron source for these pathogens (Archibald and DeVoe, 1980; Calver, Kenny and Kushner 1979).

Perhaps one of the most significant features regarding the acquisition of iron from iron-binding proteins by the *Neisseria* is the highly specific nature of the process (Table 5). This is in contrast to the known siderophore-mediated iron-uptake systems which appear to be able to take iron from any one of the three iron-binding proteins. All gonococci and meningococci seem able to obtain the iron required for growth from human transferrin, whereas most commensal species of *Neisseria* are unable to do so; their growth was inhibited by this particular iron-binding protein (Mickelsen and Sparling, 1981; Simonson, Brener and DeVoe, 1982). Similarly, Mickelsen, Blackman and Sparling (1982) found that all meningococci could obtain iron from human lactoferrin but only about 50 per cent of the gonococcal isolates and 25 per cent of

Table 5 The ability of *Neisseria* species to acquire iron from iron-binding glycoproteins

Organism	Lactoferrin (%)	Transferrin (%)	Ovotransferrin (%)
Neisseria gonorrhoeae	53	100	0
Neisseria meningitidis	100	100	0
Commensal *Neisseria* sp.	24	22	0

From Mickelsen and Sparling (1981), Mickelsen, Blackman and Sparling (1982), and Simonsen, Brener and DeVoe (1982).

commensal *Neisseria* species were able to do so; strains which were unable to remove the iron from lactoferrin were unable to multiply in the presence of this protein. The inhibitory effect of lactoferrin was abolished when sufficient iron was added to saturate the iron-binding capacity of the protein, thus showing that the growth-inhibiting property of lactoferrin was due to its iron-binding property. In contrast to human transferrin and lactoferrin, chicken ovotransferrin was bacteriostatic for all *Neisseria* species tested, suggesting that it could not act as a source of iron for any of these organisms (Archibald and DeVoe, 1979; Mickelsen and Sparling, 1981). Since transferrin and ovotransferrin are closely related glycoproteins having similar amino acid compositions, physical characteristics and iron-binding properties (Aisen and Listowsky, 1980; see also Chapter 2), these observations suggest that the mechanism by which gonococci and meningococci obtain iron from host iron-binding proteins is extremely protein specific. It should also be noted, however, that these proteins do differ in their carbohydrate moieties (see Chapter 2). A similar specificity exists in the case of the reticulocyte. For example, rabbit reticulocytes can distinguish between ovotransferrin, transferrin and lactoferrin and will remove iron only from transferrin (Zapolski and Princiotto, 1976; Morgan, 1981). Reticulocytes and other mammalian cells remove iron from transferrin by a process which involves a direct association between the iron-binding protein and a specific cell surface receptor (Aisen and Listowsky, 1980; Newman *et al.*, 1982; Octave *et al.*, 1983; see also Chapters 2 and 8). The results of several investigations suggest that a direct association between host iron-binding glycoproteins and the surface of *N.meningitidis*, and between *N.gonorrhoeae* and lactoferrin, is also required for the utilization of protein-bound iron (Archibald and DeVoe, 1979; Simonson, Brener and DeVoe, 1982; Mietzner *et al.*, 1984). However, the means by which iron is removed from the iron-binding protein remains unknown. Simonson, Brener and DeVoe (1982) have shown that apotransferrin is bound by the meningococcus to the same extent as 30 per cent iron-saturated transferrin, suggesting that *N.meningtidis* is unable to distinguish between iron-loaded and iron-free transferrin. Indeed, excess apotransferrin impeded the acquisition of iron from transferrin. Simonson,

Brener and DeVoe (1982) also showed that the uptake of iron from transferrin depending on a functional respiratory chain, although the amount of transferrin bound to the surface of cyanide-treated meningococci was similar to that bound by metabolically active cells. The fact that iron-replete *N.meningitidis* was capable of binding approximately the same number of transferrin molecules as the iron-starved cells also points to the fact that the ability of meningococci at least to bind transferrin is independent of their capacity to incorporate iron from this protein (Simonson, Brener and DeVoe, 1982). However, iron-replete meningococci, in contrast to the iron-starved organisms, were ineffective in taking iron from transferrin.

As has been discussed in Section 2.1 of this chapter, outer membrane proteins whose synthesis is induced specifically as a result of iron limitation are integral components of iron-uptake mechanisms involving siderophores. Even though the high affinity iron-uptake mechanisms of the gonococcus and meningococcus do not appear to involve siderophores, both organisms do synthesize new outer membrane proteins during iron restriction. Norqvist *et al.* (1978) were the first to show that iron-limited *N.gonorrhoeae* produced several new outer membrane proteins with apparent molecular weights in the range 70,000–100,000. Mietzner *et al.* (1984) and West and Sparling (1985) confirmed this observation and also detected an additional iron-regulated protein with a molecular weight of about 37 kDa. This additional protein is interesting since it stains poorly with Coomassie blue stain but reacts well with silver stain. When silver stain is used to stain gels the protein appears as a major component of the outer membrane of iron-restricted *N.gonorrhoeae* (Mietzner *et al.*, 1984). Yet more iron-regulated proteins were detected by West and Sparling (1985) when they examined crude membrane preparations consisting of both inner and outer membranes. Interestingly enough, the expression of iron-regulated proteins in *N.gonorrhoeae* varies slightly, not only with the strain used but also with the source of iron. For example, a particular subset of iron-regulated proteins were expressed when the bacteria were grown in the presence of transferrin or lactoferrin (West and Sparling, 1985). Iron-limited growth of *N.meningitidis* also leads to the expression of new iron-regulated proteins, the expression of which is also affected by lowering the pH from 7.4 to 6.6 (Brener, DeVoe and Holbein, 1981; Mietzner *et al.*, 1984).

The role, if any, of the iron-regulated proteins of *Neisseria* species in iron transport remains to be determined, and it is likely that a genetic approach will be needed to extend our understanding of these iron-related phenotypic changes. Clearly, though, as far as the gonococcus and meningococcus are concerned, the iron-binding proteins seem to provide specific sources of iron. Indeed, Holbein (1980) has shown that the level of iron in the circulating transferrin pool of mice determines the course of experimental *N.meningitidis* infection. Meningococcal infection in mice leads to hypoferraemia. This hypoferraemia controls the infection by depriving the pathogen of iron since the organism appears to depend on transferrin iron for growth in the host (Holbein, 1981; Letendre and Holbein, 1983, 1984). Whether an ability to take iron from lactoferrin contributes to the pathogenicity of either the gonococcus or meningococcus is not clear. An ability to use the iron in lactoferrin does not seem to be required for the survival of *Neisseria* on mucosal surfaces since most commensal species cannot use lactoferrin iron. Mickelsen, Blackman and Sparling (1982) suggest that since these organisms are able to use haem as an iron source, the haem released by dying cells sloughed from the epithelium may be one source of iron on mucosal surfaces. However, pathogenic species may need to multiply more rapidly than the commensals and an ability to use the iron in lactoferrin might help.

Other pathogenic bacteria

It seems that some other pathogens may also obtain iron *in vivo* via a mechanism involving direct contact between the pathogen and the iron-binding protein. The ability of one particular strain of *A.salmonicida* to obtain iron in this way has already been discussed in Section 2.1. It may be that *Haemophilus influenzae* can obtain iron in this way too. The fact that this organism utilizes only one type of iron-binding protein as a source of iron indicates a protein-specific iron-uptake mechanism. Herrington and Sparling (1985) have shown that *H.influenzae* type b can obtain iron from 30 per cent iron-saturated human transferrin but not from 30 per cent iron-saturated lactoferrin. Although it has been considered that *H.influenzae* has an absolute requirement for haem, which was thought to supply both the iron requirement of the cell and essential porphyrin (Biberstein, Mini and Gills, 1963; White and Granick, 1963; Coulton and Pang, 1983), it now appears that, in most cases, only protoporphyrin IX is required, provided iron is available from another source. Each of 33 *H.influenzae* type b isolates, and 28 of 35 isolates of nontypeable *H.influenzae*, including 2 of 3 systemic isolates, were able to utilize the iron of transferrin. Not one of 18 *H.parainfluenzae* isolates could do so, and this might be responsible for reducing their ability to invade the bloodstream. *H.parainfluenzae* isolates are only rarely pathogenic. Neither *H.influenzae* nor *H.parainfluenzae* strains could use 30 per cent iron-saturated lactoferrin as a source of iron *in vitro*. However, since both pathogenic and non-pathogenic *Haemophilus* strains are able to survive and grow on human mucosal surfaces they must be able to acquire iron *in vivo* from some source. It is possible that they use haem released by dying cells sloughed from the epithelium.

The mechanism whereby *H.influenzae* removes iron from transferrin is not known, nor indeed is it known if the ability to use transferrin iron is important *in vivo*. During iron restriction *H.influenzae* type b has been reported to increase the amount of three membrane proteins but no siderophores have been found (Herrington and Sparling, 1985). Williams and Brown (1986), however, found that iron restriction had little effect on the outer membrane protein profile of their isolate of *H.influenzae* type b. They did find that *H.parainfluenzae* responded to iron restriction by inducing several new proteins in the range 70–86 kDa. Clearly, more work is needed to clarify the response of different isolates of *H.influenzae* to iron restriction.

2.3 Acquisition of iron from haem or haemoglobin

In addition to obtaining iron from the iron-binding proteins, transferrin, lactoferrin or ovotransferrin, a number of pathogenic bacteria may also, under certain conditions, obtain sufficient iron *in vivo* from cell free haem or haemoglobin. In general it seems that this iron is more readily available than that bound to iron-binding proteins. It has been suggested that the increased availability of iron in haem abolishes the need for organisms such as *E.coli* to adapt to the otherwise iron-restricted environment found in host tissues and allows them to multiply more rapidly (Griffiths, 1981). However, the mechanisms whereby bacterial pathogens are able to utilze the iron in haem or haemoglobin is unknown, and this is an aspect which needs investigation.

Normally, there is only a trace of free haem in serum and this is bound to haemopexin or serum albumin (Morgan, 1981); similarly, the small amount of haemoglobin which is released into blood during red cell breakdown is bound to haptoglobin (Laurell and Gronvall, 1962; Eaton *et al.*, 1982). Even though the level of free haem might be too low to support the growth of most pathogens, there may be enough present in blood to promote the growth of pathogens like *Yersinia pestis* (Perry and Brubaker, 1979; Bullen, 1981). It is not yet clear whether *Y.pestis* produces soluble siderophores. Indirect evidence suggests that iron chelators are produced during iron restriction (Wake, Misawa and Matsui, 1975), but Perry and Brubaker (1979) failed to detect siderophore activity. Indeed, the iron-restricted strains of *Y.pestis* studied by Perry and Brubaker (1979) were unable to use exogenously supplied aerobactin, desferal, enterobactin or shizokinen, although these chelators stimulated the growth of iron-limited *Y.pseudotuberculosis* and *Y.enterocolitica* Haem was found to be the most effective nutritional source of iron for *Y.pestis*, 0.5 pmol being sufficient to allow growth of the organism in an otherwise inhibitory medium containing ovotransferrin. This extremely low requirement for haem may mean that the organism takes advantage of circulating haem bound to haemopexin or serum albumin. Bullen (1981) also raised the interesting possibility that sufficient haem to initiate an infection might be injected along with *Y.pestis* by the rat flea, *Xenopsylla cheopis*, during the transmission of plague.

For most organisms, however, it seems that it is necessary first to liberate haemoglobin from the erythrocyte by haemolysis in order to provide sufficient material to promote bacterial growth. The effect of haemolysis produced experimentally, or by injury or diseases such as sickle cell anaemia, bartonellosis and malaria, on the susceptibility of the host to infection is discussed in Chapter 7. Generally, increasing the availability of haem or haemoglobin leads to increased susceptibility to infections of various kinds. Experimental work has shown that it is the iron in haemoglobin that is responsible for stimulating bacterial growth (Lee *et al.*, 1979). In some instances, such as with *E.coli* (Eaton *et al.*, 1982) the administration of haptoglobin protects against experimental infections promoted by haemoglobin, and such work has suggested the possible use of haptoglobin in treating potentially fatal haemoglobin-mediated bacterial infections (Eaton *et al.*, 1982). However, this may not apply in all cases. *Vibrio vulnificus*, for example, can utilize the haemoglobin in the haemoglobin–haptoglobin complex (Helms, Oliver and Travis, 1984).

Since haemolysis resulting from the clinical conditions mentioned above leads to an increased susceptibility to bacterial infections, it might be expected that increasing the level of available haem or haemoglobin by haemolysin-induced lysis of erythrocytes might achieve the same result, and there is evidence that this is the case. Haemolysins are bacterial toxins that can cause the lysis of erythrocytes, and colonies of haemolytic bacteria are easily identified by the clear zone of haemolysis that surrounds them on blood agar plates. Perhaps the best understood haemolysins are those of *E.coli* (Cavalieri, Bohach and Snyder, 1984). An association of haemolytic *E.coli* with disease has long been recognized (Dudgeon, Wordley and Bawtree, 1921) and several studies have shown that a high proportion of strains isolated from various sites of extraintestinal infection in humans are haemolytic (Fried and Wong, 1970; Cooke and Ewins, 1975; Minshew *et al.*, 1978; DeBoy, Wachsmith and Davis, 1980; Green and Thomas, 1981). Many enteropathogenic *E.coli* of porcine origin also produce haemolysin (Smith and Linggood, 1971) and haemolytic strains have been found to be much more virulent for mice and rats than non-haemolytic ones (Smith and Linggood, 1971; Emody *et al.*, 1980; van den Bosch *et al.*, 1979, 1981, 1982; Welch *et al.*, 1981). About 80 per cent of strains which are virulent for chicken embryos are also haemolytic (Minshew *et al.*, 1978). Lovell and Rees (1960) were the first to describe a filterable haemolysin produced by haemolytic *E.coli* and Smith (1963) called this toxin α-haemolysin; this distinguishes it from another cell-bound haemolysin which he called β-haemolysin. The α-haemolysins produced by *E.coli* from a variety of sources are antigenically cross-reactive and have similar but not identical physical properties. They are heat-labile, acidic proteins and they require Ca^{2+} for full activity (Smith, 1963; Short and Kurtz, 1971; Rennie and Arbuthnott, 1974; Rennie, Freer and Arbuthnott, 1974; Williams, 1979b; Cavalieri, Bohach and Snyder, 1984). *E.coli* α-haemolysins lyse the erythrocytes of several animal species (Smith, 1963), although differences in the sensitivities of red blood cells from different animals have been noted (Rennie and Arbuthnott, 1974). The broad susceptibility pattern of erythrocytes from different species suggests that α-haemolysin reacts with residues common to many types of red blood cell membranes. Proposed mechanisms for the lytic reaction have been discussed by Cavalieri, Bohach and Snyder (1984).

The genes encoding α-haemolysin production in *E.coli* have, in many instances, been found to be carried by plasmids and a large number of haemolysin, Hly, plasmids have been characterized (Goebel *et al.*, 1985; Griffiths, 1985; Smith, Scotland and Rowe, 1985). These Hly plamids belong to a number of different incompatability groups and range in size from 60 to over 160 kb. DNA hybridization experiments and restriction enzyme cleavage patterns show clearly their diverse nature. However, even those Hly plasmids which are structurally unrelated share extensive homology in the region which encodes haemolysin production (Royer-Pokora and Goebel, 1976; de la Cruz *et al.*, 1980; Noegel, Rdest and Goebel, 1981; Waalwijk *et al.*, 1982; Goebel *et al.*, 1985; Smith, Scotland and Rowe, 1985). Detailed genetic analysis of certain Hly plasmids has shown that the region responsible for α-haemolysin synthesis and export consists of four cistrons: *hly*A, *hly*C, *hly*Ba, and *hly*Bb; in most Hly plasmids these regions also seem to share common flanking regions (Goebel *et al.*, 1985; Gonzalez-Carrero *et al.*, 1985; Nicaud *et al.*, 1985; Smith, Scotland and Rowe, 1985). The *hly*A gene codes for a protein which is the precursor of α-haemolysin; *hly*C encodes a protein necessary for processing the precursor to active haemolysin, although its precise function is not yet understood; *hly*Ba and *hly*Bb gene products are found predominantly in the outer membrane and seem to be involved in the transport of haemolysin from the periplasm to the exterior of the cell.

However, not all α-haemolysin determinants are carried on plasmids and there are several instances, especially in haemolytic *E.coli* isolated from human extraintestinal infections, where the haemolysin determinant is not transferred from strain to strain (Smith and Linggood, 1970; Minshew *et al.*, 1978, Hull *et al.*, 1982). In such cases, the Hly determinant could be located either on a non-conjugative plasmid or in the chromosome. It now seems that most haemolytic *E.coli* strains isolated from humans, especially those from patients with urinary tract infections, carry the haemolysin determinant in the chromosome (Berger *et al.*, 1982; Hull *et al.*, 1982; Goebel *et al.*, 1985). Chromosomal haemolysin determinants have been cloned and hybridization experiments using plasmid encoded *hly* genes have shown extensive homology in the four structural *hly* genes, which have also been shown to be functionally exchangeable (Berger *et al.*, 1982; Hacker *et al.*, 1983; Goebel *et al.*, 1985). Furthermore, it has been shown that uropathogenic *E.coli* strains carry at least two complete sets of *hly* genes in the chromosome, in contrast to some other human haemolytic *E.coli* isolates which possess only one (Knapp *et al.*, 1984).

The distance between the *hly* determinants in the chromosome is unknown, although it does seem that a tandem duplication mechanism which has been shown to be responsible for increasing the number of cholera toxin genes in the chromosome of *V.cholerae* (Mekalanos, 1983) is unlikely to be operating in this case. Detailed analysis of the *hly* determinants in the chromosome of one haemolytic *E.coli* strain suggested that the two *hly* systems present were not indentical. Indeed, more precise restriction mapping of various determinants, particularly in *hly*A, has shown that small differences exist between chromosomal and plasmid *hly* genes; obvious differences exist between the flanking regions of the plasmid and chromosomal *hly* determinants. These differences may be responsible for the differences in pathogenicity that have been observed not only between strains with plasmid and chromosomal *hly* determinants, but also among those carrying chromosomal *hly* genes (Welch *et al.*, 1981; Hacker *et al.*, 1983; Welch and Falkow, 1984; Goebel *et al.*, 1985). It is not yet known if these differences reflect alterations in the amount of haemolysin produced or subtle variations in the activity of the toxin, as suggested by Goebel *et al.*, (1985). Whether such changes might be responsible for quantitative differences in the amount of haem or haemoglobin liberated is unknown.

Although a considerable amount of information has accumulated about the nature of *E.coli* haemolysins and the genetic locus for their production, their role in pathogenesis is still not entirely clear. It is clear that haemolysin activity itself contributes towards virulence (Welch *et al.*, 1981) and that it may do so by enabling haemolytic strains of *E.coli* to obtain the iron needed for growth from the haemoglobin or haem liberated from lysed erythorcytes. Linggood and Ingram (1982) found that transferring an Hly plasmid to a non-haemolytic strain of *E.coli* increased the virulence of the strain for mice. Injection of non-toxic amounts of α-haemolysin, phenylhydrazine (which causes haemolysis), iron or haemoglobin simulated the effect of the Hly plasmid by stimulating bacterial growth. Active or passive immunization against α-haemolysin protected mice from challenge with the haemolytic *E.coli in vivo*; this protection was overcome by administering iron salts at the time of challenge. An iron-sequestering mechanism depending upon the utilization of liberated haem would, of course, be expected to be important only for growth of bacteria in blood, and the ability to make haemolysin should have little effect on bacterial growth on mucosal surfaces, such as in the gut, as actually seems to be the case (Smith and Linggood, 1971). It is not clear, however, why haemolysin-producing strains of *E.coli* should be associated with human pyelonephritis. Experimental work has shown a particular connection between haemolysin production and the ability of *E.coli* to produce pyelonephritis in mice and rats after intravenous injection, possibly indicating that an ability to multiply effectively in the bloodstream is an important factor related to the initiation of infection by this route (Fried *et al.*, 1971; van den Bosch, de Graaf and MacLaren, 1979; van den Bosch *et al.*, 1981). Waalwijk, MacLaren and de Graaf (1983) have shown that it is α-haemolysin itself that enhances the pathogenicity of *E.coli* in the haematogenous pyelonephritis model in mice, and this enhanced virulence is due to the lysis of erythrocytes, thus liberating haemoglobin which acts as a source of iron for the organisms. When a Tn5-induced non-haemolytic mutant strain was simultaneously injected into mice with the haemolytic parent both strains multiplied (Waalwijk, MacLaran and de Graaf 1983). The fact that the number of organisms of both types increased in the kidney suggested that the α-haemolysin produced by the haemolytic *E.coli* strain was acting as a growth factor for the non-haemolytic mutant *in vivo*; the virulence of the mutant strain was similarly enhanced by the injection of α-haemolysin, haemoglobin or iron salts. It would be interesting to see what effect passive or active immunization against α-haemolysin would have in such experimental kidney infections in mice. Anti-α-haemolysin antibodies have been found in animals and humans with infections caused by haemolytic *E.coli* and also in healthy individuals (Smith, 1963; Khan, Mehrota and Kumar, 1968; Emody *et al.*, 1982). However, the antibody titres were very much higher in the infected group which included patients with cystitis and pyelonephritis, showing that α-haemolysin is produced *in vivo* during infection. It is also interesting to note that the concentration of haptoglobin increases dramatically in the plasma of patients with both acute and chronic infections (Owen *et al.*, 1964; Chiancone *et al.*, 1968).

Although we have here considered how α-haemolysin might act as a virulence factor by enabling haemolytic strains of *E.coli* to obtain the iron needed for growth from lysed erythrocytes *in vivo*, the possibility that the α-haemolysins may also act as cytotoxins must not be overlooked. The cytotoxic activity of α-haemolysin preparations have been shown with chicken embryo fibroblasts and mouse fibroblasts, and they also affect both the activity and viability of human peripheral blood leukocytes *in vitro* (Charturvedi *et al.*, 1969; Cavalieri and Snyder, 1982a, 1982b, 1982c; Cavalieri, Behach and Snyder, 1984). However, studies on the cytotoxic effects of the *E.coli* α-haemolysins *in vitro* are not altogether satisfactory because of possible impurities in the haemolysin preparations; some of the data may reflect the presence of other cytotoxins (Cavalieri, Bohach and Snyder, 1984). Nevertheless, the possibility that the α-haemolysins themselves are cytotoxic *in vivo* cannot be excluded. Smith and Huggins (1985) have actually shown a toxic effect of *E.coli* α-haemolysin in mice. It may well be that the haemolytic and cytotoxic functions of haemolysins both operate *in vivo*, possibly independently of each other and at different body sites. This is clearly an aspect needing further investigation, as does the *in vivo* function of the haemolytic activities produced by other pathogens.

3. ADAPTATION TO IRON RESTRICTION

In addition to expressing new outer membrane proteins and, in many cases, synthesizing siderophores, other more fundamental changes also take place in bacteria as they adapt to and grow under the iron-restricted conditions imposed by host iron-binding proteins. Of particular interest are the changes which occur in transfer RNA (tRNA) molecules. In *E.coli*, as in other cells, tRNA genes are transcribed as polynucleotide precursor molecules. These molecules then undergo a maturation process before finally assuming their correct functional tertiary structures. This involves both a reduction in the size of the transcribed polynucleotide chain by a cleavage reaction and the modification of certain key nucleotides in the molecule.

The growth of *E.coli in vitro* in the presence of transferrin, lactoferrin or ovotransferrin results in the generation of specifically undermodified tRNA molecules (Griffiths, 1972; Griffiths and Humphreys, 1975, 1976, 1978). These altered tRNAs lack the methylthio (ms^2) moiety of the 2-methylthio-N^6-(Δ^2-isopentenyl)-adenosine (ms^2i^6A) which occurs adjacent to the 3′ end of the anticodons of the tRNAs when isolated from iron-replete *E.coli* (Griffiths and Humphreys, 1978; Buck and Griffiths, 1982). The tRNAs which are altered in this way during iron restriction are those which recognize codons with a 5′-uridine (UXY codons) and include the tRNAs for phenylalanine, tyrosine, tryptophan and serine. The altered tRNAs elute earlier on chromatography than do the same tRNAs from iron-replete cells (Wettstein and Stent, 1968; Rosenberg and Gefter, 1969; Griffiths, 1972; Griffiths and Humphreys, 1978). The change in structure which occurs during iron-restricted growth is shown for $tRNA^{phe}$ in Fig. 11.

It was originally thought that the altered tRNAs were associated with the inhibition of bacterial growth. They were found in strains of pathogenic *E.coli* inhibited by human milk, bovine colostrum or serum, bacteriostasis being induced by the combined action of antibody and iron-binding protein (Griffiths, 1972; Griffiths and Humphreys, 1975, 1977, 1978). However, not all strains of *E.coli* were inhibited by these body fluids; this was thought to be due to the lack of appropriate antibody (Griffiths and Humphreys, 1976, 1978; see also Chapter 5). The fact that the altered tRNA population was also found in pathogenic *E.coli* which grew well in human milk or bovine colostrum, or in synthetic media containing iron-binding protein, led to the idea that these alterations were connected not with the inhibition of growth but with the

Figure 11 Effect of iron on the post-transcriptional modification of phenylalanine tRNA of *E.coli*. *From E. Griffiths (1981), Iron and the susceptibility to bacterial infection, in* Nutritional Factors: Modulating Effects on Metabolic Processes (*Eds. R.F. Beers and E.G. Bassett), pp. 463–476. Reproduced by permission of Raven Press, New York*

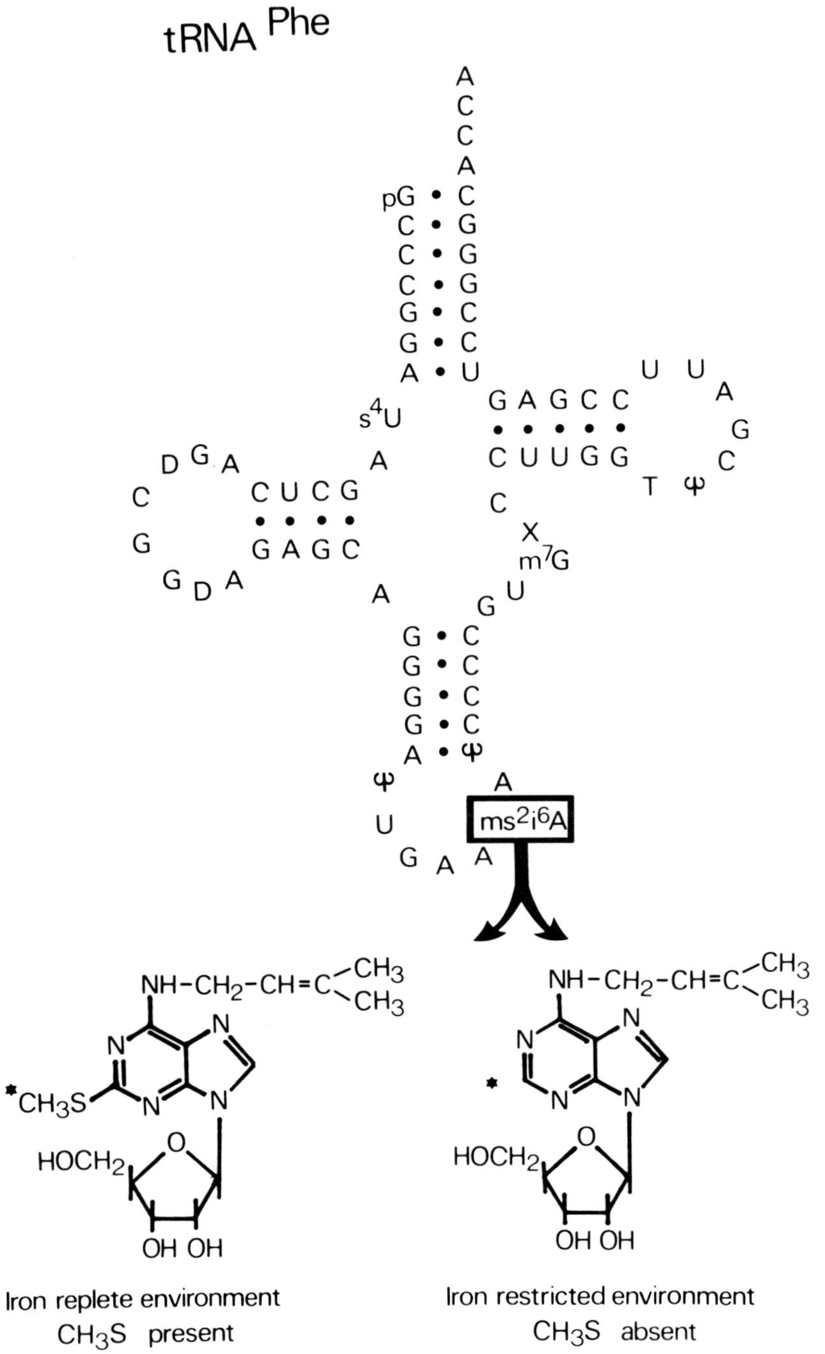
tRNA Phe
ms^2i^6A
Iron replete environment
CH_3S present
Iron restricted environment
CH_3S absent

adaptation of *E.coli* to a low iron environment (Griffiths and Humphreys, 1976, 1978; Griffiths, 1983 a, 1983 b). A regulatory role for the changes in tRNAs was proposed, possibly controlling some aspect of bacterial metabolism essential for pathogenicity. One obvious candidate for this control was the production of enterobactin (Griffiths and Humphreys, 1976, 1978).

Subsequent work showed that a direct link did exist between the iron-related post-transcriptional methylthiolation of tRNA and the function of the tRNA in regulation (Buck and Griffiths, 1981, 1982; Griffiths, 1983a, 1983b). The modification of nucleotides located immediately 3′ to the anticodon appears to be particularly important and there are data which suggest that this position is involved in tRNA function during translation (Yarus, 1982). Certainly variations in the extent of modification of the adenosine located next to the anticodon of tRNAs which read UXY codons affect codon–anticodon interaction and lead to changes in the translational efficiency of the tRNA molecule (Buck and Griffiths, 1982). Furthermore, the evidence suggests that ms^2-deficient tRNAs, with their lowered translational efficiencies, relieve transcription termination at the attenuators of certain operons of the aromatic amino acid biosynthetic pathway and that this leads to the increased expression of these operons under iron-restricted conditions (Buck and Griffiths, 1982). It is now known that a number of amino acid biosynthetic operons, including the phenylalanine and tryptophan operons, as well as the operon coding for phenylalanyl-tRNA synthetase, are regulated by attentuation of transcription (Yanofsky, 1981; Fayat *et al.*, 1983; Springer *et al.*, 1983, 1985; Trudel *et al.*, 1984). According to this mechanism, the efficiency of the transcription of one of these structural genes is controlled by the speed of translation of certain codons in a short coding sequence located in the leader sequence. These codons are sometimes called modulating codons and often consist of a run of several contiguous codons for the particular regulatory amino acid(s). For example, in the tryptophan operon leader sequence, there are two tryptophan codons in tandem; in the leader of the phenylalanine operon there are seven phenylalanine codons and in that for phenylalanyl-tRNA synthetase, there are five (Fig. 12). Efficient translation of these codons leads to the termination of transcription before the structural gene under attenuator control, whereas pauses in the translation of the so-called leader peptide favour terminator readthrough, allowing transcription to continue into the following gene. This regulatory process depends upon the formation of mutually exclusive stem and loop structures in the leader mRNA transcript; these structures are the protector and preemptor or antiterminator structures, details of which have been discussed by Yanofsky (1981). The alternative secondary structures either allow or prevent, respectively, formation of the terminator which prevents transcription from continuing into the structural genes.

Originally, attentuation was shown to be regulated by the level of aminoacyl-tRNA present, which in turn depended upon the availability of the amino acid.

1. --- AUG AAA GCA AUU UUC GUA CUG AAA GGU UGG UGG CGC ACU UCC UGA ---
met-lys-ala-ile-phe-val-leu-lys-gly-trp-trp-arg-thr-ser

2. --- AUG AAA CAC AUA CCG UUU UUC UUC GCA UUC UUU UUU ACC UUC CCC UGA ---
met-lys-his-ile-pro-phe-phe-phe-ala-phe-phe-phe-thr-phe-pro

3. --- AUG AAU GCU GCU AUU UUC CGC UUC UUU UUU UAC UUU AGC ACC UGA ---
met-asn-ala-ala-ile-phe-arg-phe-phe-phe-tyr-phe-ser-thr

Figure 12 Nucleotide sequence encoding the predicted regulatory peptide in the 5′ end of the mRNA of (1) the tryptophan operon; (2) the phenylalanine operon; (3) the phenylalanyl-tRNA synthetase operon. The amino acids which regulate the respective operons, encoded by the modulating codons, are underlined

However, the evidence now suggests that ms²-deficient tRNAs, with their lowered translational efficiencies, can also relieve transcription termination and promote expression of the genes concerned (Buck and Griffiths, 1982; Buck and Ames, 1984) (Fig. 13). It is thought that such regulatory features in the phenylalanine and tryptophan operons, and possibly other operons in the common aromatic amino acid biosynthetic pathway, may be involved with adapting *E.coli* for growth in iron-restricted environments (Buck and Griffiths,

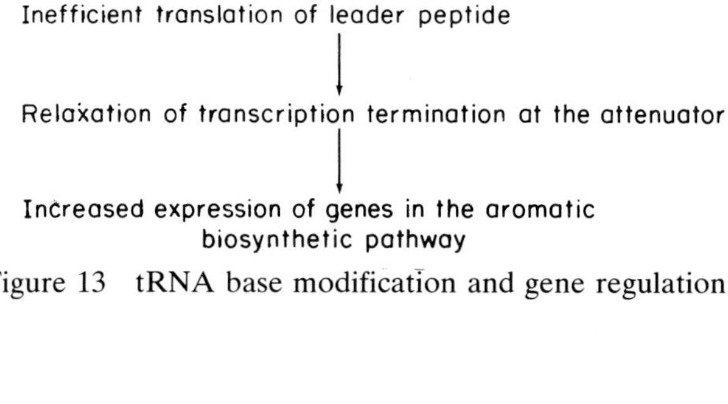

Figure 13 tRNA base modification and gene regulation

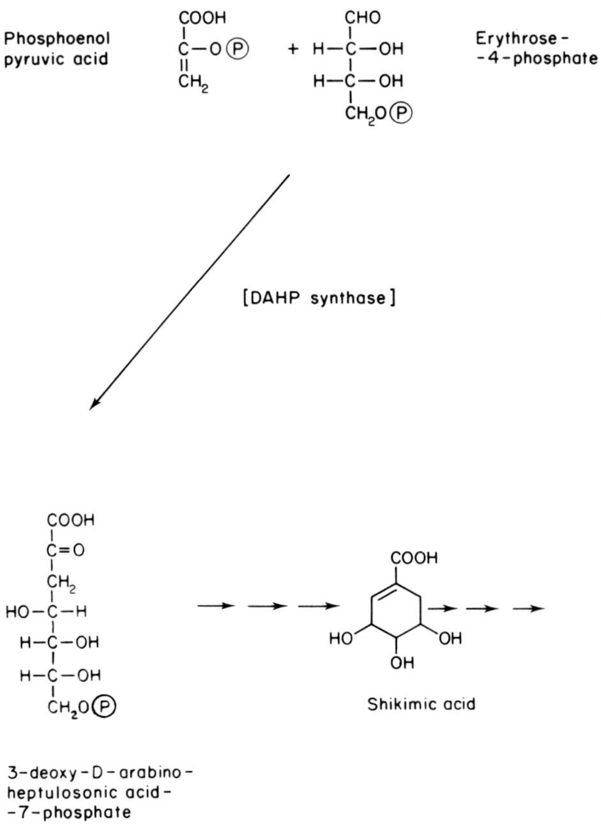

Figure 14 The aromatic biosynthetic pathway in *E.coli*

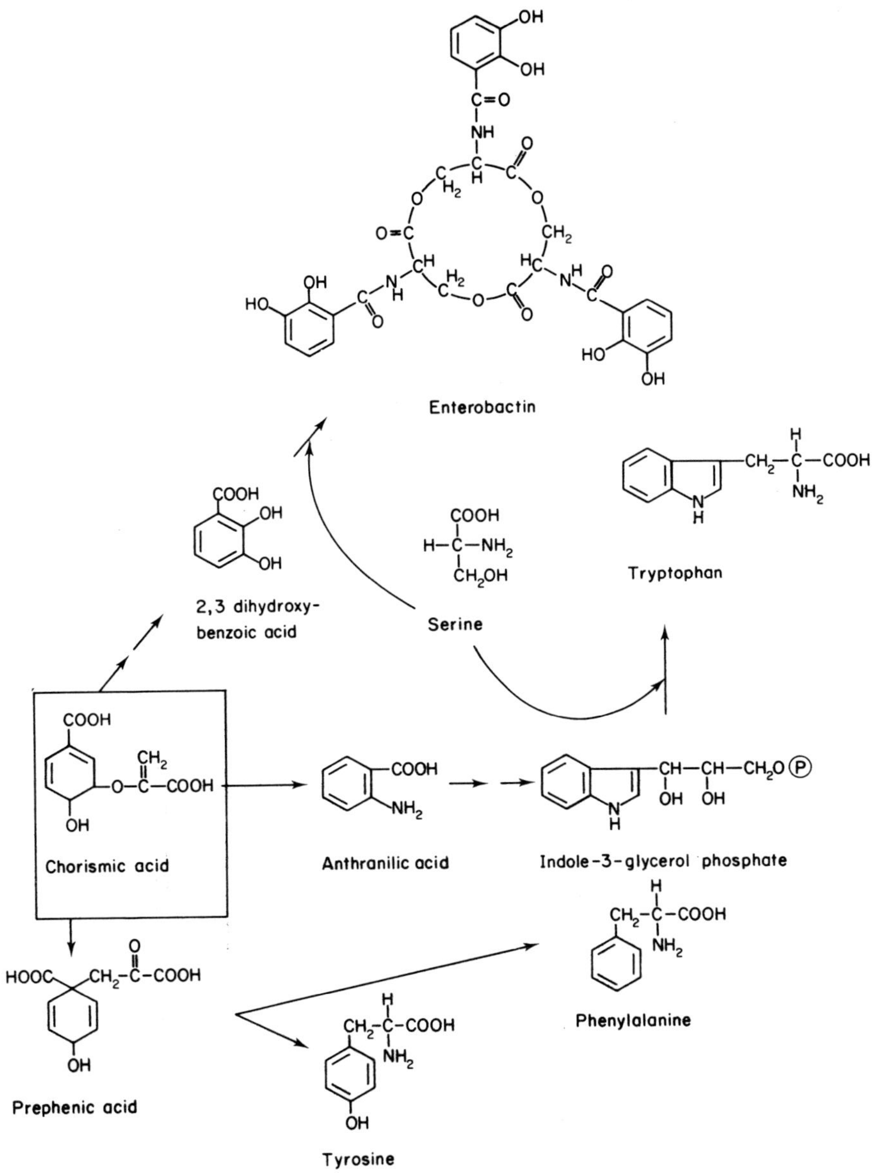

Enterobactin
2,3 dihydroxy-benzoic acid
Serine
Tryptophan
Chorismic acid
Anthranilic acid
Indole-3-glycerol phosphate
Phenylalanine
Prephenic acid
Tyrosine

1982). Since enterobactin is synthesized from chorismic acid by way of a branch of the aromatic amino acid biosynthetic pathway, derepression of the enterobactin system will require adjustments to the whole aromatic pathway to ensure production of amino acids and other aromatic compounds, if required (Fig. 14). In addition, iron itself is an essential component of the first enzyme of the common pathway (McCandliss and Herrmann, 1978). Multiple control of these operons through the level of charged tRNA and by the degree of post-transcriptional modification of tRNA, in turn dependent upon iron levels, could provide the cell with considerable regulatory flexibility which may be important for growth under iron-restricted conditions (Buck and Griffiths, 1982; Griffiths, 1983a, 1983b, 1985).

It is also interesting to note that serine is required for the biosynthesis of enterobactin and that alterations do occur in two $tRNA^{ser}$ molecules during iron restriction (McLennan *et al.*, 1981). It is not known if alterations in $tRNA^{ser}$ have a regulatory role. However, it has recently been discovered that in *S.typhimurium* the gene *ser*C, which encodes the enzyme phosphoserine aminotransferase, and the gene *aro*A, which specifies 3-enol-pyruvate-shikimate-5-phosphate synthase, an essential enzyme in the common aromatic biosynthetic pathway, are to be found in a single operon, with *ser*C being promotor proximal (Hoiseth and Stocker, 1985) (Fig. 15). These two genes are also located very close together on the linkage map of *E.coli*, at 20′ (Bachmann, 1983). It is possible that the grouping of one gene concerned with a step in the common aromatic biosynthetic pathway (*aro*A) and one concerned with serine biosynthesis (*ser*C) into a single operon may allow their co-regulation according to the iron status of the bacterial cell; this might involve regulation through attentuation by $tRNA^{ser}$. Detailed sequence analyses of serine tRNAs have shown that only two of the $tRNA^{ser}$ molecules which read the four codons UCN (where N = C,U,G or A) have a methylthioisopentenyl modification on the adenosine adjacent to the anticodon (Grosjean *et al.*, 1985). It was originally thought that ms^2i^6A was to be found adjacent to the anticodons of all tRNAs reading UXY codons, but clearly this is not the case and it explains why McLennan *et al.* (1981) found that iron restriction altered only two $tRNA^{ser}$ molecules. The reason why two of the four possible $tRNA^{ser}$ molecules are not hypermodified at position 37, even though there is an A at this location, is not clear, although it is thought that it may be due to perturbations in the conformation of the anticodon loop which prevent it being recognized by the isopentenylating enzymes (Grosjean *et al.*, 1985). This fact has important implications for the reading of the U(XY) family of serine codons. Table 6 shows codon and anticodon usage by serine tRNAs. From this it can be seen that only the reading of the UCA and UCG codons might be expected to be affected by the loss of the ms^2 group during iron restriction; the other serine codons, UCC, UCU, as well as AGC and AGU, would be unaffected. Codons UCA and UCG are rarely used codons in *E.coli* and could well function as

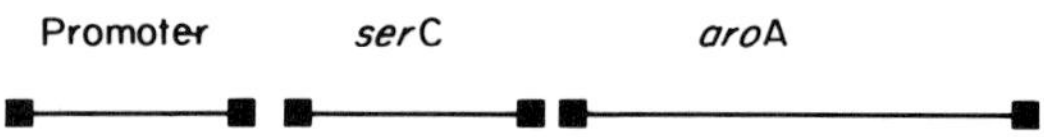

Figure 15 The *aro*A and *ser*C genes of *S.typhimurium* constitute one operon.

modulating codons in attenuation. It is interesting to note that in one system at least, that of the *ilv* GEDA operon of *Serratia marcescens*, even a single codon acts as a modulating codon and tandem or runs of codons are, therefore, not always necessary (Hsu, Harms and Umbarger, 1985).

Methylthiolation of tRNA also influences aromatic amino acid transport in *E.coli* (Buck and Griffiths, 1981), although it is not known how undermodified tRNAs function to increase the uptake of phenylalanine, tryptophan and tyrosine from the medium. The ability of the bacterial cell to scavenge the environment for these amino acids rather than synthesize them may, however, be a helpful feature of cellular economy when enterobactin synthesis is necessary for continued growth in an iron-restricted environment. Whether other metabolic consequences arise as a result of changes in the methylthiolation of tRNAs remains to be seen (Kersten, 1984).

In some operons like the His operon of *E.coli*, transcription termination at the attenuator is the major controlling element and there is no repressor molecule (Yanofsky, 1981). However, the absence of the ms^2 moiety in tRNA does not seem to be the major controlling signal regulating enterobactin synthesis nor the synthesis of the iron-regulated outer membrane proteins in *E.coli* (Griffiths and Buck, 1979). The synthesis of enterobactin and of some of the iron-regulated outer membrane proteins appear to be coordinately regulated by iron even though the genes are not all included in the same transcriptional unit (McIntosh and Earhart, 1977; Klebba, McIntosh and Neilands, 1982; Bachman, 1983; Fleming, Nahlik and McIntosh, 1983). The 83, 81 and 74 kDa proteins have been reported to be regulated together but the synthesis of the 78 kDa protein is controlled separately (Plastow, Pratt and Holland, 1981; Klebba, McIntosh and Neilands, 1982). Induction of the FecA protein depends not only on low levels of iron but, in addition, on a relatively high concentration of exogenous citrate (Hussein, Hantke and Braun, 1981; Zimmermann, Hantke and Braun, 1984). However, constitutive mutants of *E.coli* K12 which express the iron-transport genes in iron-rich media have been produced (Hantke, 1981). This shows that a regulatory mechanism exists which covers all iron-uptake systems, including the aerobactin system, and which is superimposed upon the regulation of the individual systems (Hantke, 1981, 1984; Braun and Burkhardt, 1982; Fecker and Braun, 1983; Gross, Engelbrecht and Braun, 1984). These constitutive mutants have been called *fur* mutants and are similar to those found in *S.typhimurium* (Ernst, Bennett and Rothfield, 1987). The nature of the regulatory mechanism affected by the *fur* mutation is unknown although the *fur* gene region has now been cloned and there is

Table 6 Codon and anticodon usage in serine tRNA

Relative amount (%)	Anticodon + adjacent 3′ base	Expected codon recognized
40	GGA . A	UCC
5	GGA . A	UCU
19	VGA . ms^{2}i^{6}A	UCA ●
5	CGA . ms^{2}i^{6}A	UCG ●
13	GCU. t^{6}A	AGC
19	GCU. A	AGU

● = codons expected to be read inefficiently during iron restriction.
Large letters correspond to the 'wobble' base of the anticodon or to the corresponding third base of the codon.
V = uridine-5-oxyacetic acid.
t^{6}A = *N*-(9-(β-D-ribofuranosyl)purin-6-ylcarbamoyl)threonine.
Data taken from Grosjean *et al.* (1985).

evidence to suggest that the *fur* gene determines a protein which acts as a repressor at high iron concentration (Hantke, 1982, 1984).

In any work in infection it is essential to show, as far as is possible, that biochemical mechanisms studied *in vitro* really do apply to conditions in the host during infection. It is significant, therefore, that the iron-related tRNA changes seen in *E.coli* grown *in vitro* in the presence of iron-binding proteins are indeed found in pathogenic *E.coli* recovered directly without subculture from infected animals (Griffiths *et al.*, 1978; Fig. 16). Iron-regulated tRNA alterations have also been seen in *S.typhimurium, K.pneumoniae* and *Ps.aeruginosa* (McLennan *et al.*, 1981). Transfer RNAs that recognize codons starting with uridine almost always contain a hydrophobic modified nucleoside, such as isopentenyl-adenosine (i^{6}A) or a derivative, adjacent to the 3′ end of the anticodon (Sprinzl *et al.*, 1985; but see tRNA^{ser} above). In *E.coli* this is ms^{2}i^{6}A, but the tRNAs of *Ps.aeruginosa, S.typhimurium* and *K.pneumoniae*

Figure 16 Chromatography of tryptophanyl-tRNA (trp-tRNA^{trp}) on benzoylated–DEAE–cellulose: (a) (^{3}H)-trp-tRNA^{trp} extracted from iron-replete, broth-grown *E.coli* 0111; (b) co-chromatography of (^{14}C)-trp-tRNA^{trp} (o) isolated from *E.coli* 0111 grown *in vivo* during infection and (^{3}H)-trp-tRNA^{trp} (●) from *E.coli* 0111 grown in trypticase soy broth containing ovotransferrin. (a) was chromatographed separately but on the same column. *From Griffiths* et al. (1978). *Reproduced by permission of the American Society for Microbiology*

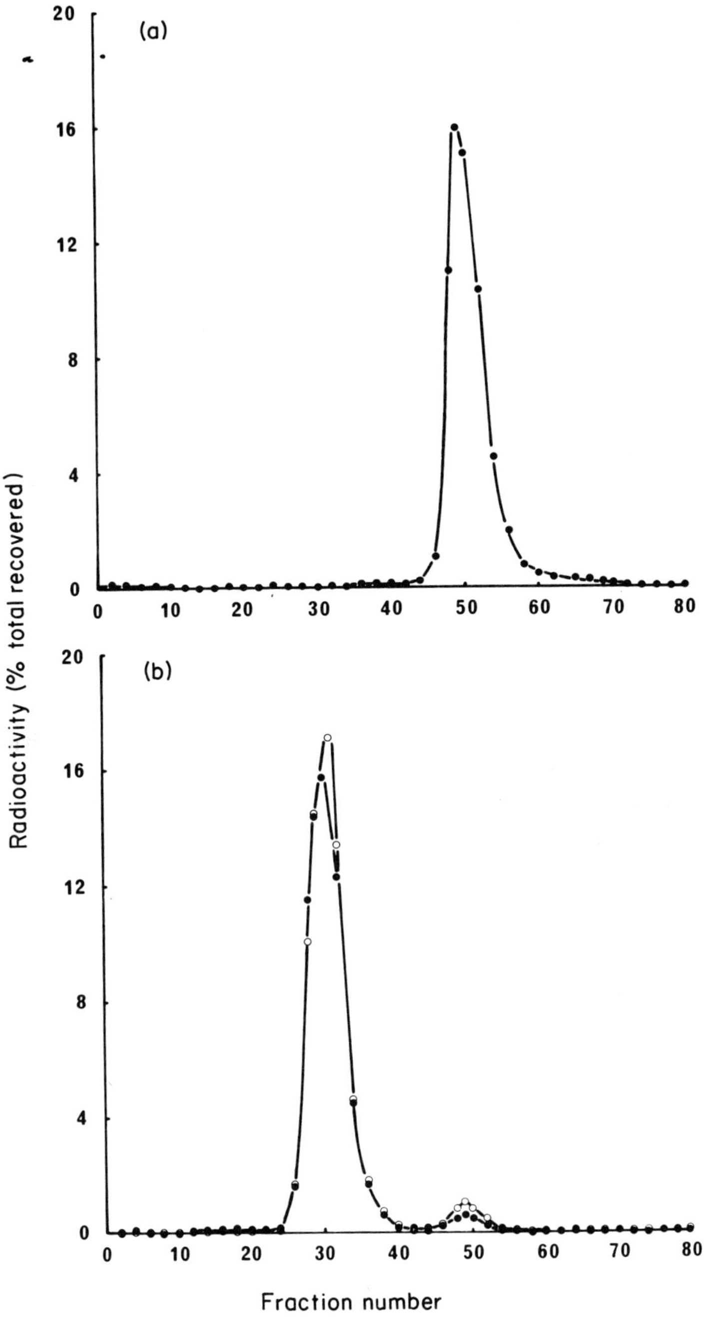
(a)
(b)
Radioactivity (% total recovered)
Fraction number
0
4
8
12
16
20
0
10
20
30
40
50
60
70
80

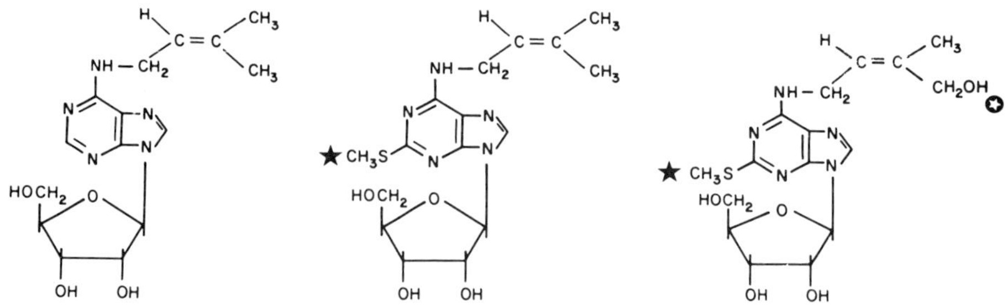

Figure 17 Structural formulae of the hypermodified nucleosides found adjacent to the 3′ end of the anticodon of certain tRNA molecules: (**1**) isopentenyl-adenosine; (**2**) 2-methylthio-N^6-(Δ^2-isopentenyl)-adenosine; (**3**) *cis*-methylthioribosylzeatin. The positions of the relevant modifications are indicated by ★ for the methylthio moiety *(CH_3S-) and by* ✪ for the hydroxyl group (OH). *From Griffiths (1983a). Reproduced by permission of The Royal Society, London*

contain another i^6A derivative, a hydroxylated form of ms^2i^6A called *cis*-methylthioribosylzeatin (ms^2io^6A) (Fig. 17) (Thimmappaya and Cherayil, 1974; Buck *et al.*, 1982; Janzer, Raney and McLennan, 1982). Although ms^2io^6A is the major hypermodified nucleoside present in *S.typhimurium* and *K.pneumoniae*, small amounts of ms^2i^6A have also been seen; *E.coli* does not contain any ms^2io^6A. The synthesis of ms^2io^6A in *Salmonella* has been shown to require the presence of high levels of oxygen; ms^2i^6A predominates in the anaerobically grown organisms (Buck and Ames, 1984).

Furthermore, the hydroxylation of the isopentenyl side-chain only occurs after methylthiolation of i^6A to ms^2i^6A has taken place. Both the methylthiolation and hydroxylation modifications of i^6A in tRNA are, therefore, greatly reduced in iron-restricted *S.typhimurium*. Buck and Ames (1984) suggest that the change in tRNA modification with anerobiosis may be involved in regulating the switching of anaerobic pathways to aerobic ones. Although the regulatory significance of the ms^2io^6A modification in *Salmonella* tRNA remains to be demonstrated, the work does show how alterations in the bacterial environment, in this case in the level of oxygen and in the availability of iron, can have subtle but quite fundamental effects on cellular machinery.

4. CONCLUDING REMARKS

Much of our understanding of what may be happening as pathogenic bacteria adapt to and grow in the iron-restricted extracellular environment of the host (Table 7) has come from studies with Gram-negative organisms, in particular with *E.coli*. This is because *E.coli* provides an ideal experimental model; a great deal is already known about its biochemistry and its genetics and it is also the causative agent of important infections in both man and animals. The work

Table 7 Alterations in the metabolism of bacterial pathogens during growth under iron restriction *in vitro* or during growth *in vivo*

Synthesis of siderophores		Expression of iron-regulated membrane proteins	Changes in tRNAs
Escherichia coli		*Escherichia coli*	*Escherichia coli*
Klebsiella	Enterobactin	*Klebsiella*	*Klebsiella*
Shigella	Aerobactin	*Shigella*	*Salmonella*
Salmonella		*Salmonella*	
		Proteus	
Vibrio cholerae	Vibriobactin	*Vibrio cholerae*	
Pseudomonas	Pyochelin	*Pseudomonas*	*Pseudomonas*
	Pyoverdin		
Mycobacteria	Mycobactin	*Neisseria meningitidis*	
	Exochelin	*Neisseria gonorrhoea*	

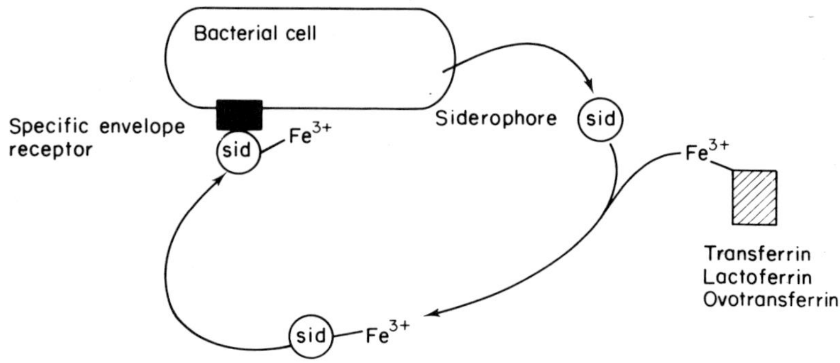

(a)

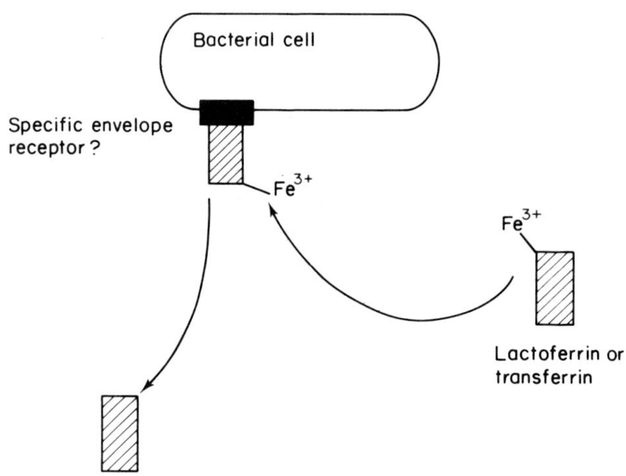

(b)

Figure 18 Schematic representation of two ways by which pathogenic bacteria obtain iron from iron-binding proteins: (a) siderophore-mediated iron uptake; (b) iron uptake by direct interaction with host iron-binding glycoproteins

with *E.coli* has established the principle that pathogenic bacteria can undergo considerable phenotypic changes in both their metabolism and in the composition of their outer membranes when growing *in vivo* during infection. This information is now serving as a guideline for the often more difficult investigation of other pathogens. To date, two main types of mechanisms have been identified by which pathogenic bacteria acquire essential iron *in vivo*; these are shown schematically in Fig.18. However, except for the relatively recent work on *C.diphtheriae*, little is known about how Gram-positive pathogens, such as stapylococci and streptococci, acquire iron *in vivo* or about the changes they may undergo in these circumstances. Schade (1963) found that several strains of coagulase-negative *Staphylococcus albus* were inhibited by human serum although growth was restored by adding iron. A coagulase-positive strain of *S.aureus*, however, grew well in human serum suggesting that it was able to remove iron from transferrin. It is known, of course, that many Gram-positive organisms can synthesize siderophores during iron restriction *in vitro* (Lankford, 1973). For example, *Bacillus megaterium* produces shizokinen, a dihydroxamate siderophore based on citric acid and closely related to aerobactin (Lankford, 1973; Neilands, 1981). However, it is not known if siderophores play any part in the virulence of Gram-positive pathogens other than *C.diphtheriae*. It could well be that mechanisms involving direct contact with the iron-binding protein are involved in some cases; such mechanisms may be more widespread than is thought at present. The Gram-negative *Legionella* species, for example, do not appear to produce siderophores and there is a possibility that a direct-contact mechanism may function in this case (Reeves *et al.*, 1983). Recently, it has been shown that *Bordetella pertussis* absorbs host iron-binding proteins into its outer membrane, although it is not known if this process is connected with iron uptake (K. Redhead, personal communication). The mechanisms whereby non-bacterial pathogens, such as *Candida albicans*, acquire iron *in vivo* are also very poorly understood at present; what is known is discussed in Chapter 8. Much of what is already known about the conditions encountered by bacterial pathogens in host tissues concerns the extracellular environment. Little is known about the environment encountered by intracellular pathogens, nor about the availability of iron inside cells such as polymorphs and macrophages. Although something is already known about the ability of microorganisms to survive intracellularly (Smith, 1976; Draper, 1981), much less is known about their capability to multiply inside host cells. It will therefore be important in future work to compare the ability of certain pathogens, such as *Shigella* and *Salmonella*, to multiply both extracellularly and intracellularly, as well as to consider the availability of intracellular iron.

REFERENCES

Ainscough, E.W., Brodie, A.M., Plowman, J.E., Bloor, S.J., Loehr, J.S., and Loehr, T.M. (1980). Studies on human lactoferrin by electron paramagnetic resonance, fluorescence and resonance Raman spectroscopy. *Biochemistry*, **19**, 4072–4079.

Aisen, P. (1980). The transferrins. In *Iron in Biochemistry and Medicine* (Eds. A. Jacobs and M. Worwood), Vol.II, pp.87–129. Academic Press, New York and London.

Aisen, P., and Listowsky, I. (1980). Iron transport and storage proteins. *Annual Review of Biochemistry*, **49**, 357–392.

Anderson, E.S., Threlfall, E.J., Carr, J.M., McConnell, M.M., and Smith, H.R. (1977). Clonal distribution of resistance plasmid-carrying *Salmonella typhimurium* mainly in the Middle East. *Journal of Hygiene (Cambridge)*, **79**, 425–448.

Ankenbauer, R., Sriyosachati, S., and Cox, C.D. (1985). Effects of siderophores on the growth of *Pseudomonas aeruginosa* in human serum and transferrin. *Infection and Immunity*, **49**, 132–140.

Anwar, H., Brown, M.R.W., Day, A., and Weller, P.H. (1984). Outer membrane antigens of mucoid *Pseudomonas aeruginosa* isolated directly from the sputum of a cystic fibrosis patient. *FEMS Microbiology Letters*, **24**, 235–239.

Archibald, F.S., and DeVoe, I.W. (1979). Removal of iron from human transferrin by *Neisseria meningitidis*. *FEMS Microbiology Letters*, **6**, 159–162.

Archibald, F.S., and DeVoe, I.W. (1980). Iron acquisition by *Neisseria meningitidis in vitro*. *Infection and Immunity*, **27**, 322–334.

Bachmann, B.J. (1983). Linkage map of *Escherichia coli* K12, Edition 7. *Microbiology Reviews*, **7**, 180–230.

Baker, P.J., and Wilson, J.B. (1965). Hypoferremia in mice and its application to the assay of endotoxin. *Journal of Bacteriology*, **90**, 903–910.

Barclay, R., and Ratledge, C (1983). Iron-binding compounds of *Mycobacterium avium*, *M.intracellulare*, *M.scrofulaceum* and mycobactin-dependent *M.paratuberculosis* and *M.avium*. *Journal of Bacteriology*, **153**, 1138–1146.

Barksdale, L. (1970). *Corynebacterium diphtheriae* and its relatives. *Bacteriological Reviews*, **34**, 378–422.

Beaumier, D.L., Caldwell, M.A., and Holbein, B.E. (1984). Inflammation triggers hypoferremia and de novo synthesis of serum transferrin and ceruloplasmin in mice. *Infection and Immunity*, **46**, 489–494.

Benjamin, Jr., W.H., Turnbough, Jr., C.L., Posey, B.S., and Briles, D.E. (1985). The ability of *Salmonella typhimurium* to produce the siderophore enterobactin is not a virulence factor in mouse typhoid. *Infection and Immunity*, **50**, 392–397.

Berger, H., Hacker, J., Juarez, A., Hughes, C., and Goebel, W. (1982). Cloning of the chromosomal determinants encoding haemolysin production and mannose-resistant haemagglutination in *Escherichia coli*. *Journal of Bacteriology*, **152**, 1241–1247.

Biberstein, E.L., Mini, P.D., and Gills, M.G. (1963). Action of *Haemophilus* cultures on δ-aminolevulinic acid. *Journal of Bacteriology*, **86**, 814–819.

Bindereif, A., Braun, V., and Hantke, K. (1982). The cloacin receptor of ColV-bearing *Escherichia coli* is part of the Fe^{3+}-aerobactin transport system. *Journal of Bacteriology*, **150**, 1472–1475.

Bindereif, A., and Neilands, J.B. (1985). Aerobactin genes in clinical isolates of *Escherichia coli*. *Journal of Bacteriology*, **161**, 727–735.

Bjorn, M.J., Pavlovski, O.R., Thompson, M.R., and Iglewski, B.H. (1979). Production of exoenzymes during *Pseudomonas aeruginosa* infections of burned mice. *Infection and Immunity*, **24**, 837–842.

Blake, P.A., Merson, M.H., Weaver, R.E., Hollis, D.G., and Heublein, P.C. (1979). Disease caused by a marine vibrio: clinical characteristics and epidemiology. *New England Journal of Medicine*, **300**, 1–5.

Braun, V. (1981). *Escherichia coli* cells containing the plasmid ColV produce the iron ionophore aerobactin. *FEMS Microbiology Letters*, **11**, 225–228.

Braun, V., Brazel-Faisst, C., and Schneider, R. (1984). Growth stimulation of *Escherichia coli* in serum by iron(III)–aerobactin: recycling of aerobactin. *FEMS Microbiology Letters*, **21**, 99–103.

Braun, V., and Burkhardt, R. (1982). Regulation of the ColV-plasmid determined iron(III)–aerobactin transport system in *Escherichia coli*. *Journal of Bacteriology*, **152**, 233–231.

Braun, V., Burkhardt, R., Schneider, R., and Zimmermann, L. (1982). Chromosomal genes for ColV plasmid-determined iron(III)–aerobactin transport in *Escherichia coli*. *Journal of Bacteriology*, **151,** 553–559.

Braun, V., Gross, R., Koster, W., and Zimmermann, L. (1983). Plasmid and chromosomal mutants in the iron(III)–aerobactin transport system of *Escherichia coli*. Use of streptonigrin for selection. *Molecular and General Genetics*, **192**, 131–139.

Braun, V., Hancock, R.E.W., Hantke, K., and Hartmann, A. (1976). Functional organization of the outer membrane of *Escherichia coli*: phage and colicin receptors as components of iron uptake systems. *Journal of Supramolecular Structure*, **5,** 37–58.

Braun, V., and Hantke, K. (1981). Bacterial cell surface receptors. In *Organization of Prokaryotic Cell Membranes* (Ed. B.K. Ghosh), Vol. II, pp. 1–73. CRC Reviews, Boca Raton, Florida.

Brener, D., DeVoe, I.W., and Holbein, B.E. (1981). Increased virulence of *Neisseria meningitidis* after *in vitro* iron-limited growth at low pH. *Infection and Immunity*, **33,** 59–66.

Brock, J.H., Esparza, I., and Logie, A.C. (1984). The nature of iron released by resident and stimulated mouse peritoneal macrophages. *Biochimica et Biophysica Acta*, **797**, 105–111.

Brown, M.R.W., Anwar, H., and Lambert, P.A. (1984). Evidence that mucoid *Pseudomonas aeruginosa* in the cystic fibrosis lung grows under iron-restricted conditions. *FEMS Microbiology Letters*, **21,** 113–117.

Buck, M., and Ames, B.N. (1984). A modified nucleotide in tRNA as a possible regulator of anaerobiosis: synthesis of *cis*-2-methythio-ribosylzeatin in the tRNA of *Salmonella, Cell*, **36**, 523–531.

Buck, M., and Griffiths, E. (1981). Regulation of aromatic amino acid transport by tRNA: role of 2-methylthio-N^6- (Δ^2-isopentenyl)-adenosine. *Nucleic Acids Research*, **9**, 401–414.

Buck, M., and Griffiths, E. (1982). Iron mediated methylthiolation of tRNA as a regulator of operon expression in *Escherichia coli. Nucleic Acids Research*, **10,** 2609–2624.

Buck, M., McCloskey, J.A., Basile, B., and Ames, B.N. (1982). *cis*-2-Methylthioribosylzeatin (ms^2io^6A) is present in the transfer RNA of *Salmonella typhimurium* but not *Escherichia coli. Nucleic Acids Research*, **10,** 5649–5662.

Bullen, J.J. (1981). The significance of iron in infection. *Reviews of Infectious Diseases*, **3,** 1127–1137.

Bullen, J.J., Rogers, H.J., and Griffiths, E. (1978). Role of iron in bacterial infections. *Current Topics in Microbiology and Immunology*, **80,** 1–35.

Calver, G.A., Kenny, C.P., and Kushner, D.J. (1979). Inhibition of the growth of *Neisseria meningitidis* by reduced ferritin and other iron-binding agents. *Infection and Immunity*, **25,** 880–890.

Carlsson, J., Hofling, J.F., and Sundqvist, G.K. (1984). Degradation of albumin, haemopexin, haptoglobin and transferrin by black-pigmented *Bacteriodes* species. *Journal of Medical Microbiology*, **18,** 39–46.

Carrano, C.J., and Raymond, K.N. (1979). Ferric iron sequestering agents. 2. Kinetics and mechanisms of iron removal from transferrin by enterochelin and synthetic tricatechols. *Journal of the American Chemical Society*, **101,** 5401–5404.

Cartwright, G.E., Lauritsen, A., Humphreys, S., Jones, P.J., Merrill, I.M., and Wintrobe, M.M (1946). The anaemia of infection.II. The experimental production of hypoferremia and anemia in dogs. *Journal of Clinical Investigation*, **25,** 81–86.

Cavalieri, S.J., Bohach, G.A., and Snyder, I.S. (1984). *Escherichia coli*-haemolysin: characteristics and probable role in pathogenicity. *Microbiology Reviews*, **48,** 326–343.

Cavalieri, S.J., and Snyder, I.S. (1982a). Cytotoxic activity of a partially purified *Escherichia coli* alpha-haemolysin. *Journal of Medical Microbiology*, **15**, 11–21.

Cavalieri, S.J., and Snyder, I.S. (1982b). Effect of *Escherichia coli* alpha-haemolysin on human peripheral leukocyte viability *in vitro*. *Infection and Immunity*, **36,** 455–461.

Cavalieri, S.J., and Synder, I.S. (1982c). Effect of *Escherichia coli* alpha-haemolysin on human peripheral leukocyte function *in vitro*. *Infection and Immunity*, **37,** 966–974.

Chart, H., Buck, M., Stevenson, P., and Griffiths, E. (1986). Iron regulated outer membrane proteins of *Escherichia coli*: variations in expression due to the chelator used to restrict the availability of iron. *Journal of General Microbiology*, **132,** 1373–1378.

Chart, H., and Griffiths, E. (1985a). The availability of iron and the growth of *Vibrio vulnificus* in sera from patients with haemochromatosis. *FEMS Microbiology Letters*, **26,** 227–231.

Chart, H., and Griffiths, E. (1985b). Antigenic and molecular hormology of the ferric–enterobactin receptor protein of *Escherichia coli*. *Journal of General Microbiology*, **131,** 1503–1509.

Chart, H., and Trust, T.J. (1983). Acquisition of iron by *Aeromonas salmonicida*. *Journal of Bacteriology*, **156,** 758–764.

Chaturvedi, U.C., Mathur, A., Khan, A.M., and Mehrotra, R.M.L. (1969). Cytotoxicity of filtrates of haemolytic *Escherichia coli*. *Journal of Medical Microbiology*, **2,** 211–218.

Chiancone, E., Alfsen, A., Ioppolo, C., Vecchini, P., Finazzi-Agro, A., Wyman, J., and Antonini, E. (1968). Studies on the reaction of haptoglobin with haemoglobin and haemoglobin chains. I:stoichiometry and affinity. *Journal of Molecular Biology*, **34,** 347–356.

Colonna, B., Nicoletti, M., Visca, P., Casalino, M., Valenti, P., and Maimone, F. (1985). Composite IS1 elements encoding hydroxamate-mediated iron uptake in FI*me* plasmids from epidemic *Salmonella* spp. *Journal of Bacteriology*, **162,** 307–316.

Cooke, E.M., and Ewins, S.P. (1975). Properties of strains of *Escherichia coli* isolated from a variety of sources. *Journal of Medical Microbiology*, **8,** 107–111.

Cooper, S.R., McArdle, J.V., and Raymond, K.N. (1978). Siderophore electrochemistry: relation to intracellular release mechanism. *Proceedings of the National Academy of Sciences* (USA), **75,** 3551–3554.

Coulton, J.W., and Pang, J.C.S. (1983). Transport of hemin by *Haemophilus influenzae* type b. *Current Microbiology*, **9,** 93–98.

Cowart, R.E., and Foster, B.G. (1985). Differential effects of iron on the growth of *Listeria monocytogenes*: minimum requirements and mechanism of acquisition. *Journal of Infectious Diseases*, **151,** 721–730.

Cox, C.D. (1980). Iron uptake with ferripyochelin and ferric citrate by *Pseudomonas aeruginosa*. *Journal of Bacteriology*, **142,** 581–587.

Cox, C.D. (1982). Effect of pyochelin on the virulence of *Pseudomonas aeruginosa*. *Infection and Immunity*, **36,** 17–23.

Cox, C.D., and Adams, P. (1985). Siderophore activity of pyoverdin for *Pseudomonas aeruginosa*. *Infection and Immunity*, **48,** 130–138.

Cox, C.D., and Graham, R. (1979). Isolation of an iron-binding compound from *Pseudomonas aeruginosa*. *Journal of Bacteriology*, **137,** 357–364.

Cox, C.D., Rinehart, K.L., Moore, M.L., and Cooke, J.C. (1981). Pyochelin: novel structure of an iron-chelating growth promoter for *Pseudomonas aeruginosa*. *Proceedings of the National Academy of Sciences* (USA), **78,** 4256–4260.

Crosa, J.H. (1980). A plasmid associated with virulence in the marine fish pathogen *Vibrio anguillarum* specifies an iron sequestering system. *Nature*, **284,** 556–568.

Crosa, J.H. (1984). The relationship of plasmid mediated iron transport and bacterial virulence. *Annual Reviews of Microbiology*, **38,** 69–89.

Crosa, J.H., and Hodges, L.L. (1981). Outer membrane proteins induced under conditions of iron limitation in the marine fish pathogen *Vibrio anguillarum*. *Infection and Immunity*, **31**, 223–227.

DeBoy, II, J.M., Wachsmith, K.I., and Davis, B.R. (1980). Hemolytic activity in enterotoxigenic and non-enterotoxigenic strains of *Escherichia coli*. *Journal of Clinical Microbiology*, **12,** 193–198.

de la Cruz, F., Muller, D., Ortiz, J.M., and Goebel, W. (1980). Hemolysis determinant common to *Escherichia coli* hemolytic plasmids of different incompatability groups. *Journal of Bacteriology*, **143,** 825–833.

Draper, P. (1981). Mycobacterial inhibition of intracellular killing. In *Microbial Perturbation of Host Defences* (Eds. F. O'Grady and H. Smith), pp. 143–157. Academic Press, London.

Dudgeon, L.S., Wordley, E., and Bawtree, F. (1921). On bacillus coli infections of the urinary tract, especially in relation to haemolytic organisms. *Journal of Hygiene*, **20,** 137–164.

Eaton, J.W., Brandt, P., Mahoney, J.R., and Lee. J.T. (1982). Haptoglobin: a natural bacteriostat. *Science*, **215,** 691–693.

Emody, L., Batai. Jr., I., Kerenyi, M., Szekely, Jr., J., and Polyak, L. (1982). Anti-*Escherichia coli* alpha-haemolysin antibodies in control and patient sera. *Lancet*, **2,** 986.

Emody, L., Pal., T., Safonova, N.V., Kuch, B., and Golutra, N.K. (1980). Alpha-haemolysin: an additive virulence factor in *Escherichia coli*. *Acta Microbiologica Academiae Scientorum Hungaricae*, **27,** 333–342.

Ernst, J.F., Bennett, R.L., and Rothfield, L.I. (1978). Constitutive expression of the iron-enterochelin and ferrichrome uptake systems in a mutant strain of *Salmonella typhimurium*. *Journal of Bacteriology*, **135,** 928–934.

Fayat, G., Mayaux, J.F., Sacerdot, C., Fromant, M., Springer, M., Grunberg-Manago, M., and Blanquet, S., (1983). *Escherichia coli* phenylalanyl-tRNA synthetase operon region: evidence for an attenuation mechanism. Identification of the gene for the ribosomal protein L20. *Journal of Molecular Biology*, **171,** 239–261.

Fecker, L., and Braun, V. (1983). Cloning and expression of the *fhu* genes involved in iron(III)-hydroxamate uptake by *Escherichia coli*. *Journal of Bacteriology*, **156,** 1301–1314.

Fiss, E.H., Stanley-Samuelson, P., and Neilands, J.B. (1982). Properties and proteolysis of ferric enterobactin outer membrane receptor in *Escherichia coli* K12. *Biochemistry*, **21,** 4517–4522.

Fitzgerald, S.P., and Rogers, H.J. (1980). Bacteriostatic effect of serum: role of antibody to lipopolysaccharide. *Infection and Immunity*, **27,** 302–308

Fleming, T.P., Nahlik, M.S., and McIntosh, M.A. (1983). Regulation of enterobactin iron transport in *Escherichia coli*: characterization of ent:: Mu*d* (Ap^r*lac*) operon fusions. *Journal of Bacteriology*, **156,** 1171–1177.

Fleming, T.P., Nahlik, M.S., Neilands, J.B., and McIntosh, M.A. (1985). Physical and genetic characterization of cloned enterobactin genomic sequences from *Escherichia coli* K12. *Gene*, **34,** 47–54.

Formal, S.B., Hale, T.L., and Boedeker, E.C. (1983). Interactions of enteric pathogens and the intestinal mucosae. *Philisophical Transactions of the Royal Society, London*, Series B, **303**, 65–73.

Formal, S.B., Hale, T.L., and Sansonetti, P.J. (1983). Invasive enteric pathogens. *Reviews in Infectious Diseases*, **5**, S702–S707.

Fried, F.A., Vermuelen, C.W., Ginsburg, M.J., and Cone, C.M. (1971). Etiology of

pyelonephritis: further evidence associating the production of experimental pyelonephritis and haemolysin in *Escherchia coli. Journal of Urology*, **106,** 351–354.
Fried, F.A., and Wong, R.J. (1970). Etiology of pyelonephritis: significance of hemolytic *Escherichia coli. Journal of Urology*, **103,** 718–721.
Frost, G.E., and Rosenberg, H. (1973). The inducible citrate-dependent iron transport system in *Escherichia coli* K12. *Biochimica et Biophysica Acta*, **330**, 90–101.
Gibson, F., and Magrath, D.I. (1969). The isolation and characterization of a hydroxamic acid (aerobactin) formed by *Aerobacter aerogenes* 62–1. *Biochimica et Biophysica Acta*, **192,** 175–184.
Goebel, W., Hacker, J., Knapp, S., Then, I., Wagner, W., Hughes, C., and Juarez, A. (1985). Structure, function and regulation of the plasmid encoded haemolysin determinants of *Escherichia coli.* In *Plasmids and Bacteria* (Eds. D.R. Helinski, S.N. Cohen, D.B. Clewell, D.A. Jackson and A. Hollander, pp. 791–805. Plenum Press, New York.
Gonzalez-Carrero, M.I., Zabala, J.C., de la Cruz, F., and Ortiz, J.M. (1985). Purification of α-haemolysin from an over producing *Escherichia coli* strain. *Molecular and General Genetics*, **199,** 106–110.
Green, C.P., and Thomas, V.L. (1981). Haemagglutination of human type O erythrocytes, haemolysin production and serogrouping of *Escherichia coli* isolates from patients with acute pyelonephritis, cystitis and asymptomatic bacteruria. *Infection and Immunity*, **31,** 309–315.
Greenwood, K.T., and Luke, R.K.J. (1978) Enzymic hydrolysis of enterochelin and its iron complex in *Escherichia coli* K12. *Biochimica et Biophysica Acta*, **525**, 209–218.
Grewal, K.K., Warner, P.J., and Williams, P.H. (1982). An inducible outer membrane protein involved in aerobactin mediated iron transport by ColV strains of *Escherchia coli. FEBS Letters*, **140,** 27–30.
Griffiths, E. (1972). Abnormal phenylalanyl-tRNA found in serum inhibited *Escherchia coli* strain 0111. *FEBS Letters*, **25,** 159–164.
Griffiths, E. (1981). Iron and the susceptibility to bacterial infection. In *Nutritional Factors: Modulating Effects on Metabolic Processes* (Eds. R.F. Beers and E.G. Bassett), pp. 463–476. Raven Press, New York.
Griffiths, E. (1983a). Adaptation and multiplication of bacteria in host tissues. *Philosophical Transactions of the Royal Society, London,* Series B, **303,** 85–96.
Griffiths, E. (1983b). Bacterial adaptation to a low iron environment. In *Microbiology-1983*, pp. 329–333. American Society for Microbiology.
Griffiths, E. (1985). Candidate virulence markers. In *The Virulence of Escherichia coli* (Ed. M. Sussman), Society for General Microbiology Special Publication No. 13, pp. 193–226. Academic Press, London.
Griffiths, E., and Buck, M. (1979). tRNA alteration and adaptation of pathogenic *Escherichia coli* to growth *in vivo. Society for General Microbiology Quarterly*, **7,** 10.
Griffiths, E., and Humphreys, J. (1975). Changes in aminoacyl-tRNAs associated with the inhibition of *Escherichia coli* 0111 by bovine colostrum. *Proceedings of the Society for General Microbiology*, **3,** 61.
Griffiths, E., and Humphreys, J. (1976). Alterations in *Escherchia coli* tRNAs: a possible relationship with pathogenicity. *Proceedings of the Society for General Microbiology*, **4,** 11–12.
Griffiths, E., and Humphreys, Janice (1977). Bacteriostatic effect of human and bovine colostrum on *Escherichia coli*: the importance of bicarbonate. *Infection and Immunity*, **15,** 396–401.
Griffiths, E., and Humphreys, J. (1978). Alterations in tRNAs containing 2-methylthio-N^6-(Δ^2isopentenyl)-adenosine during growth of enteropathogenic

Escherichia coli in the presence of iron-binding proteins. *European Journal of Biochemistry*, **82,** 503–513.

Griffiths, E., and Humphreys, J. (1980). Isolation of enterochelin from the peritoneal washings of guinea-pigs lethally infected with *Escherichia coli*. *Infection and Immunity*, **28,** 286–289.

Griffiths, E., Humphreys, J., Leach, A., and Scanlon, L. (1978). Alerations in the tRNAs of *Escherichia coli* recovered from lethally infected animals. *Infection and Immunity*, **22,** 312–317.

Griffiths, G.L., Sigel, S.P., Payne, S.M., and Neilands, J.B. (1984). Vibriobactin, a siderophore from *Vibrio cholerae*. *Journal of Biological Chemistry*, **259,** 383–385.

Griffiths, E., Stevenson, P., and Joyce, P. (1983). Pathogenic *Escherichia coli* express new outer membrane proteins when growing *in vivo*. *FEMS Microbiology Letters*, **16,** 95–99.

Griffiths, E., Stevenson, P., Thorpe, R., and Chart, H. (1985a). Naturally occurring antibodies in human sera that react with the iron-regulated outer membrane proteins of *Escherichia coli*. *Infection and Immunity*, **47,** 808–813.

Griffiths, E., Stevenson, P., Hale, T.L., and Formal, S.B. (1985b). The synthesis of aerobactin and a 76000 dalton iron-regulated outer membrane protein by *Escherichia coli* K12–*Shigella* hybrids and by enteroinvasive strains of *Escherichia coli*. *Infection and Immunity*, **49,** 67–71.

Grosjean, H., Nicoghosian, K., Haumont, E., Soll, D., and Cedegren, R. (1985). Nucleotide sequences of two serine tRNAs with a GGA anticodon: the structure–function relationships in the serine family of *E.coli* tRNAs. *Nucleic Acids Research*, **13,** 5697–5706.

Gross, R., Engelbrecht, F., and Braun, V. (1984). Genetic and biochemical characterization of the aerobactin synthesis operon on pColV. *Molecular and General Genetics*, **196,** 74–80.

Gutteridge, J.M.C., Rowley, D.A., Griffiths, E., and Halliwell, B. (1985). Low-molecular-weight iron complexes and oxygen radical reactions in idiopathic haemochromatosis. *Clinical Sciences*, **68,** 463–467.

Hacker, J., Hughes, C., Hof, H., and Goebel, W. (1983). Cloned hemolysin genes from *Escherichia coli* that cause urinary tract infection determine different levels of toxicity in mice. *Infection and Immunity*, **42,** 57–63.

Hall, R.M., and Ratledge, C. (1984). Mycobactins as chemotaxonomic characters for some rapidly growing mycobacteria. *Journal of General Microbiology*. **130,** 1883–1892.

Hall, R.M., and Ratledge, C. (1985). Mycobactins in the classification and identification of armadillo-derived mycobacteria. *FEMS Microbiology Letters*, **28,** 243–247.

Hancock, R.E.W., Hantke, K., and Braun, V. (1976). Iron transport in *Escherichia coli* K12: involvement of the colicin B receptor and of a citrate-inducible protein. *Journal of Bacteriology*, **127,** 1370–1375.

Hantke, K. (1981). Regulation of ferric iron transport in *Escherichia coli* K12: isolation of a constitutive mutant. *Molecular and General Genetics*, **182,** 288–292.

Hantke, K. (1982). Negative control of iron uptake systems in *Escherichia coli*. *FEMS Microbiology Letters*, **15,** 83–86.

Hantke, K. (1984). Cloning of the repressor protein gene of iron-regulated systems in *Escherichia coli* K12. *Molecular and General Genetics*, **197,** 337–341.

Harbell, S.O., Hodgins, H.O., and Schiewe, M.H. (1979). Studies on the pathology of vibriosis on the coho salmon (*Oncorhynchus kisutch*). *Journal of Fish Diseases*, **2,** 527–535.

Harris, W.R., Carrano, C.J., Cooper, S.R., Sofen, S.R., Avdeef, A.E., McArdle,

J.V., and Raymond, K.N. (1979).Co-ordination chemistry of microbial iron transport compounds. 19: Stability constants and electrochemical behaviour of ferric enterobactin and model complexes. *Journal of the American Chemical Society*, **101,** 6097–6104.

Harris, W.R., Carrano, C.J., and Raymond, K.N. (1979a). Spectrophotometric determination of the proton dependent stability constant of ferric enterochelin. *Journal of the American Chemical Society*, **101,** 2213–2214.

Harris, W.R., Carrano, C.J., and Raymond, K.N. (1979b). Co-ordination chemistry of microbial iron transport compounds. 16: Isolation, characterization and formation constants of ferric aerobactin. *Journal of the American Chemical Society*, **101,** 2722–2727.

Hartmann, A., and Braun, V. (1980). Iron transport in *Escherichia coli*: uptake and modification of ferrichrome. *Journal of Bacteriology*, **143,** 246–255.

Helms, S.D., Oliver, J.D., and Travis, J.C. (1984). Role of heme compounds and haptoglobin in *Vibrio vulnificus* pathogenicity. *Infection and Immunity*, **45,** 345–349.

Herman, R.L. (1968). Fish furunculosis 1952–1966. *Transactions of the American Fish Society*, **97,** 221–230.

Herrington, D.A., and Sparling, P.F. (1985). *Haemophilus influenzae* can use human transferrin as a sole source of required iron. *Infection and Immunity*, **48,** 248–251.

Hider, R.C., Silver, J., Neilands, J.B., Morrison, I.E.G., and Rees, L.V.C. (1979). Identification of iron(II)–enterobactin and its possible role in *Escherichia coli* iron transport. *FEBS Letters*, **102,** 325–328.

Hoiseth, S.,K., and Stocker, B.A.D. (1985). Genes *aro*A and *ser*C of *Salmonella typhimurium* constitute an operon. *Journal of Bacteriology*, **163,** 355–361.

Holbein, B.E. (1980). Iron controlled infection with *Neisseria meningitidis* in mice. *Infection and Immunity*, **29,** 886–891.

Holbein, B.E. (1981). Enhancement of *Neisseria meningitidis* infection in mice by addition of iron bound to transferrin. *Infection and Immunity*, **34,** 120–125.

Hollifield, Jr., W.C., and Neilands, J.B. (1978). Ferric enterobactin transport system in *Escherichia coli* K12: extraction, assay and specificity of the outer membrane receptor. *Biochemistry*, **17,** 1922–1928.

Hsu, J.H., Harms, E., and Umbarger, H.E. (1985). Leucine regulation of the *ilv* GEDA operon of *Serratia marcescens* by attenuation is modulated by a single leucine codon. *Journal of Bacteriology*, **164,** 217–222.

Hull, S.I., Hull, R.A., Minshew, B.H., and Falkow, S. (1982). Genetics of hemolysin of *Escherichia coli*. *Journal of Bacteriology*, **151,** 1006–1012.

Hunter, R.L., Bennett, B., Towns, M., and Vogler, W.R. (1984). Transferrin in disease.II: Defects in the regulation of transferrin saturation with iron contribute to susceptibility to infection. *American Journal of Clincial Pathology*, **81,** 748–753.

Hussein, S., Hantke, K., and Braun, V. (1981). Citrate-dependent iron transport system in *Escherichia coli* K12. *European Journal of Biochemistry*, **117,** 431–437.

Janzer, J.J., Raney, J.P., and McLennan, B.D. (1982). Isolation and identification of a hydroxylated isopentenyl adenosine derivative from tRNA of enteric bacteria. *Nucleic Acids Research*, **10,** 5663–5672.

Jones, R.L., Peterson, C.M., Grady, R.W., Kumbaraci, T., and Cerami, A. (1977). Effects of iron chelators and iron overload on *Salmonella* infection. *Nature*, **267,** 63–64.

Kay, W.W., Buckley, J.T., Ishiguro, E.E., Phipps, B.M., Monette, J.P.L., and Trust, T.J. (1981). Purification and disposition of a surface protein associated with virulence of *Aeromonas salmonicida*. *Journal of Bacteriology*, **147,** 1077–1084.

Kay, W.W., and Cameron, M. (1978). Citrate transport in *Salmonella typhimurium*. *Archives of Biochemistry and Biophysics*, **190,** 270–280.

Kersten, H. (1984). On the biological significance of modified nucleosides in tRNA. *Progress in Nucleic Acid Research and Molecular Biology*, **31,** 59–114.

Khan, A.M., Mehrota, R.M.L., and Kumar, R. (1968). Antigenicity and toxicity of alpha-haemolysins of *Escherichia coli*. *Indian Journal of Medical Research*, **56,** 1241–1246.

Khimji, P.L., and Miles, A.A. (1978). Microbial iron-chelators and their action on *Klebsiella* infections in the skin of guinea-pigs. *British Journal of Experimental Pathology*, **59,** 137–147.

Klebba, P.E., McIntosh, M.A., and Neilands, J.B. (1982). Kinetics of biosynthesis of iron regulated membrane proteins in *Escherichia coli*. *Journal of Bacteriology*, **149,** 880–888.

Klempner, M.S., Dinarello, C.A., and Gallin, J.I. (1978). Human leukocytic pyrogen induces release of specific granule contents from human neutrophils. *Journal of Clinical Investigation*, **61,** 1330–1336.

Knapp, S., Hacker, J., Then, I., Muller, D., and Goebel, W. (1984). Multiple copies of hemolysin genes and associated sequences in the chromosomes of uropathogenic *Escherichia coli* strains. *Journal of Bacteriology*, **159,** 1027–1033.

Kochan, I. (1973). The role of iron in bacterial infections with special consideration of host–tubercle bacillus interaction. *Current Topics in Microbiology and Immunology*, **60,** 1–30.

Kochan, I., Pellis, N.R., and Golden, C.A. (1971). Mechanism of tuberculostasis in mammalian serum. III: Neutralization of serum tuberculostasis by mycobactin. *Infection and Immunity*, **3,** 553–558.

Kojima, N., and Bates, G.W. (1979). The reduction and release of iron from Fe^{3+}–transferrin–$CO_3{}^{2-}$. *Journal of Biological Chemistry*, **254,** 8847–8854.

Konisky, J. (1979). Specific transport systems and receptors for colicins and phages. In *Bacterial Outer Membranes; Biogenesis and Functions* (Ed. M. Inouye), pp. 319–359. J. Wiley and Sons, New York.

Konopka, K., Bindereif, A., and Neilands, J.B. (1982). Aerobactin-mediated utilization of transferrin iron. *Biochemistry*, **21,** 6503–6508.

Konopka, K., and Neilands, J.B. (1984). Effect of serum albumin on siderophore-mediated utilization of transferrin iron. *Biochemistry*, **23,** 2122–2127.

Krone, W.J.A., Stegehuis, F., Koningstein, G., van Doarn, C., Roosendaal, B., de Gray, F.K., and Oudega, B. (1985). Characterization of the pColV-K30 encoded cloacin DF13/aerobactin outer membrane receptor protein of *Escherichia coli*; isolation and purification of the protein and analysis of its nucleotide sequence and primary structure. *FEMS Microbiology Letters*, **26,** 153–161.

Laird, A.J., Ribbons, D.W., Woodrow, G.C., and Young, I.G. (1980). Bacteriophage Mu-mediated gene transposition and *in vitro* cloning of the enterochelin gene cluster of *Escherichia coli*. *Gene*, **11,** 347–357.

Lam, C., Turnowsky, F., Schwarzinger, E., and Neruda, W., (1984). Bacteria recovered without subculture from infected human urines expressed iron regulated outer membrane proteins. *FEMS Microbiology Letters*, **24,** 255–259.

Langman, L., Young, I.G., Frost, G., Rosenberg, H., and Gibson, F. (1972). Enterochelin system of iron transport in *Escherichia coli*: mutations affecting ferric–enterochelin esterase. *Journal of Bacteriology*, **112,** 1142–1149.

Lankford, C.E. (1973). Bacterial assimilation of iron, *CRC Critical Reviews in Microbiology*, **2,** 273–331.

Laurell, C.B., and Gronvall, C. (1962). Haptoglobins. *Advances in Clinical Chemistry*, **5,** 135–172.
Lawlor, K.M., and Payne, S.M. (1984). Aerobactin genes in *Shigella* spp. *Journal of Bacteriology*, **160,** 266–272.
Lee, Jr., J.T., Ahrenhoz, D.H., Nelson, R.D., and Simmons, R.L. (1979). Mechanisms of the adjuvant effect of hemoglobin in experimental peritonitis V. The significance of the co-ordinated iron component. *Surgery*, **86,** 41–48.
Leffell, M.S., and Spitznagel, J.K. (1974). Intracellular and extracellular degranulation of human polymorphonuclear azurophil and specific granules induced by immune complexes. *Infection and Immunity*, **10,** 1241–1249.
LeMinor, S. (1972). Apparition en France d'une epidemie a *Salmonella wien*. *Medecine et Maladies Infectieuses*, **2**, 441–448.
Leong, J., and Neilands, J.B. (1976). Mechanisms of siderophore iron transport in enteric bacteria. *Journal of Bacteriology*, **126,** 823–830.
Letendre, E.D., and Holbein, B.E. (1983). Turnover in the transferrin iron pool during the hypoferremic phase of experimental *Neisseria meningitidis* infection in mice. *Infection and Immunity*, **39,** 50–59.
Letendre, E.D. and Holbein, B.E. (1984). Mechanism of impaired iron release by the reticuloendothelial system during the hypoferraemic phase of experimental *Neisseria meningitidis* infection in mice. *Infection and Immunity*, **44,** 320–325.
Linggood, M.A., and Ingram, P.L. (1982). The role of alpha haemolysin in the virulence of *Escherichia coli* for mice. *Journal of Medical Microbiology*, **15,** 23–30.
Liu, P.V. (1966). The roles of various fractions of *Pseudomonas aeruginosa* in its pathogenesis. III: Identity of the lethal toxins produced *in vitro* and *in vivo*. *Journal of Infectious Diseases*, **116,** 481–489.
Liu, P.V., and Shokrani, F. (1978). Biological activities of pyochelins: iron-chelating agents of *Pseudomonas aeruginosa*. *Infection and Immunity*, **22,** 878–890.
Lovell, R., and Rees, T.A. (1960). A filterable haemolysin from *Escherichia coli*. *Nature (London)*, **188,** 755–756.
Lowrie, D.B., Aber, U.B., and Carrol, M.E.W. (1979). Division and death rates of *Salmonella typhimurium* inside macrophages: use of penicillins as a probe. *Journal of General Microbiology*, **110,** 409–419.
McCandliss, R.J., and Herrmann, K.M. (1978). Iron, an essential element for biosynthesis of aromatic compounds. *Proceedings of the National Academy of Sciences* (USA), **75,** 4810–4813.
McClelland, D.B.L., and van Furth, R. (1976). Antimicrobial factors in the exudates of skin windows in human subjects. *Clinical and Experimental Immunology*, **25,** 442–448.
McIntosh, M.A., and Earhart, C.F. (1977). Co-ordinated regulation by iron of the synthesis of phenolate compounds and three outer membrane proteins in *Escherichia coli*. *Journal of Bacteriology*, **131,** 331–339.
Mackaness, G.B., Blanden, R.V., and Collins, F.M. (1966). Host-parasite relations in mouse typhoid. *Journal of Experimental Medicine*, **124**, 573–583.
McLennan, B.D., Buck, M., Humphreys, J., and Griffiths, E. (1981). Iron related modification of bacterial tRNA. *Nucleic Acids Research,* **9,** 2629–2640.
Mekalanos, J.J. (1983). Duplication and amplification of toxin genes in *Vibrio cholerae*. *Cell*, **35,** 253–263.
Merriman, C.R., Pulliam, L.A., and Kampschmidt, R.F. (1977). Comparison of leukocytic pyrogen and leukocytic endogenous mediator. *Proceedings of the Society for Experimental Biology and Medicine*, **154,** 224–227.

Messenger, A.J.M., and Ratledge, C. (1982). Iron transport in *Mycobacteria smegmatis*: uptake of iron from ferric citrate. *Journal of Bacteriology*, **149,** 131–135.

Meyer, J.M., Mock, M., and Abdallah, M.A. (1979). Effect of iron on the protein composition of the outer membrane of fluorescent pseudomonas. *FEMS Microbiology Letters*, **5,** 395–398.

Mickelsen, P.A., and Sparling, P.F. (1981). Ability of *Neisseria gonorrhoeae*, *Neisseria meningitidis* and commensal *Neisseria* species to obtain iron from transferrin and iron compounds. *Infection and Immunity*, **33,** 555–564.

Mickelsen, P.A., Blackman, E., and Sparling, P.F. (1982). Ability of *Neisseria gonorrhoeae*, *Neisseria meningitidis* and commensal *Neisseria* species to obtain iron from lactoferrin. *Infection and Immunity*, **35,** 915–920.

Mietzner, T.A., Luginbuhl, G.H., Sandstrom, E., and Morse, S.A. (1984). Identification of an iron-regulated 37000 dalton protein in the cell envelope of *Neisseria gonorrhoeae*. *Infection and Immunity*, **45,** 410–416.

Miles, A.A., and Khimji, P.L. (1975). Enterobacterial chelators of iron: their occurrence, detection and relation to pathogenicity. *Journal of Medical Microbiology*, **8,** 477–490.

Minshew, B.H., Jorgensen, J., Counts, G.W., and Falkow, S. (1978). Association of hemolysin production, hemagglutination of human erythrocytes and virulence for chicken embryos of extraintestinal *Escherichia coli* isolates. *Infection and Immunity*, **20,** 50–54.

Montgomerie, J.Z., Bindereif, A., Neilands, J.B., Kahmanson, G.M., and Guze, L.B. (1984). Association of hydroxamate siderophore (aerobactin) with *Escherichia coli* isolated from patients with bacteraemia. *Infection and Immunity*, **46,** 835–838.

Moore, D.G., and Earhart, C.F. (1981). Specific inhibition of *Escherichia coli* ferrienterochelin uptake by a normal human serum immunoglobulin. *Infection and Immunity*, **31,** 631–635.

Moore, D.G., Yancey, R.J., Lankford, C.E., and Earhart, C.F. (1980). Bacteriostatic enterochelin-specific immunoglobulin from normal human serum. *Infection and Immunity*, **27,** 418–423.

Morgan, E.H. (1981). Transferrin, biochemistry, physiology and clinical significance. *Molecular Aspects of Medicine*, **4,** 1–123.

Moulder, J.W. (1979). The cell as an extreme environment. *Proceedings of the Royal Society, London*, Series B, **204,** 199–210.

Munn, C.B., Ishiguro, E.E., Kay, W.W., and Trust, T.J. (1982). Role of surface components in serum resistance of virulent *Aeromonas salmonicida*. *Infection and Immunity*, **36,** 1069–1075.

Neilands, J.B. (1981). Microbial iron compounds, *Annual Review of Biochemistry*, **50,** 715–731.

Neilands, J.B. (1982). Microbial envelope proteins related to iron. *Annual Review of Microbiology*, **36,** 285–309.

Newman, R., Schneider, C., Sutherland, R., Vodinelech, L., and Greaves, M. (1982). The transferrin receptor. *Trends in Biochemical Sciences*, **7,** 397–400.

Nicaud, J.M., Mackman, N., Gray, L., and Holland, I.B. (1985). Regulation of haemolysin synthesis in *Escherichia coli* determined by HLY genes of human origin. *Molecular and General Genetics*, **199,** 111–116.

Nikaido, H. (1979). Non specific transport through the outer membrane. In *Bacterial Outer Membranes, Biogenesis and Functions* (Ed. M. Inouye), pp. 361–407. J. Wiley and Sons, New York.

Noegel, A., Rdest, U., and Goebel, W. (1981). Determination of the functions of hemolytic plasmid pHly 152 of *Escherichia coli*. *Journal of Bacteriology*, **145,** 233–247.

Norqvist, A., Davies, J. Norlander, L., and Normark, S., (1978). The effect of iron starvation on the outer membrane protein composition of *Neisseria gonorrhoeae*. *FEMS Microbiology Letters*, **4,** 71–75.

Norrod, P., and Williams, R.P. (1978). Growth of *Neisseria gonorrhoeae* in media deficient in iron without detection of siderophores. *Current Microbiology*, **1**, 281–284.

O'Brien, A.D. (1982). Innate resistance of mice to *Salmonella typhi* infection. *Infection and Immunity*, **38,** 948–952.

O'Brien, I.G., and Gibson, F. (1970). The structure of enterochelin and related 2,3-dihydroxy-*N*-benzoylserine conjugates from *Escherichia coli*. *Biochimica et Biophysica Acta*, **215,** 393–402.

Octave, J.N., Schneider, Y.J., Trouet, A., and Crichton, R.R. (1983). Iron uptake and utilization by mammalian cells, I. Cellular uptake of transferrin and iron. *Trends in Biochemical Sciences*, **8,** 217–220.

Oliver, J.B., Warner, R.A., and Cleland, D.R. (1983). Distribution of *Vibrio vulnificus* and other lactose fermenting vibrios in the marine environment. *Environmental Microbiology*, **45,** 985–988.

Ong, S.A., Peterson, T., and Neilands, J.B. (1979). Agrobactin, a siderophore from *Agrobacterium tumefacians*. *Journal of Biological Chemistry*, **254,** 1860–1865.

Oudega, B., Oldziel-Werner, W.J.M., Klaasen-Bloor, P., Rezee, A., Glas, J., and de Graaf, F.K. (1979). Purification and characterization of cloacin DF13 receptor from *Enterobacter cloacae* and its interaction with cloacin DF13 *in vitro*. *Journal of Bacteriology*, **138,** 7–16.

Owen, J.A., Smith, R., Padaya, R., and Martin, J. (1964). Serum haptoglobin in disease. *Clinical Science*, **26,** 1–6.

Pappenheimer, Jr., A.M. (1977). Diphtheria toxin. *Annual Review of Biochemistry*, **46,** 69–94.

Payne, S.M., and Finkelstein, R.A. (1978a). Siderophore production by *Vibrio cholerae*. *Infection and Immunity*, **20,** 310–311.

Payne, S.M., and Finkelstein, R.A. (1978b). The critical role of iron in host-bacterial interactions. *Journal of Clinical Investigation*, **61,** 1428–1440.

Payne, S.M., Niesel, D.W., Peixotto, S.S., and Lawlor, K.M. (1983). Expression of hydroxamate and phenolate siderophores by *Shigella flexneri*. *Journal of Bacteriology*, **155,** 949–955.

Perry, R.D., and Brubaker, R.R (1979). Accumulation of iron by *Yersiniae*. *Journal of Bacteriology*, **137,** 1290–1298.

Perry, R.D., and San Clemente, C.L. (1979) Siderophore synthesis in *Klebsiella pneumoniae* and *Shigella sonnei* during iron deficiency. *Journal of Bacteriology*, **140,** 1129–1132.

Peterson, T., Falk, K.E., Leong, S.A., Klein, M.P., and Neilands, J.B. (1980). Structure and behaviour of spermidine siderophores. *Journal of the American Chemical Society*, **102,** 7715–7718.

Phipps, B.M., Trust, T.J., Ishiguro, E.E., and Kay, W.W. (1983). Purification and characterization of the cell-surface virulent A-protein from *Aeromonas salmonicida*. *Biochemistry*, **22,** 2934–2939.

Plastow, G.S., Pratt, J.M., and Holland, I.B. (1981). The ferrichrome receptor protein (tonA) of *Escherichia coli* is synthesized as a precursor *in vitro*. *FEBS Letters*, **131,** 262–264.

Pollack, J.R., and Neilands, J.B. (1970). Enterobactin, an iron transport compound from *Salmonella typhimurium*. *Biochemical and Biophysical Research Communications*, **38,** 989–992.

Pollack, S., Aisen, P., Lasky, F.D., and Vanderhoff, G. (1976). Chelate mediated transfer of iron from transferrin to desferrioxime. *British Journal of Haematology*, **34,** 231–235.

Prody, C.A., and Neilands, J.B. (1984). Genetic and biochemical characterization of the *Escherichia coli* K12 *fhu* B mutation. *Journal of Bacteriology*, **157,** 874–880.

Rangneker, V.M., Banker, D.D., and Jhala, H.I. (1983). Antimicrobial resistance and incompatability groups of R plasmids in *Salmonella typhimurium* isolated from human sources in Bombay from 1978 to 1980. *Antimicrobial Agents and Chemotherapy*, **23,** 54–58.

Ransom, D.P., Lannon, C.N., Rohovec, J.S., and Fryer, J.L. (1984). Comparison of histopathology caused by *Vibrio anguillarum* and *Vibrio ordallii* in three species of Pacific salmon. *Journal of Fish Diseases*, **7,** 107–115.

Ratledge, C., and Hall, M.J. (1971). Influence of metal ions on the formation of mycobactin and salicylic acid in *Mycobacterium smegmatis* grown in static culture. *Journal of Bacteriology*, **108,** 314–319.

Ratledge, C., Patel, C.V., and Mundy, J. (1982). Iron transport in *Mycobacterium smegmatis*; the localization of mycobactin by electron microscopy. *Journal of General Microbiology*, **128,** 1559–1565.

Raymond, K.N., and Carrano, C.J. (1979). Co-ordination chemistry of microbial iron transport. *Accounts of Chemical Research*, **12,** 183–190.

Reeves M.W., Pine, L., Neilands, J.B., and Balows, A. (1983). Absence of siderophore activity in *Legionella* species grown in iron-deficient media. *Journal of Bacteriology*, **154,** 324–329.

Rennie, R.P., and Arbuthnott, J.P. (1974). Partial characterization of *Escherichia coli* haemolysin. *Journal of Medical Microbiology*, **7,** 179–188.

Rennie, R.P., Freer, J.H., and Arbuthnott, J.P. (1974). The kinetics of erythrocyte lysis by *Escherichia coli* haemolysin. *Journal of Medical Microbiology*, **7,** 189–195.

Rogers, H.J. (1973). Iron-binding catechols and virulence in *Escherichia coli*. *Infection and Immunity*, **7,** 445–456.

Rogers, H.J. Bullen, J.J., and Cushnie, G.H. (1970). Iron compounds and resistance to infection: further experiments with *Clostridium welchii* type A *in vivo* and *in vitro*. *Immunology*, **19,** 521–538.

Rogers, H.J., Synge, C., Kimber, B., and Bayley, P.M. (1977). Production of enterochelin by *Escherichia coli* 0111. *Biochimica et Biophysica Acta*, **497,** 548–557.

Rosenberg, A.H., and Gefter, M.L. (1969). An iron-dependent modification of several transfer RNA species in *Escherichia coli*. *Journal of Molecular Biology*, **46,** 581–584.

Rosenberg, H., and Young, I.G. (1974). Iron transport in the enteric bacteria. In *Microbial Iron Metabolism* (Ed. J.B. Neilands), pp. 67–82. Academic Press, New York.

Royer-Pokora, B., and Goebel, W. (1976). Plasmids controlling synthesis of hemolysin in *Escherichia coli*.II. Polynucleotide sequence relationships among hemolytic plasmids. *Molecular and General Genetics*, **144,** 177–183.

Russell, L.M., Cryz, Jr., S.J., and Holmes, R.K. (1984). Genetic and biochemical evidence for a siderophore dependent iron transport system in *Corynebacterium diphtheriae*. *Infection and Immunity*, **45**, 143–149.

Russell, L.M., and Holmes, R.K. (1983). Initial characterisation of the ferric iron transport system of *Corynebacterium diphtheriae*. *Journal of Bacteriology*, **155,** 1439–1442.

Russell, L.M., and Holmes, R.K. (1985). Highly toxigenic but avirulent Park-Williams 8 strain of *Corynebacterium diphtheriae* does not produce siderophore. *Infection and Immunity*, **47,** 575–578.

Schade, A.L. (1963). Significance of serum iron for growth, biological characteristics

and metabolism of *Staphylococcus aureus*. *Biochemische Zeitschrift*, **338,** 140–148.
Sciortino, C.V., and Finkelstein, R.A. (1983). *Vibrio cholerae* expresses iron-regulated outer membrane proteins *in vivo*. *Infection and Immunity*, **42,** 990–996.
Shand, G.H., Anwar, H., Kaduruganuwa, J., Brown, M.R.W., Silverman, S.H., and Melling, J. (1985). *In vivo* evidence that bacteria in urinary tract infection grow under iron-restricted conditions. *Infection and Immunity*, **48,** 35–39.
Short, Jr., E.C., and Kurtz, H.J. (1971). Properties of the hemolytic activities of *Escherichia coli*. *Infection and Immunity*, **3,** 678–687.
Sigel, S.P., and Payne, S.M. (1982). Effect of iron limitation on growth, siderophore production and expression of outer membrane proteins of *Vibrio cholerae*. *Journal of Bacteriology*, **150,** 148–155.
Sigel, S.P., Stoebner, J.A., and Payne, S.M. (1985). Iron–vibriobactin transport system is not required for virulence of *Vibrio cholerae*. *Infection and Immunity*, **47,** 360–362.
Simonson, C., Brener, D., and DeVoe, I.W. (1982). Expression of a high-affinity mechanism for acquisition of transferrin iron by *Neisseria meningitidis*. *Infection and Immunity*, **36,** 107–113.
Simpson, L.M., and Oliver, J.D. (1983). Siderophore production by *Vibrio vulnificus*. *Infection and Immunity*, **41,** 644–649.
Smith, H. (1976). Survivial of vegetative bacteria in animals. Society for General Microbiology, Symposium No. 26, pp. 299–326.
Smith, H.R., Scotland, S.M., and Rowe, B. (1985). Genetics of *Escherichia coli* virulence. In *The Virulence of Escherichia coli* (Ed. M. Sussman), Society for General Microbiology Special Publication No. 13, pp. 227–269. Academic Press, London.
Smith, H.W. (1963). The haemolysins of *Escherichia coli*. *Journal of Pathology and Bacteriology*, **85,** 197–211.
Smith, H.W., and Huggins M.B. (1980). The association of the 018 K1 and H7 antigens and the ColV plasmid of a strain of *Escherichia coli* with its virulence and immunogenicity. *Journal of General Microbiology*, **121,** 387–400.
Smith, H.W., and Huggins, M.B. (1985). The toxic role of alpha-haemolysin in the pathogenesis of experimental *Escherichia coli* infection in mice. *Journal of General Microbiology*, **131,** 395–403.
Smith, H.W., and Linggood, M.A. (1970). Transfer factors in *Escherichia coli* with particular regard to their incidence in enteropathogenic strains. *Journal of General Microbiology*, **62,** 287–299.
Smith, H.W., and Linggood, M.A. (1971). Observations on the pathogenic properties of the K88, Hly and Ent plasmids of *Escherichia coli* with particular reference to porcine diarrhoea. *Journal of Medical Microbiology*, **4,** 467–485.
Smith, H.W., Parsell, Z., and Green, P. (1978). Thermosensitive Hl plasmids determining citrate utilization. *Journal of General Microbiology*, **109,** 305–311.
Snow, G.A. (1970). Mycobactins: iron-chelating growth factors from mycobacteria. *Bacteriological Reviews*, **34,** 99–125.
Snow, G.A., and White, A.J. (1969). Chemical and biological properties of mycobactins isolated from various mycobacteria. *Biochemical Journal*, **115,** 1031–1045.
Sokol, P.A. (1984). Production of the ferripyochelin outer membrane receptor by *Pseudomonas* species. *FEMS Microbiology Letters*, **23,** 313–317.
Sokol, P.A., and Woods, D.E., (1983). Demonstration of an iron siderophore binding protein in the outer membrane of *Pseudomonas aeruginosa*. *Infection and Immunity*, **40,** 665–669.
Soucek, S., and Konisky, J. (1977). Normal iron–enterochelin uptake in mutants lacking the colicin I outer membrane receptor protein of *Escherichia coli*. *Journal of Bacteriology*, **130,** 1399–1401.

Springer, M., Mayaux, J.F., Fayat, G., Plumbridge, J.A., Graffe, M., Blanquet, S., and Grunberg-Manago, M. (1985). Attenuation control of the *Escherichia coli* phenylalanyl-tRNA synthetase operon. *Journal of Molecular Biology*, **181,** 467–478.

Springer, M., Trudel, M., Graffe, M., Plumbridge, J.A., Fayat, G., Mayaux, J.F., Sacerdot, C., Blanquet, S., and Grunberg-Manago, M. (1983). *Escherichia coli* phenlalanyl-tRNA synthetase operon is controlled by attenuation *in vivo. Journal of Molecular Biology*, **171,** 263–279.

Sprinzl, M., Moll, J., Meissener, F., and Hartmann, T. (1985). Compilation of tRNA sequences. *Nucleic Acids Research*, **13,** rl-r49.

Stephenson, M.C., and Ratledge, C. (1979). Iron transport in *Mycobacterium smegmatis*: uptake of iron from ferriexochelin. *Journal of General Microbiology*, **110,** 193–202.

Stevenson, P., and Griffiths, E. (1985) Growth of *Escherichia coli* under iron restricted conditions. In *The Virulence of Escherichia coli* (Ed. M. Sussman), Special Publication of the Society for General Microbiology No. 13, pp. 413–417.

Stuart, S.J., Greenwood, J.K.T., and Luke, R.K.J. (1980). Hydroxamate-mediated transport of iron controlled by ColV plasmids. *Journal of Bacteriology*, **143,** 35–42.

Stuart, S.J., Greenwood, J.K.T., and Luke, R.K.J. (1982). Iron-suppressible production of hydroxamate by *Escherichia coli* isolates. *Infection and Immunity*, **36,** 870–875.

Thimmappaya. B., and Cherayil, J.D. (1974). Unique presence of 2-methylthioribosylzeatin in the transfer ribonucleic acid of the bacterium *Pseudomonas aeruginosa. Biochemical and Biophysical Research Communications*, **60,** 665–672.

Tidmarsh, G.F., Klebba, P.E., and Rosenberg, L.T. (1983). Rapid release of iron from ferritin by siderophores. *Journal of Inorganic Biochemistry*, **18,** 161–168.

Tidmarsh, G.F., and Rosenberg, L.T. (1981). Acquisition of iron from transferrin by *Salmonella paratyphi* B. *Current Microbiology*, **6,** 217–220.

Tolmasky, M.E., Actis, L.A., Toranzo, A.E., Barja, J.L., and Crosa, J.H. (1985). Plasmid-mediated iron uptake system in *Vibrio anguillarum* strains isolated from turbot in Spain. *Journal of General Microbiology*, **131,** 1989–1997.

Tolmasky, M.E., and Crosa, J.H. (1984). Molecular cloning and expression of genetic determinants for the iron uptake system mediated by the *Vibrio anguillarum* plasmid pJM1. *Journal of Bacteriology*, **160,** 860–866.

Toranzo, A.E., Barja, J.L., Potter, S.A., Colwell, R.R., Hetrich, F.M., and Crosa, J.H. (1983). Molecular factors associated with virulence of marine vibrios isolated from striped bass in Chesapeake Bay. *Infection and Immunity*, **39,** 1220–1227.

Trudel, M., Springer, M., Graffe, M., Fayat, G., Blanquet, S., and Grunberg-Manago, M. (1984). Regulation of *E.coli* phenylalanyl-tRNA synthetase operon *in vivo. Biochimica et Biophysica Acta*, **782,** 10–17.

Trust, T.J., Kay, W.W., Ishiguro, E.E., Buckley, J.T., and Pearson, T.W. (1982). Properties of A protein, a virulence factor on the surface of *Aeromonas salmonicida. Developmental and Comparative Immunology*, Supplement 2, 175–180.

Udey, L.R., and Fryer, J.L. (1978). Immunization of fish with bacterins of *Aeromonas salmonicida. Marine Fish Reviews*, **40,** 12–17.

Valvano, M.A., and Crosa, J.H. (1984). Aerobactin iron transport genes commonly encoded by certain ColV plasmids occur in the chromosome of a human invasive strain of *Escherichia coli* K1. *Infection and Immunity*, **46,** 159–167.

van den Bosch, J.F., de Graaf, F., and MacLaren, D.M. (1979). Virulence of *Escherichia coli* in experimental hematogenous pyelonephritis in mice. *Infection and Immunity*, **25,** 68–74.

van den Bosch, J.F., Emody, L., and Ketyi, I. (1982). Virulence of haemolytic strains of

Escherichia coli in various animal models. *FEMS Microbiology Letters*, **13,** 427–430.

van den Bosch, J.F., Postma, P., de Graaf, F., and Maclaren, D.M. (1981). *Haemolysis* by urinary *Escherichia coli* and virulence in mice. *Journal of Medical Microbiology*, **14,** 321–331.

van Snick, J.L., Masson, P.L., and Heremans, J.F. (1974). The involvement of lactoferrin in the hyposideremia of acute inflammation. *Journal of Experimental Medicine*, **140,** 1068–1084.

van Tiel-Menkveld, C.J., Mentjox-Vervuust, J.M., Oudega, B., and de Graaf, F.K. (1982). Siderophore production by *Enterobacter cloacae* and a common receptor protein for the uptake of aerobactin and cloacin DF13. *Journal of Bacteriology*, **150,** 490–497.

Waalwijk, C., MacLaren, D.M., and de Graaf, J. (1983). *In vivo* function of hemolysin in the nephropathogenicity of *Escherichia coli*. *Infection and Immunity*, **42,** 245–249.

Waalwijk, C., van den Bosch, J.F., MacLaren, D.M., and de Graaf, J. (1982). Hemolysin plasmid coding for the virulence of a nephropathogenic *Escherichia coli* strain. *Infection and Immunity*, **35,** 32–37.

Wagegg, W., and Braun, V. (1981). Ferric citrate transport in *Escherichia coli* requires outer membrane receptor protein FecA. *Journal of Bacteriology*, **145,** 156–163.

Wake, A., Misawa, M., and Matsui, A. (1975). Siderochrome production by *Yersiniae pestis* and its relation to virulence. *Infection and Immunity*, **12,** 1211–1213.

Warner, P.J., Williams, P.H., Bindereif, A., and Neilands, J.B. (1981). ColV plasmid-specified aerobactin synthesis by invasive strains of *Escherichia coli*. *Infection and Immunity*, **33,** 540–545.

Welch, R.A., Dellinger, E.P., Minshew, B., and Falkow, S. (1981). Hemolysin contributes to virulence of extraintestinal *Escherichia coli* infections. *Nature*, **294**, 665–667.

Welch, R.A., and Falkow, S. (1984). Characterization of *Escherichia coli* haemolysins conferring quantitiative differences in virulence. *Infection and Immunity*, **43,** 156–160.

Wendenbaum, S., Demange, P., Dell, A., Meyer, J.M., and Abdallah, M.A. (1983). The structure of pyoverdine Pa, the siderophore of *Pseudomonas aeruginosa*. *Tetrahedron Letters*, **24,** 4877–4880.

West, S.E.H., and Sparling, P.F. (1985). Response of *Neisseria gonorrhoeae* to iron limitation: alteration in expression of membrane proteins without apparent siderophore production. *Infection and Immunity*, **47,** 388–394.

Wettstein, F.O., and Stent, G.S. (1968). Physiologically induced changes in the property of phenylalanine tRNA in *Escherichia coli*. *Journal of Molecular Biology*, **38,** 25–40.

White, D.C., and Granick, S. (1963). Hemin biosynthesis in *Haemophilus*. *Journal of Bacteriology*, **85,** 842–850.

Williams, P.H. (1979a). Novel iron uptake system specified by ColV plasmids: an important component in the virulence of invasive strains of *Escherichia coli*. *Infection and Immunity*, **26,** 925–932.

Williams, P.H. (1979b). Determination of the molecular weight of *Escherichia coli* α-haemolysin. *FEMS Microbiology Letters*, **5,** 21–24.

Williams, P., and Brown, M.R.W. (1986). Influence of iron restriction on growth and the expression of outer membrane proteins by *Haemophilus influenzae* and *H.parainfluenzae*. *FEMS Microbiology Letters*, **33,** 153–157.

Williams, P., Brown, M.R.W., and Lambert, P.A. (1984). Effect of iron deprivation on the production of siderophores and outer membrane proteins in *Klebsiella aerogenes*. *Journal of General Microbiology*, **130,** 2357–2365.

Williams, P.H., and Warner, P.J. (1980). ColV-plasmid-mediated, Colicin V-independent iron uptake system of invasive strains of *Escherichia coli*. *Infection and Immunity*, **29,** 411–416.

Woodrow, G.C., Langman, L., Young, I.G., and Gibson, F. (1978). Mutations affecting the citrate-dependent iron uptake systems in *Escherichia coli*. *Journal of Bacteriology*, **133,** 1524–1526.

Worsham, P.L., and Konisky, J. (1985). Locus affecting regulation of the Colicin I receptor by iron. *Journal of Bacteriology*, **161,** 428–431.

Wright, A.C., Simpson, L.M., and Oliver, J.D. (1981). Role of iron in the pathogenesis of *Vibrio vulnificus* infection. *Infection and Immunity*, **34,** 503–507.

Yancey, R.J., Breeding, S.A.L., and Lankford, C.E. (1979). Enterochelin (enterobactin): virulence factor for *Salmonella typhimurium*. *Infection and Immunity*, **24**, 174–180.

Yancey, R.J., and Finkelstein, R.A. (1981a). Siderophore production by pathogenic *Neisseria* spp. *Infection and Immunity*, **32,** 600–608.

Yancey, R.J., and Finkelstein, R.A. (1981b). Assimilation of iron by pathogenic *Neisseria* spp. *Infection and Immunity*, **32,** 592–599.

Yang, C., and Leong, J. (1984). Structure of pseudobactin 7 SR1, a siderophore from a plant-deleterious *Pseudomonas*. *Biochemistry*, **23,** 3534–3540.

Yanofsky, C. (1981). Attenuation in the control of expression of bacterial operons. *Nature*, **289,** 751–758.

Yarus, M. (1982). Translational efficiency of transfer RNAs: uses of an extended anticodon. *Science*, **218,** 646–652.

Young, L.S. (1980). The role of exotoxins in the pathogenesis of *Pseudomonas aeruginosa* infection. *Journal of Infectious Diseases*, **142**, 626–630.

Zapolski, E.J., and Princiotto, J.V. (1976). Failure of rabbit reticulocytes to incorporate conalbumin or lactoferrin iron. *Biochimica et Biophysica Acta*, **421,** 80–86.

Zimmermann, L., Hantke, K., and Braun, V. (1984). Exogenous induction of the iron dicitrate transport system of *Escherichia coli* K12. *Journal of Bacteriology*, **159,** 271–277.

Iron and Infection
Edited by J.J. Bullen and E. Griffiths

Chapter 4
Bacterial iron metabolism, plasmids and other virulence factors

J. H. CROSA
Department of Microbiology and Immunology,
School of Medicine,
The Oregon Health Sciences University,
3181 SW Sam Jackson Park Road,
Portland, Oregon 97201, USA

1. INTRODUCTION

It must now be very clear to the reader that the availability of iron plays an important role in the ability of bacteria to cause infections. Consequently, it may not come as a surprise that bacterial uptake of the vertebrate host iron, which is largely bound to high affinity iron-binding proteins, becomes an important virulence factor, heavily dependent on the presence of active iron-transport systems.

Chromosome-mediated iron-transport systems have been discussed in the previous chapter and evidence presented for their possible contribution to bacterial pathogenicity. Analysis of the subject of siderophores, iron transport and bacterial virulence can also be found in several published reviews (Bullen, 1981; Bullen, Rogers and Griffiths 1978; Crosa, 1984; Griffiths 1983a, 1983b; Neilands, 1981; Weinberg, 1978).

Dedicated to Luis F. Leloir on the occasion of his 80th birthday, 6th September 1986.

In this chapter, I shall discuss more specialized iron transport or iron-regulated extrachromosomal systems which are intimately associated with the ability of bacteria to cause disease. I shall begin by briefly reviewing the relationship of plasmids and bacterial virulence, then focus on the plasmid-mediated iron-transport systems present in invasive strains of *Vibrio anguillarum* and *Escherichia coli* and conclude with the analysis of one other virulence factor which is also regulated by the iron concentration of the cells, namely, the production of *Corynebacterium* β-phage-mediated diphtheria toxin. I hope that by the end the reader will realize that there are indeed some common features in this apparent smorgasbord of subjects.

2. PLASMIDS AND VIRULENCE

With the advent of new methods for detection, it is now clear that many species of bacteria possess plasmids. There are many functions that can be associated with the presence of particular classes of plasmids, ranging from antibiotic resistance to the ability to degrade or utilize organic compounds. A number of plasmids have been found to carry genetic determinants encoding bacterial virulence determinants (Elwell and Shipley, 1980). Among the most well known are plasmids coding for enterotoxin production and adhesive factors in *E. coli* strains associated with diarrhoeal diseases (Gyles, Palchaudhuri and Maas, 1977; Gyles, So and Falkow, 1974; Smith and Halls, 1986; Smith and Linggood, 1972; So, Crosa and Falkow, 1975). In order to achieve full pathogenic potential, *E. coli* strains must be able to colonize the small intestine effectively. Plasmid-mediated, adhesive, proteinaceous pili are, thus required for the bacteria to adhere to the wall of the vertebrate small intestine. At this site the organisms synthesize enterotoxins which act on the adenylate cyclase system of the epithelial cells and stimulate the production of fluids, which results in diarrhoea (Evans *et al.*, 1975; Ørskov and Ørskov, 1966; Smith and Lingood, 1972). Plasmids have also been shown to be associated with many other virulence mechanisms in *E. coli*, such as haemolysin production and resistance to the bactericidal activity of non-immune serum of the host (Berger *et al.*, 1982; Minshew *et al.*, 1978; Moll, Manning and Timmis 1980; Smith and Halls, 1967; Taylor and Hughes, 1978; van den Bosch *et al.*, 1981; Welch *et al.*, 1981). Plasmids are necessary for the virulence of *Shigella* strains (Hale *et al.*, 1983; Kopecko, Washington and Formal, 1980; Sansonetti, David and Toucas, 1980; Sansonetti *et al.*, 1983; Sansonetti, Kopecko and Formal, 1981, 1982) and are associated with invasiveness in both *Yersinia pestis* and *Y. enterocolitica* (Gemski, Lazere and Casey, 1980; Portnoy, Moseley and Falkow, 1981; Portnoy and Falkow, 1981; Zink *et al.*, 1980).

Specific plasmid classes have been linked with the ability of two types of bacteria to cause septicaemic diseases. *E. coli* strains causing bacteraemias in humans and domestic animals harbour ColV plasmids, which code for the antibacterial protein colicin V. Highly virulent strains of the marine fish pathogen *Vibrio anguillarum*, which cause a disease characterized as a haemorrhagic septicaemia, carry the pJMl plasmid. Elimination of either of these two plasmids from their bacterial hosts invariably reduces their pathogenicity for experimental animals. In the case of the ColV plasmids, virulence could be regained simply by reintroducing the plasmids into the *E. coli* strains. However, the pJMl plasmid could not be reintroduced into the avirulent *V. anguillarum* strains although, as will be discussed later, cloned pJM1 DNA segments carrying the iron-uptake region could be, whereupon the organism regained virulence.

2.1 The *V. anguillarum* pJM1 plasmids

Vibriosis caused by infection with *V. anguillarum* is one of the most devastating diseases affecting salmonids and other species of fish important in aquaculture (Canestrini, 1893; Cisar and Fryer, 1969; Evelyn, 1971; Rucker, Earp and Ordal, 1953). However, the actual molecular nature of the virulence factors present in *V. anguillarum* is poorly understood. The sequence of events in an episode of vibriosis is similar to that found in invasive septicaemic diseases in man. Experimental infections caused by avirulent strains of *V. anguillarum* do not proceed beyond initial stages, but if the infecting strain is virulent, the disease progresses with the appearance of the characteristic bloody lesions in the musculature and generalized septicaemia. Death is a consequence of hypoxia and dysfunction of various organs (Harbell, Hodgins and Schiewe 1979; Ransom *et al.*, 1984). Clearly, the virulent strains of *V. anguillarum* have developed the ability to evade or overcome both the specific and non-specific defence mechanisms of the fish.

Many of the virulent strains isolated from epizootics harbour a specific plasmid class of 65 kb, which is absent from avirulent strains (Crosa, Schiewe and Falkow, 1977). Curing experiments, where the plasmid is experimentally eliminated from the cell, demonstrated that the specific plasmid, designated pJMl, carries genetic determinants for an important component of the virulence complex of *V. anguillarum* (Crosa, Hodges and Schiewe, 1980). Recently, I showed that this plasmid specifies a very efficient iron-sequestering system which enables the virulent, plasmid-carrying strains of *V. anguillarum* to survive and grow *in vitro* under conditions of limited iron availability. This occurrred in culture media containing high concentrations of the iron-binding protein transferrin or other non-assimilable iron chelators (Crosa, 1979, 1980). Under the same conditions, avirulent cured strains (plasmidless) were completely inhibited. Experimental infections of fish with a mixture of a plasmid-carrying virulent strain and its cured isogenic avirulent derivative, showed that there was a selective advantage for the plasmid-carrying virulent strain. However, when iron was included in the inoculum, this advantage was greatly diminished and the plasmidless, avirulent strains grew at a rate similar to the virulent strains carrying the pJM1 plasmid (Crosa, 1979, 1980).

The efficient uptake of iron by plasmid-carrying strains of *V. anguillarum* is associated with the induction of two new outer membrane proteins. At least one of them, OM2, an 86KDa protein, is induced only when the virulence plasmid pJMl is present (Crosa and Hodges, 1981). This outer membrane protein may play a role as a receptor for a putative plasmid-mediated siderophore. Further characterization of the pJMl plasmid-mediated iron-uptake system was achieved by using transposition sequences to generate iron-uptake deficient mutants by insertional inactivation of the pJMl iron-transport region. Transportation sequences are DNA segments that can insert into several sites in a genome and are thus excellent tools to introuduce specific mutations in the genome under study (Shapiro, 1983). These sequences behave formally like insertion (IS) elements but contain additional genes unrelated to insertion functions; they are generally larger than 2 kb. A number of transposition sequences are known that could be used as mutagenic agents, as long as the donor genome could be transferred to the bacterium where the genome to be mutated resides. The R plasmid (resistance plasmid) RP4, which carries the transposition sequences Tn*1* (Hedges and Jacob, 1974) coding for β-lactamase resistance, can be easily conjugated to *V. anguillarum* (Crosa, Hodges and Schiewe, 1980). Thus, by using this R plasmid as a donor of Tn*1*, a series of mutants of *V. anguillarum* were generated which were either proficient or deficient in iron uptake (Crosa, Walter and Potter, 1983a, 1983b; Walter, Potter and Crosa, 1983). In these derivatives the transposition sequence Tn*l* was inserted at different sites on the pJM1 plasmid (shown in Fig. 1). In some cases, the inserted Tn*1* sequence generated deletions beginning in regions adjacent to the site of insertion. Mutants obtained by this method were subdivided into two classes. One class consisted of those mutants which were able to be cross fed only by supernatants from wild-type strains. It is likely that members of this class were affected in plasmid genes responsible for the biosynthesis or activity of a putative plasmid-mediated siderophore, but still possessed an active gene for the biosynthesis of the membrane receptor. This mutant class was designated sid$^-$rec$^+$. The other class consisted of those derivatives which could not be cross-fed by supernatants from wild-type strains; nor could they themselves cross-feed members of the sid$^-$rec$^-$ class. Thus, these derivatives not only had a lesion in genes involved in siderophore biosynthesis or activity, but also in DNA regions associated with the biosynthesis or activity of a membrane receptor for the iron-siderophore complex.

Restriction endonuclease cleavage analysis of the pJMl plasmids carrying the Tn*l* insertions permitted the iron-uptake genes on plasmid pJM1 to be located to a region within 20–25 kb (Fig. 1). Tn*l* insertions that affected the production of the siderophore did not affect receptor activity, nor the biosynthesis of the OM2 protein (Walter, Potter and Crosa, 1983). In the case of the strain

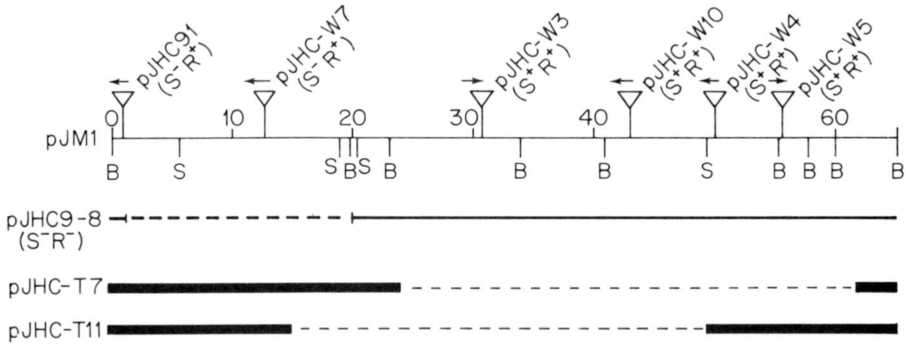

Figure 1 Physical location of pJMl iron-uptake regions cloned in the cosmid vector pVK102

Vibrio anguillarum stains containing Tn*1* derivatives were classified as iron proficient or deficient by a cross-feeding assay. Iron-uptake proficient derivatives are indicated as S^+R^+: production of siderophore (S) and receptor (R); iron-uptake deficient derivatives are classified depending on whether the Tn*1* insertions or deletions affected the genes associated with the production or activity of either siderophore (S^-R^+) or receptor (S^+R^-) or both (S^-R^-). The dashed lines correspond to pJMl DNA regions that were deleted (i.e. in pJHC9-8) or that were not included in the cloned DNA (i.e. in pJHC-T7 and pJHC-T11). Thicker lines represent the pJMl DNA cloned in pVK102

The symbol Y shows the sites of Tn*1* insertions on the pJM1 genome. The arrows over this symbol indicate the orientation of the Tn*1* sequence with respect to β-lactamase gene transcription. The cleavage sites for the restriction endonucleases *Bam*H1(B) and *Sal*I(S) are also shown. The numbers correspond to the coordinates in kb in this linearized map of the pJMl plasmid

harbouring the pJM1 deletion derivative pJHC9-8 (Fig. 1), both siderophore and receptor activity were affected, and the OM2 protein was no longer induced under conditions of iron limitation. Instead, a 69KDa protein was synthesized (Walter, Potter and Crosa, 1983). This protein could possibly be either a truncated OM2 protein or a fusion product generated by Tn*1*-mediated deletion of pJMl DNA. These results support the hypothesis that OM2 could be the plasmid-mediated receptor. That the OM2 protein is encoded on the pJM1 plasmid was recently demonstrated by transferring to *E. coli*, a recombinant clone obtained from pJM1 that actually endowed *E. coli* with the ability to synthesize OM2 (Actis, Potter and Crosa, 1985). Immunological and radioiodination experiments have also shown that the OM2 protein is exposed on the outside of the bacterial outer membrane (Actis, Potter and Crosa, 1985). These results are consistent with its possible role as a receptor for complexes of iron with a plasmid-mediated siderophore. Recently, by using transposition mutagenesis and complementation analysis it was demonstrated that the OM2 protein is essential for the pJM1-mediated iron-uptake process. However, another pJM1-mediated component, in addition to OM2, is required for the transport of iron into the cell cytosol (Actis, Tolmasky and Crosa, submitted for publication).

To date, the production of the putative plasmid-mediated siderophore has been demonstrated *in vitro* only by the cross-feeding experiments with the sid$^-$rec$^+$ Tn*1* insertion mutants. The preliminary characterization of this plasmid-mediated siderophore, named anguibactin, indicates that it is a catecholate with a molecular weight of 348, but it is not related to enterochelin (Actis *et al.*, 1986). Recent experiments have indicated that the plasmid-mediated siderophore is also produced *in vivo* during infection. Mixtures of the wild-type strain carrying an intact pJM1 plasmid, and thus possessing a sid$^+$rec$^+$ phenotype with either the sid$^-$rec$^+$ strain carrying the Tn*1* insertion plasmid pJHC91 or the sid$^-$rec$^-$ derivative carrying the deletion plasmid, pJHC 9-8, were injected into fish. After sufficient time to allow for bacterial proliferation, but before death occurred, the fish were killed and samples taken from different organs and blood, were inoculated onto appropriate culture media. By using differential antibiotic resistance markers the proportion of wild type to either of the two mutants in the respective recovered samples was assessed. Table 1 shows that in the case of those fish injected with the mixture of the wild-type 775(pJMl) strain and the sid$^-$rec$^-$ derivative, the wild-type strain is the only bacterial type recovered from blood and kidney after infection. Conversely, the recovery ratios of bacteria, obtained by sampling the blood and kidney of fish infected with the mixture of the wild-type strain and the sid$^-$rec$^+$ derivative, indicated that a higher proportion of the sid$^-$rec$^+$ mutant was recovered compared with that injected. These results strongly suggest that the plasmid-mediated siderophore is produced *in vivo* by the wild-type strain allowing for the proliferation of the sid$^-$rec$^+$ strain. Since only those mutants having an active receptor could be recovered after infection, the experiments described here also suggest that the siderophore is not only being synthesized *in vivo* but is also being excreted (Wolf and Crosa, 1986). With other bacteria such as *Neisseria gonorrhoeae* and *N. meningitidis*, the bacterial surface appears to

Table 1 Infection experiments with mutants of *V. anguillarum* in fish: cross-feeding of sid$^-$rec$^+$ mutants

Mixture injected	Strains in mixture	Percentage in mixture	Phenotype	Recovery (%)	
				Blood	Kidney
I	775(pJM1)	2	sid$^+$ rec$^+$	17	19
	775::Tr*1*-5(pJHC-91)	98	sid$^-$ rec$^+$	83	81
II	775(pJM1)	4	sid$^+$ rec$^+$	100	100
	775::Tr*1*-6(pJHC9-8)	96	sid$^-$ rec$^-$	0	0

interact directly with iron bound to the high affinity iron-binding proteins lactoferrin or transferrin (Mickelsen and Sparling, 1981; Mickelsen, Blackman and Sparling, 1982; Norrod and Williams, 1978). Incorporation of iron into the bacterial cell appears to occur without the involvement of a siderophore (see Chapter 3). It is clear that this is not the case in *V. anguillarum* where a plasmid-mediated siderophore is produced in a diffusible form. Furthermore, these results show that this siderophore is an important virulence factor.

In order to characterize further the pJMl plasmid-mediated iron-transport system in *V. anguillarum*, it was necessary to clone molecularly specific regions of the pJM1 plasmid. The pJM1 plasmid-mediated iron-uptake system is not expressed in *E. coli*, as assessed by transformation of plasmid DNA obtained from iron-proficient Tn*1* insertion derivatives. Since the R plasmid RP4 can be conjugated from *E. coli* to *V. anguillarum*, it seemed logical to use a cloning vector derived from RP4 to initiate the genetic dissection of the pJMl iron-uptake system. The cosmid vector pVK102 was chosen for this purpose. This plasmid is a small non-self-transmissible cosmid cloning vector, constructed by Knauff and Nester (1982) by ligating drug resistance genes and lambda cohesive ends into the plasmid pRK290, originally constructed by Ditta *et al* (1980) from the R plasmid RK2, which is identical to RP4. The pVK102 cosmid vector can be transferred from *E. coli* to *V. anguillarum* (Tolmasky and Crosa, 1984) by mobilization with the transfer factor pRK2013, also described by Ditta *et al.* (1980). A cosmid is a vector which combines some of the useful features of phage and plasmid vectors. Cosmids are particularly useful for cloning long DNA molecules, thus increasing the probability of cloning complex genes or operons. Clones of restriction endonuclease partial digests of pJMl DNA in pVK102 were transduced to *E. coli*, after *in vitro* packaging, and then mobilized to suitable *V. anguillarum* recipients, by using a triparental mating with strains containing the mobilising plasmid pRK2013. An *E. coli* strain harbouring the pJMl DNA clones was mixed with *E. coli* (pRK2013) and the appropriate *V. anguillarum* recipients. By using this methodology, Tolmasky and Crosa (1984) transferrred several cosmids containing DNA inserts with part, or all, of the pJM1 iron-uptake region, as mapped by Tn*1* insertion mutagenesis, to various *V. anguillarum* strains to study their expression. Two cosmids, pJHC-T7 and pJHC-T11, were analysed in detail. The location of the cloned regions is included in Fig 1. Exconjugants obtained by transfer of the pJHC-T7 cosmid to the iron-uptake deficient derivative 775::Tn*1*(pJHC-91), which is sid$^-$rec$^+$, were now able to grow under conditions of iron limitation to the same extent as the wild-type 775(pJMl) strain (Table 2) and produce siderophore (Fig.2 a). These results suggested that the recombinant cosmid pJHC-T7 carried the pJMl genes necessary for siderophore biosynthesis. Mobilization of pJHC-T11 to the plasmidless *V. anguillarum* strain generated derivatives that, although not producing siderophore, could be cross-fed with supernatants from the strains carrying the cloned or wild-type

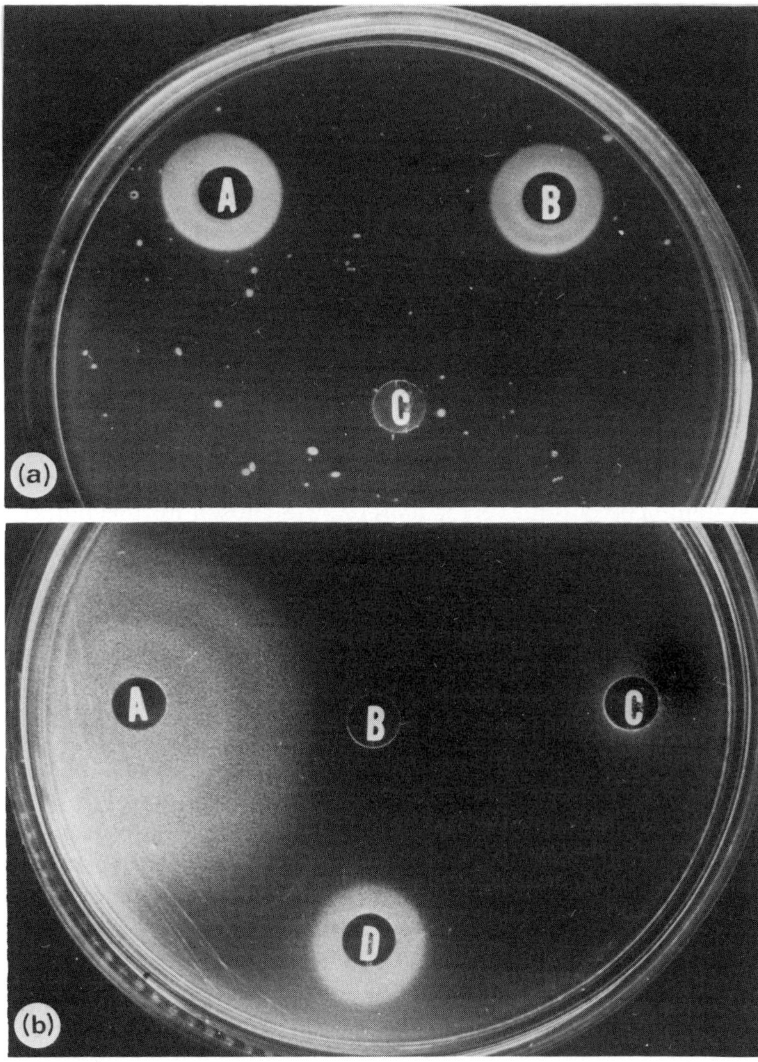

Figure 2 Siderophore activity of supernatants and cell homogenates of *V.anguillarum* strains carrying the clone pJHC-T7.

Strains were cultured in M9 minimal medium during 48 hours at 24°C. (a) Supernatants. After centrifugation of the cells, the supernatants were filter sterilized. 10 μl samples were then loaded onto sterile filter paper disks placed on the surface of an M9 minimal medium 0.7% agarose plate containing 20 μ*M* EDDA that had been seeded with approximately 10^8 cells of an overnight culture of the indicator strain *V.anguillarum* 775::Tn*1*-5(pJHC-91). Supernatant from *V.anguillarum* strains: A, 775::Tn*1*-5(pJHC-91, pJHC-T7); B, 775(pJMl); C, 775::Tn*1*-5(pJHC-91). (b) Cell homogenates. I ml cultures, grown as described in (a), were centrifuged, the cells resuspended in 0.5 ml of M9 minimal medium and sonically treated. 10 μl of the homogenates were loaded onto filter disks placed on the surface of minimal agarose plates as specified in (a). Homogenates from *V.anguillarum* strains: A, 775(pJMl); B, H775-3; C, H775-3B(pJHC-T7). Disk D is a control of sonically treated supernatant from 775(pJM1)

Table 2 Properties of *Vibrio anguillarum* strains harbouring recombinant plasmids

V. anguillarum strain	*Plasmid*	*Siderophore* production[a]	*Presence of* receptor[b]	*Growth in* 10 μM EDDA[c]	*Virulence*[d]
775	pJM1	+	+	+	High
775-3	—	−	−	−	Low
775-3C	pJHC-T11	−	+	−	NT
775-Tn*1*::5	pJHC91	−	+	−	Low
775-Tn*1*::5A	pJHC91 and pJHC-T7	+	+	+	High
775-Tn*1*::5C	pJHC91 and pJHC-T11	−	+	−	Low

[a,b] Siderophore production and presence of receptor were determined as previously described (Walter, Potter and Crosa, 1983).
[c] Growth in minimal medium containing the non-assimilable iron chelator EDDA (ethylenediamine-di (*o*-hydroxyphenyl acetic acid) was measured by reading OD_{590} at several time points.
[d] Virulence was measured by determination of LD_{50} values (mean lethal doses) as previously described (Crosa, 1980). High virulence correspond to LD_{50} values of about 10^2–10^3 bacterial cells whereas LD_{50} values of about 10^8 cells are classified as low virulence. NT = not tested.

siderophore genes (Table 2). Hence, the recombinant cosmid pJHC-T11 must carry genes for iron transport. Strains carrying the cosmid clone, when grown under iron-restriction conditions, synthesized an outer membrane protein of the same molecular weight as the OM2 protein (Fig.3 and Tolmasky and Crosa, 1984). Exconjugants obtained by transfer of the cosmid pJHC-T7 to a plasmid-less derivative could also be cross-fed with supernatants from strains carrying wild-type siderophore genes, suggesting that pJHC-T7 must also contain genes for iron transport in addition to the genetic information for siderophore production. Cells harbouring both pJHC-T7 and pJHC-91 (sid^-rec^+) became iron-uptake proficient and produced siderophore (Table 2 and Fig. 2a); however, the exconjugants obtained by transfer of pJHC-T7 into the plasmid-less strain of *V. anguillarum* produced only barely detectable levels of siderophore activity (Fig. 2b and Tolmasky and Crosa, 1984). Figure 2(b) also shows the results obtained with homogenates of *V. anguillarum* cells. The siderophore activities in supernatants of the wild-type *V. anguillarum* and the strain carrying only pJHC-T7 were similar to those obtained with the homogenates. These results suggested that another product encoded by pJHC-91 but absent from the cloned DNA may be required for efficient synthesis of siderophore activity. One explanation for these results is the existence of a *trans*-acting factor(s) that regulates the transcription or translation, or both, of the siderophore genes. This genetic information must be encoded on a plasmid pJM1 DNA region different from the regions cloned. An alternative explanation for

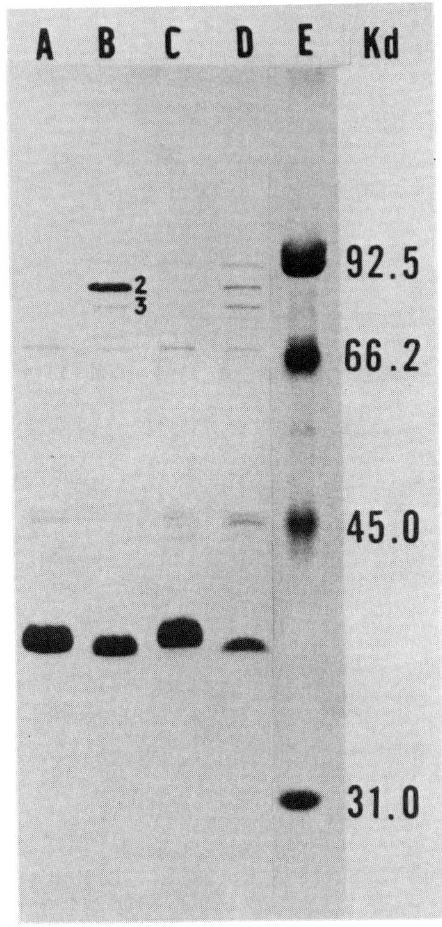

Figure 3 Sodium dodecyl sulphate-polyacrylamide gel electrophoresis analysis of outer membrane proteins of *V. anguillarum* strains harbouring recombinant plasmids.

Vibrio anguillarum cells were cultured under either iron-sufficient or iron-limiting conditions. Lanes A and C: outer membranes obtained from cultures growing under iron sufficient conditions; lanes B and D: outer membrane proteins obtained from cultures growing under iron limitation conditions; lanes A and B, 775 (pJMl); lanes C and D, H775-3 (pJHC-T7); lane E: molecular weight standards

this finding, that the clones are deficient in genetic information for export of the siderophore outside the cell, was ruled out by determining the amount of siderophore present in bacterial sonicates (Tolmasky and Crosa, 1984).

However, other models could explain these results. For instance, the clones may lack one or more of the genes encoding enzymes of the siderophore biosynthetic pathway, resulting in a siderophore which cannot form stable complexes with iron, or the complexes once formed cannot interact properly with the bacterial cell receptor complex. Results obtained with *V. anguillarum* strains carrying the plasmid pJHC9-8, which has an extensive deletion of the pJMl iron-uptake region, suggest that this is not the case. The pJHC-T7 recombinant clone, when introduced into this strain, yields iron-uptake proficient derivatives despite the lack of most of the pJMl iron uptake region on the indigenous plasmid pJHC9-8 (Tolmasky and Crosa, 1984). Determination of whether the *trans*-acting factor(s) is either a regulatory substance or a biosynthetic enzyme necessary for the generation of a complete siderophore molecule will require detailed knowledge of the structure of the pJM1-mediated siderophore. Experiments to determine its molecular nature are currently under way in our laboratory. Furthermore, a pJM1 region containing the *trans*-acting factor genes was recently cloned (Tolmasky and Crosa, submitted for publication). Possession of this clone will undoubtedly help in the elucidation of the role played by the *trans*-acting factor(s) in the pJMl-mediated iron-uptake process.

An important result, also shown in Table 2, is that the sid$^+$rec$^+$ derivative carrying both the pJHC91 plasmid as well as the pJHC-T7 recombinant cosmid not only grew well under conditions of iron limitation but had also acquired virulence, unlike the original iron-uptake deficient recipient harbouring only the pJHC91 plasmid, or exconjugants carrying the recombinant cosmid pJHC-T11, in addition to pJHC91.

The restoration of virulence by introduction of cloned pJMl iron–siderophore regions into an avirulent strain clearly demonstrates the intimate relationship which exists between the presence of an active pJM1 plasmid-mediated iron-uptake system, and the high virulence phenotype of *V. anguillarum*.

2.2 The *E. coli* ColV plasmids

Certain invasive strains of *E. coli* responsible for generalized infections in livestock and humans, harbour plasmids which enhance their virulence (Smith, 1974; Smith and Huggins, 1976). Although these plasmids are rather heterogeneous in size and in general restriction endonuclease patterns, they do have two properties in common, in addition to their ability to enhance virulence. They are usually members of the FI incompatibility group and they also possess genetic determinants for the synthesis of the small antibacterial protein colicin V (Kahn and Helinski, 1964; Nagel de Zwaig and Anton, 1964). The elimination of these ColV plasmids invariably reduces the pathogenicity of the *E. coli* strains for experimental animals and this virulence can be restored simply by reintroducing the plasmid into the cured strains (Smith, 1974; Smith and Huggins, 1976). A considerable amount of work has been carried out to determine the nature of the virulence determinants carried by the ColV plasmids (Frederick, 1951; Frederick and Joiris, 1950; Gratia 1925; Smith, 1974; Smith and Huggins, 1976). Because it is frequently present in clinical strains, colicin V itself was originally considered to be a potential candidate for the virulence factor encoded by the ColV plasmids. However, it is now clear that there is no correlation between the production of colicin V and virulence. Transposition mutagenesis of a ColV plasmid showed that insertions inactivating colicin V production did not affect the virulence phenotype of the *E. coli* strain harbouring the now-mutated plasmid (Quackenbush and Falkow, 1979).

At least three genetic determinants have been reported to be associated with virulence in different ColV plasmids. One of these virulence factors is associated with the ability of *E. coli* to withstand the bactericidal activity of non-immune serum. The plasmid pColV, I-K94 which also codes for the bacteriocin colicin I (Binns, Davies and Hardy, 1979; Kahn and Helinski, 1964; Nagel de Zwaig and Anton, 1964; Smith, 1974) is an example of this type of ColV plasmids. Cloning experiments permitted the localization of the genetic determinants for the phenotype, expressed as an increased survival in serum (*iss*), to within a 5.3 kb sequence of the pColV,I-K94 plasmid DNA (Binns, Davies and Hardy, 1979).

Another phenotype present in certain ColV plasmids which may enhance bacterial virulence is related to bacterial adhesion. Strains harbouring these ColV plasmids adhere *in vitro* to mouse intestinal epithelium in two- to three-fold greater numbers than isogenic strains without the plasmid. By using male-specific phages, pili could be demonstrated by electron microscopy only in those strains harbouring these ColV plasmids (Clancy and Savage, 1981).

The third potential virulence factor associated with ColV plasmids is connected with the assimilation of iron. Bacteria possessing these plasmids can relieve the effect of iron limitation imposed on *E. coli* strains deficient in the biosynthesis of enterobactin. The plasmids pColV-K30, pRJ100 and pColV-K311 are examples of ColV plasmids possessing iron-uptake genes (Braun, 1981; Stuart, Greenwood and Luke, 1980; Williams, 1979). Experimental infections of mice, carried out with mixtures of *E. coli* strains harbouring the pColV-K30 plasmid and its isogenic plasmidless derivative, were also carried out. As was the case for the pJMl plasmid in *V. anguillarum*, possession of the pColV-K30 plasmid conferred selective advantage only if iron was not included in the inoculum (Williams and George, 1979).

Identification of important plasmid-mediated components of the pColV-K30 iron-uptake system was carried out by chemical mutagenesis (Williams and Warner, 1980). The pColV-K30 plasmid can relieve the effects of iron restriction imposed on enterochelin-deficient strains of *E. coli*. Mutants of an enterochelin defective strain of *E. coli* carrying the pColV-K30 plasmid which were defective in iron uptake due to mutations of the pColV-K30 plasmid were isolated and indentified as being considerably attenuated in their pathogenicity. Cross-feeding experiments between the different plasmid iron-uptake deficient mutants identified two plasmid-mediated components: a diffusible iron-chelating compound and a non-diffusible membrane associated substance. The two components were sufficient for the efficient transport of iron into the bacterial cell in the absence of an operating enterochelin system. Recent studies have clarified the nature of these two components. The non-diffusible component was characterized as an outer membrane receptor for the iron–siderophore complex and identified as a 74KDa protein (Bindereiff, Braun and Hantke, 1982; Grewal, Warner and Williams 1982; van Tiel-Menkveld *et al.*, 1981, 1982). This protein receptor also serves as the binding site for the bacteriocin cloacin produced by *Enterobacter cloacae* DF13 (Oudega *et al.*, 1979; van Tiel-Menkveld *et al.*, 1981, 1982). The soluble iron-chelating compound produced by strains carrying this type of ColV plasmids was shown to be a siderophore of the hydroxamate type (Stuart, Greenwood and Luke, 1980). Hydroxamate-type siderophores were also detected in clinical strains of *E. coli* carrying ColV plasmids and associated with septicaemia in man and animals (Stuart, Greenwood and Luke, 1982). The hydroxamate siderophore mediated by the pColV-K30 plasmid was later indentified as aerobactin (Braun, 1981; Warner *et al.*, 1981). The siderophore aerobactin was orginally isolated from the supernatants of iron-limited cultures of *Aerobacter aerogenes* (Gibson and McGrath, 1969). Ferric aerobactin has an association constant many orders of magnitude below that of enterochelin, but it is nonetheless equipped with structural properties that may enhance its ability to remove iron from transferrin (Konopka, Bindereif and Neilands, 1982). Furthermore, in contrast to enterochelin, aerobactin is not destroyed after delivery of iron to the cell and thus it may be recycled (Braun, Brazel-Faisst and Schneider, 1984). As discussed in Chapter 3 these characteristics, as well as the presence of antibodies against enterochelin (Moore and Earhardt 1981) and the enterochelin receptor in vertebrate serum (Griffiths, 1983a, and 1983b), may contribute to the status of aerobactin as a virulence determinant in *E. coli* which also produce enterochelin.

In this regard, it was recently reported that growth of *E. coli* strains in calf serum was greatly enhanced if they harboured ColV plasmids specifying the aerobactin system (Braun, Brazel-Faisst and Schneider, 1984).

In addition to those functions mediated by the ColV plasmid several chromosomal genes in *E. coli* also appear to be necessary for aerobactin utilization (Braun *et al.*, 1982, 1983). For instance, the *ton*A (*fhu*A), *fhu*B, *fhu*C, *fhu*D and *exb*B genes are required for ferric aerobactin uptake. Some of these genes are also required for uptake of ferrichrome and other hydroxamate siderophores (Neilands, 1981, 1982). By insertion of phage Mu d1 (Ap *lac*) into the plasmid pColV-K311, Braun and Burkhardt (1982) placed the expression of the β-galactosidase gene under the control of the iron in the cells. In *fur* mutants, which have impaired regulation of all iron-supply systems (Hantke, 1981), β-galactosidase was synthesized independently of the cellular iron concentration, suggesting that is was no longer regulated by the iron supply (Braun and Burkhardt, 1982). Thus, at least in the pColV-K311 plasmid, there is an iron-controlled promoter which is subject to regulation by one other chromosomal determinant, the *fur* gene, although the nature of this regulation is still unclear (see Chapter 3).

In more recent work, Braun and colleagues (1983) used insertion mutagenesis with both the Mu dl (Ap *lac*) and the transposition sequence Tn*5* to show that the aerobactin genes in the plasmid pColV-K311 are transcribed from a locus that determines not only aerobactin synthesis itself but also encodes the ferric aerobactin outer membrane receptor.

Different regions of the aerobactin-mediated iron-uptake system present in the pColV-K30 plasmid have been cloned into multicopy vectors (Bindereiff and Neilands, 1983; Krone *et al.*, 1983a, 1983b). Figure 4 shows the cloned regions, the products synthesized and the designation of the recombinant plasmids. The plasmid pABN1 is one of such recombinant derivatives containing the iron-uptake region in a cloned 16.3 kb Hind III fragment of pColV-K30. Enterochelin-deficient strains of *E. coli* harbouring pABN1 could grow under conditions of iron limitation when producing the siderophore aerobactin. The aerobactin receptor was also synthesized as assessed by the cloacin sensitivity of the strain harbouring the recombinant plasmid and by the production of the 74KDa outer membrane protein as seen in polyacrylamide gels. Trans-

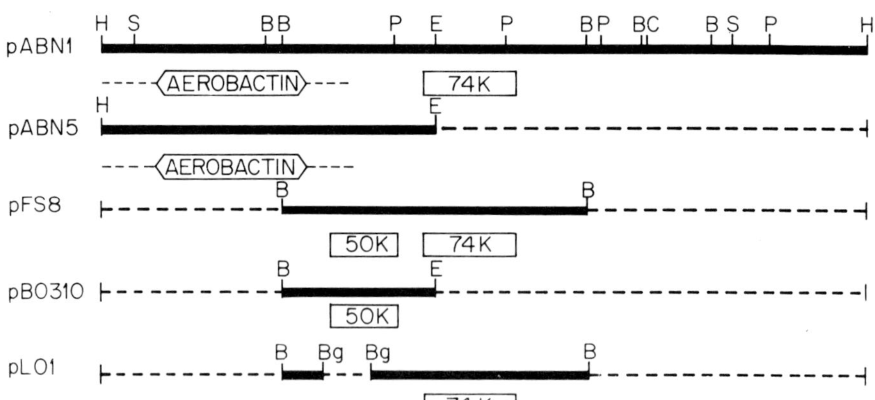

Figure 4 Physical map of the cloned iron-uptake regions from the pColV-K30 plasmid. This diagram is a summary of previously published maps for the cloned iron-uptake regions of pColV-K30. The cleavage sites for various restriction endonucleases are shown. *Bam*H1: B; *Hind*III: H; *Sal*I: S; *Bgl*II: *Bg; Pvu*II: P; *Cla*I: C; *Eco*RI: E. The cloning vehicle used was pBR322 in all recombinant derivatives, with the exception of pABN1 and pABN5, which were generated by using the cloning vector pPlac

formation of *E. coli* cells with subclones of pABN1 in which the *lac* promoter present in the cloning vector was eliminated, generated derivatives in which aerobactin was still being synthesized, suggesting the presence of at least one specific promoter in the cloned sequence (Bindereiff and Neilands, 1983). *E. coli* cells harbouring one of these subclones, pABN5, obtained by cleavage with the restriction endonucleases *Hind*III and *Eco*RI, did not synthesize the 74KDa receptor but still produced aerobactin. These results suggested that the genes for the aerobactin receptor must overlap the *Eco*R1 restriction site (see Fig. 4). By using the cloning vector pBR322 (Bolivar *et al.*, 1977), the genes for the 74KDa receptor were also cloned. The recombinant plasmid, pFS8, contains a 6.5 kb *Bam*H1 fragment which is a subset of the 16.3 kb *Hind*III fragment of the pColV-K30 plasmid (Krone *et al.*, 1983b). The 6.5 kb *Bam*H1 fragment encodes not only the 74KDa receptor but also a 50KDa protein, as determined by analysis of the proteins synthesized by the cloned fragments in minicells (Krone *et al.*, 1983a). Minicells are non-growing bodies produced by aberrant cell division at the polar ends of rod-shaped bacteria; as such they do not possess chromosomal DNA and are approximately spherical in shape. They do contain RNA and protein. Plasmid DNA in plasmid-containing minicell-producing strains segregates into minicells providing a system to study plasmid DNA replication and transcription and translation of plasmid-specified genetic information (Clark-Curtiss and Curtiss, 1983). Plasmid pBO310 carries a 3.1 kb *Eco*R1-*Bam*H1 subset of the 6.5 kb *Bam*H1 fragment. Cells harbouring this plasmid did not show cloacin or aerobactin binding and were resistant to the action of cloacin. Analysis of the polypeptides made by minicells carrying pBO310 showed that the 50KDa protein was synthesized. Although enterochelin-deficient cells of *E. coli*, harbouring the plasmid pFS8, could utilize iron complexed to aerobactin (Krone et al., 1983a), cells carrying the pLO1 plasmid, which was obtained by deletion of a *Bgl*II fragment from pFS8, were unable to take up ferric aerobactin. However, these cells were almost as sensitive to cloacin as those harbouring pFS8 or pColV-K30. Further insight into this system was obtained by complementation analysis. Transformation of a recombinant plasmid carrying the pColV-K30 fragment present in pLO1 (recloned in a different cloning vehicle) into the strain-carrying pBO310 generated transformants that were not only sensitive to cloacin but also capable of taking up ferric aerobactin, in contrast to controls containing either of the two plasmids alone. Thus, it appeared that uptake of ferric aerobactin required the expression of both the 74 and 50KDa polypeptides, while the 74KDa polypeptide was sufficient for expression of the cloacin sensitivity phenotype. However, as will be seen below, evidence from other laboratories suggests that the 50KDa protein may have a role in aerobactin biosynthesis rather than transport.

Elucidation of the functions encoded by the genetic region containing the locus for aerobactin synthesis was recently achieved by transposition mutagenesis with transposon Tn*1000* of the cloned aerobactin regions of plasmids pColV-K311 (Gross, Engelbrecht and Braun, 1984) and pColV-K30 (Carbonetti and Williams, 1984). Sites of insertion resulting in loss of aerobactin synthesis were included within a 5.5 kilobase pair region of cloned pColV-K30 DNA (Carbonetti and Williams, 1984). By using a combination of Tn*1000* mutagenesis and deletion with restriction enzymes, Gross, Englebrecht and Braun (1984) generated multicopy plasmids which complemented mutants of pColV-K311 impaired in various steps of aerobactin biosynthesis. The insertion and deletion mutants were mapped and assigned to three loci termed *aer*A, *aer*B and *aer*C (Gross, Engelbrecht and Braun, 1984). It was proposed that these genes mediate the synthesis of aerobactin by specifying functions for hydroxylation (*aer*A), acetylation of the 6-amino group of 6-hydroxylysine (*aer*B) and the coupling of *N*-acetyl-*N*-hydroxylysine with citrate (*aer*C). These investigators found that the order of transcription and polarity of these genes was *aer*B, *aer*C and *aer*A. More recent work (Gross, Engelbrecht and Braun, 1985; DeLorenzo and Neilands, 1985) indicates that there is a fourth function in charge of coupling a second *N*-acetyl-*N*-hydroxylysine with citrate. Thus, the synthetase reaction occurs through two discrete steps mediated by the products of *aer*D (*iuc*A in Neilands' nomenclature), a 63KDa polypeptide, and *aer*C (*iuc*C), a 62KDa polypeptide. The other aerobactin biosynthetic genes are : *aer*B (*iuc*B), which encodes a 32KDa polypeptide that functions in the N-acetylation of hydroxylysine; the oxygenation of L-lysine to produce -hydroxylysine is carried out by the 50–53KDa polypeptide which is the product of the *aer*A (*iuc*D) gene. Data presented by Gross *et al* (1985) and by DeLorenzo and Neilands (1986) show that the 50–53KDa polypeptide does not play any part in the transport of iron into the cell cytosol. The order of transcription of the genes is: *iuc*A, B, C, D.

Therefore, it is clear that a total of five pColV-K30 genes, *iuc*A–D and *iut*A, encoding, respectively, the 63, 33, 62, 50–53 and 74KDa polypeptides are necessary for aerobactin biosynthesis and the successful transport of iron into the cell.

2.3 Are the pJMl and pColV iron-uptake systems related?

This is an obvious question to ask. These two plasmids are found in bacteria belonging to different ecological niches, contribute to pathogenicity and code for iron-uptake systems. Since the pColV plasmids are conjugative it seems possible that pColV regions could have been transferred to *V. anguillarum* or to other bacteria. However, hybridization and cross-feeding experiments suggest that these two plasmid-mediated iron-uptake systems are unrelated (Walter *et al.*, 1984). Nevertheless, there is a precedent for the mobilization of pJM1 and pColV sequences between genomes and bacteria. Certain virulent strains of *V. anguillarum* which do not possess a pJMl-like plasmid are able to acquire iron and do possess chromosomal DNA sequences that are homologous to pJMl plasmid DNA sequences (Toranzo *et al.*, 1983). pJMl sequences are also found in several *V. anguillarum* R plasmids (Mitoma, Aoki and Crosa, 1984). The pColV iron-uptake region also appears to be mobile since the genes for aerobactin synthesis occur on plasmids from other enteric bacteria such as *Aerobacter aerogenes* (McDougall and Neilands, 1984) and in the chromosome of an *E. coli* Kl strain responsible for human neonatal infections (Valvano and Crosa, 1984). *Shigella flexneri*, a bacterium recently shown to produce aerobactin (Payne, 1980), also has chromosomal sequences in common with the cloned aerobactin regions (Lawlor and Payne, 1984). The ubiquity of the plasmid-mediated iron-uptake systems present in *V. anguillarum* and *E. coli* may thus be related to an enhanced recombinational mobility. Consequently, an important common feature of these two apparently unrelated plasmid-mediated iron- uptake systems may be that they are part of recombinational units, possibly transposition sequences, capable of epidemiological spread within their own ecological niches.

The hypothesis that these plasmid-mediated iron-transport sequences may have recombinational mobility is strengthened by the recent finding that in both the pJMl and the pColV-K30 plasmids, the iron-uptake regions are flanked by repeated sequences. Sequences that are 300-base pairs long and in direct orientation flank the iron-uptake region in the pJMl plasmid (Crosa *et al.*, 1985; Mitoma, Perez-Casal, Salinas and Crosa, submitted for publication). These sequences were also found in the chromosome of certain strains of *V. anguillarum*. In the case of pColV-K30 the sequences flanking the aerobactin genes were identified as IS*1*-like elements (Lawlor and Payne, 1984; McDougal and Neilands, 1984; Perez-Casal and Crosa, 1984). the IS*1* element found upstream of the aerobactin iron-transport genes was demonstrated to be in an inverted orientation as compared to the IS*1* sequence present at the other end of these genes (Perez-Casal and Crosa, 1984). In addition, two replication regions, REPI and REPII, were also found at each end of the IS*1*-flanked aerobactin region of pColV-K30 (Perez-Casal and Crosa, 1984). These replication regions may have contributed to the conservation of the aerobactin sequences since recombinational events that conserve one of these replication regions may also leave intact the aerobactin system, especially in deletion or insertion events in which new plasmids are generated. That this may be the case was recently demonstrated by examining the DNA environment surrounding the aerobactin genes in eleven ColV plasmids and one R plasmid found in clinical strains of *E. coli* (Waters and Crosa, 1986). The results of this work showed that the aerobactin genes together with the upstream IS*1* sequence and the REPI region were conserved in all those plasmids encoding an aerobactin-mediated iron-transport system. The conserved REPI regions were functional as assessed by transformation into a polymerase I-deficient mutant of *E. coli* K12. In contrast, the downstream IS*1* element was not always found in the same genetic location with respect to the aerobactin system genes, and the corresponding flanking region to the right, including REPII, was variable. Therefore, the upstream region including REPI must have been instrumental in the preservation and possible spread of the aerobactin genes among plasmids of the FI-incompatibility group.

This pattern of conservation does not appear to hold in the case of the chromosomal aerobactin genes from the invasive *E. coli* K1 strain (Valvano and Crosa, 1984). Molecular cloning experiments permitted isolation of these genes and comparison with those found in the pColV-K30 plasmid, and demonstrated that the aerobactin sequences *per se* were highly conserved in this chromosomal system, although neither ISl sequences nor REPII-related sequences could be detected within 10 kb of either the upstream or downstream regions from the aerobactin genes (Valvano and Crosa, submitted for publication). However, chromosomal sequences upstream of the aerobactin genes showed homology with a subset of the REPI region. In yet another chromosomal aerobactin gene, that present in *Shigella flexneri* strains, it was determined that the upstream IS*1* element is conserved while no IS*1* sequence could be detected downstream of the aerobactin genes, even after 'chromosome-walking' experiments that analysed 15 kb of DNA downstream from the aerobactin genes (Marolda, Valvano, Lawlor and Payne, personal communication).

Therefore, it appears that the chromosomal aerobactin genes may not have the same pattern of conservation of flanking sequences as that found in plasmids. This is not surprising since the combination of a replication region and virulence factor may be essential only in the preservation of these genes as an extrachromosomal element. Therefore, although the chromosome and plasmid aerobactin genes may have evolved from a common ancestral origin, recombination and selective pressures may have resulted in the conservation of different flanking sequences.

3. IRON AND TOXIN PRODUCTION

It is notable that there is a wealth of other potential virulence factors that are regulated by the iron concentration of the cell. Table 3 shows that low iron concentration enhances the production of exotoxin A in *Pseudomonas aeruginosa* and the phage-mediated diphtheria toxin in *Corynebacterium diphtheriae*. These two toxins belong to a class of bacterial ADP-ribosyl transferases that also includes cholera toxin and the *E. coli* heat-labile enterotoxin (Iglewski and Kabat, 1975). Like diphtheria toxin, exotoxin A inhibits protein synthesis in eukaryotic cells by catalysing the transfer of the ADP-ribosyl moiety of oxidized NAD onto elongation factor 2 (EF-2). Exotoxin A is similar to diphtheria toxin in other ways since it is of a similar size and it is secreted as a single polypeptide chain. Furthermore, these two toxins undergo alterations in covalent structure before ADP-ribosyl transferase activity is expressed and appear to modify the same site on EF-2 with similar binding constants for

Table 3 Bacterial toxins that are regulated by the iron concentration of culture medium

Bacteria	Toxin	References
Pseudomonas aeruginosa	Toxin A	Bjorn *et al.*, 1978
Corynebacterium diphtheriae	Diphtheria toxin	Locke and Main, 1931; Pappenheimer, 1977
Shigella dysenteriae 1	Shiga toxin	Dubos and Geiger, 1946; van Heyningen and Gladstone, 1953;
Clostidium perfringens	α-toxin	Pappenheimer and Shaskan, 1944
Clostridium tetani	Tetanus	Mueller and Miller, 1945

NAD^+. Despite these similarities, the two toxins differ considerably in other properties such as amino acid composition, mode of activation and binding of cell receptors, and show no immunological cross-reactivity (Dubos and Geiger, 1946; Eidels, Proia and Hart, 1983). Comparison of the toxins' COOH terminal and amino terminal regions as well as consecutive 60-nucleotide stretches of the exotoxin A coding region with all of the diphtheria toxin coding sequences did not show significant homologies, suggesting that the functional similarities between these two toxins are not the result of the evolution of any of their sequences from the same ancestral gene (Gray *et al.*, 1984). However, the production of these two toxins is regulated in similar fashion by the iron concentration of the cells (Bjorn *et al.*, 1978; Locke and Main, 1931; Pappenheimer, 1977).

In addition to toxin A, the yields of some other extracellular products of *Ps. aeruginosa*, such as alkaline protease and elastase, are all reduced if the iron concentration of the medium is increased (Bjorn *et al.*, 1978; Bjorn, Sokol and Iglewski, 1979). Mutant analysis suggested that the yields of these three extracellular products can be independently regulated by iron (Sokol, Cox and Iglewski, 1982). Thus, *Ps. aeruginosa* may synthesize a series of specific product repressors which, when complexed with iron, become active and bind to the specific product operators. Hence, the synthesis of the extracellular products is specifically shut off. Under conditions of iron restriction, the repressors are inactive and these genes are derepressed. Another possible model is that iron regulates post translational processing of the extracellular proteins. For instance, membrane proteins involved in the export of toxin A, alkaline protease or elastase may be specifically regulated by iron (Sokol, Cox and Iglewski, 1982).

Table 3 shows that low iron concentration enhances the production of several other toxins in addition to exotoxin A and diphtheria toxin; those affected by iron include *Clostridium tetani* (tetanus toxin), *Clostridium perfringens* (α-toxin) and *Shigella dysenteriae* (shiga toxin). It is of interest that added iron also decreased the amount of shiga-like toxin produced by an *E. coli* K12 substrain 395 lysogenized with a toxin-converting phage from the highly toxinogenic strain *E. coli* 026 H1-9 that causes haemorrhagic colitis (O'Brien *et al.*, 1984; O'Brien, personal communication). In the next section I will describe in more detail the status of the knowledge on the iron regulation of diphtheria toxin production.

3.1 The *Corynebacterium diphtheriae* β-phage-mediated toxin

Freeman (1951) and Groman and colleagues (Groman, 1953; Groman and Eaton, 1955; Groman, Eaton and Booher, 1958) originally demonstrated that the corynephage was responsible for the conversion of nontoxigenic *C. diphtheriae* to toxigenicity. Later, several investigators mapped the genetic marker *tox* as being present on the β-phage genome (Holmes and Barksdale, 1969; Matsuda, Kanai and Yoneda, 1971; Singer, 1973). The diphtheria *tox* gene may be expressed from the prophage genome, from repressed genomes and also from replicating genomes during vegetative phage growth (Matsuda and Barksdale, 1967; Murphy and Bacha, 1979). In 1971, Uchida, Gill and Pappenheimer (1971) showed that *tox* was the actual structural gene for diphtheria toxin. However, it was evident that the host bacteria played at least some role in the regulation of toxin production (Holmes and Russell, 1983). Diphtheria toxin is produced at maximum levels only when *C. diphtheriae* is grown under conditions of iron limitation. The addition of iron to starved cultures results in rapid inhibition of diphtheria toxin production (Locke and Main, 1931; Pappenheimer, 1977). Iron-mediated inhibition of toxin production was found to be linear within the range of 16 nmol – 16 μmol (Murphy, Michel and Teng, 1978). By using *E. coli* extracts for the *in vitro* synthesis of diphtheria *tox* gene products an attempt was made to identify factors that my be involved in the inhibition by iron of toxin production from the β-phage determinants (Murphy, Pappenheimer and Tayart de Borms, 1974). However, an excess of iron that would normally inhibit the synthesis of diphtheria toxin by *C. diphtheriae in vivo* had no inhibitory effect on the *in vitro* synthesis in the *E. coli* system. Conversely, specific inhibition of the expression of the *tox* gene could be achieved by adding bacterial extracts from a culture of a non-lysogenic, non-toxigenic *C. diphtheriae* (Murphy, Pappenheimer and Tayart de Borms, 1974). These results strongly suggested that there is a repressor-like activity in corynebacterial extracts and that this activity is of a chromosomal nature. Further insight into the mechanism of iron regulation of the synthesis of diphtheria toxin was obtained by analysis of mutants. Certain mutations in either the chromosome or in the β-phage result in constitutive production of diphtheria toxin, irrespective of the iron concentration in the growth medium. Mutants that were toxinogenic in high-iron medium were identified by using a passive immune haemolysis assay to detect toxin antigen production in individual plaques (Cryz, Russell and Holmes, 1983; Welkos and Holmes, 1979; 1981a, 1981b). Chromosomal mutations were responsible for the altered phenotypes of the mutant strains. Phenotypically distinct mutant strains were classified according to the production of toxin under high-iron conditions. One of these mutants possessed a phage mutation designated *tox-201*. This mutation had a cis dominant effect on the expression of the toxin structural gene of the β-phage (Welkos and Holmes, 1981a). The characteristics of the *tox-201* mutation suggests that it must be within a regulatory locus of phage β, which is involved in control of toxinogenesis by iron in *C. diphtheriae*. Murphy, Michel and Teng (1978) isolated the bacteriophage mutant $\beta^{tox+}{}_{cti}$ and demonstrated that toxin production by a *C. diphtheriae* strain C7 harbouring this phage was partially resistant to the inhibitory effect of iron. All of these results supported the hypothesis that iron may act as a corepressor in the chromosome-mediated regulation of the β-phage *tox* gene. Phage mutations such as *tox-201* may thus have occurred in an operator, promoter or attenuator involved in control of toxinogenesis by iron in *C. diphtheriae* C7. This hypothesis was strengthened by recent genetic results that demonstrated that the *tox*-201 regulatory site is closely linked to the end of the toxin structural gene corresponding to the origin of transcription (Welkos and Holmes, 1981b). Recent evidence suggests that the regulation of diphtheria toxin production may be indeed directed at the level of transcription since the inhibition kinetics of toxin production in iron-limited cultures of *C. diphtheriae* harbouring the β-phage, after the addition of iron or rifampin, an RNA polymerase inhibitor, are identical (Murphy, Michel and Teng, 1978). In addition, ^{3}H-RNA extracted from iron-limited toxigenic *C. diphtheriae* hybridized to a greater extent to β-phage DNA than ^{3}H-RNA extracted from either bacteria grown at higher concentration of iron or ^{3}H-RNA obtained from non-lysogenic, non-toxigenic *C. diphtheriae* (Murphy, Michel and Teng, 1978). An alternative hypothesis is that the inhibitory effect of iron may be at the level of toxin release from *C. diphtheriae* involving some sort of feedback control. The only problem with this hypothesis is that it is known that diphtheria toxin does not accumulate intracellularly (Smith *et al.*, 1980). In addition no appreciable levels of β-phage-hybridizing RNA were found in *C. diphtheriae* prior to toxin production (Murphy, Michel and Teng, 1978). A working model for the regulation of diphtheria toxin production by iron is shown in Fig. 5. This model assumes that irrespective of its lysogenic state the information for the synthesis of a diphtheria toxin aporepressor is on the *C. diphtheriae* chromosome. At high iron concentrations a repressor–iron complex would form. This complex would have specific affinity for the β-phage *tox* operator locus and would likely act at the level of transcription as a controlling element. Of course, under iron-restricted conditions, the repressor–iron complex would dissociate and the diphtheria *tox* gene would be expressed. Restriction endonuclease cleavage analysis of corynebacteriophages β_c and β_{vir} and hybridization experiments with toxin-specific ^{32}P-

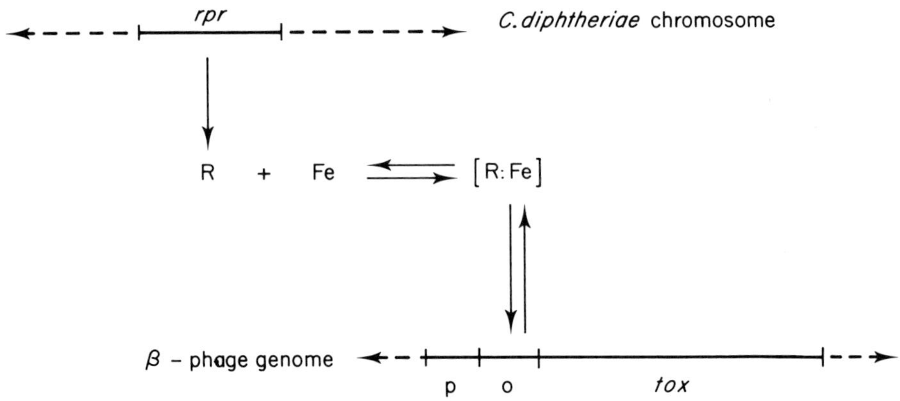

Figure 5 Model of the iron regulation of corynephage *tox* gene.
Corynebacterium diphtheriae carries the structural information (*rpr*) for the synthesis of the diphtheria toxin repressor (R). In the presence of iron, an active repressor–iron complex forms, which can bind to the corynephage *tox* operator locus. The equilibrium would shift under conditions of iron limitation, the inactive R molecule would not bind to the phage operator and the *tox* gene would become derepressed. From Murphy and Bacha (1979)

labelled mRNA suggest that the *tox* operon of the β phage is monocistronic (Costa *et al.*, 1981). The gene for diphtheria toxin fragment A, which carries the active site for ADP-ribosylation of the elongation factor EF-2, has now been cloned and expressed in *E. coli* (Leong, Coleman and Murphy, 1983). Also, the complete nucleotide sequence of the diphtheria toxin structural gene and that of the *tox*228 gene coding for the non-toxic serologically related protein CRM228 have been determined (Greenfield *et al.*, 1983; Kaczorec *et al.*, 1983). The signal peptide of prodiphtheria toxin and the putative *tox* promoter have been identified in these sequences. Analysis of sequences upstream from the *tox* structural gene may identify possible candidate sites for the *tox* operator.

Bacterial mutants that produced high yields of toxin under high iron concentrations have been recently isolated (Cryz, Russell and Holmes, 1983). These mutants were shown to possess severe defects in their iron-transport systems for ferric iron. Therefore, the altered regulation of toxinogenesis by iron in these mutants must have been caused by the defective iron-transport process, i.e. they exhibited low-iron phenotype during growth under conditions that permitted wild-type *C. diphtheriae* to exhibit a high-iron phenotype. Recent studies by Russell and Holmes (1983) were aimed at characterizing the iron-transport process in *C. diphtheriae*. These authors demonstrated that transport of ferric iron into *C. diphtheriae* C7 (β) occurred by a high affinity, active transport system with the electrochemical proton gradient as the major energy source for iron transport. Evidence was also obtained for stimulation of iron uptake at pH 8.0 by a dialysable, extracellular factor, possibly a siderophore, present in conditioned medium from low-iron cultures of *C. diphtheriae*. More recent work provided additional evidence for a corynebacterial siderophore, by using a recently isolated siderophore-deficient mutant of *C. diphtheriae* (Russell, Cryz and Holmes, 1984). Development of specific bioassays with this mutant permitted its partial purification. The corynebacterial siderophore was not related to various phenolate and hydroxamate siderophores and did not give positive reactions in the Arnow test for phenolates nor the Csaky test for hydroxamates, suggesting that it may have a novel chemical structure. An interesting finding was that the growth of the siderophore-deficient mutant HC6 was also stimulated by the hydroxamate aerobactin which is the siderophore encoded by certain ColV plasmids (see above). However, the properties of the corynebacterial siderophore were not identical to those of aerobactin. It is notable that the highly toxigenic but avirulent Park–Williams 8 strain of *C. diphtheriae* is defective in iron uptake and does not produce the corynebacterial siderophore corynebactin. Addition of partially purified corynebactin stimulated iron uptake and growth of iron-deprived cells of this mutant (Russell and Holmes, 1984). It is possible that the defect in siderophore production by this strain is responsible for its poor growth *in vivo* and for the high production of toxin *in vitro*. It is worth noting here that the regulation of diphtheria toxin production by iron has also been found in strains of *Corynebacterium ulcerans* and *C. pseudotuberculosis*, bacteria in which the existence of *tox* gene sequences has only been demonstrated by using *tox* probes from *C. diphtheriae* β-phage DNA (N. Groman, personal communication).

4. CONCLUDING REMARKS

The iron concentration of culture medium significantly affects the yield of the plasmid-mediated products involved in iron transport in *V. anguillarum* and *E. coli*, as well as the production of toxins in various bacteria. Low iron concentration enhances the production of these factors, which in all these bacteria are correlated with their ability to cause disease. Thus, at a functional level it seems likely that the regulation of these systems may be somewhat similar, i.e. via production of a repressor which is active only in the presence of a certain iron concentration. In the case of the ColV plasmid-mediated iron-uptake system there is evidence that a product of the chromosome gene *fur* may control the expression of the aerobactin operon. There is, as yet, no evidence for a similar type of chromosomal regulator gene for the pJMl plasmid-mediated iron transport system in *V. anguillarum*, but iron regulation of diphtheria toxin does indeed require a product encoded by the *C. diphtheriae* chromosome and not by the β-phage.

At the beginning of this chapter I promised that at this stage the reader would have found several common features in the extrachromosomal systems examined in this work. Albeit in a nutshell, I hope that this chapter has achieved that goal and there is now an increased awareness of the importance of iron for the universal regulation of these extrachromosomal systems, as well as several others of a chromosomal nature, which are responsible for the production of important components of the bacteria virulence repertoire.

ACKNOWLEDGEMENTS

The research from my laboratory reported in this work was supported by US Public Health Service Grant AI19018 from the National Institutes of Health.

REFERENCES

Actis, L.A., Fish, W., Crosa, J.H., Kellerman, K., Ellenberg, S.R., Hauser, F.M. and Sanders-Loehr, J. (1986). Characterization of anguibactin, a novel siderophore from *Vibrio anguillarum* 775(pJM1). *Journal of Bacteriology*, **167**, 57–65.

Actis, L.A., Potter, S.A., and Crosa, J.H. (1985) Iron-regulated outer membrane protein OM2 of *Vibrio anguillarum* is encoded by virulence plasmid pJMl. *Journal of Bacteriology*, **161**, 736–742.

Berger, H., Hacker, J., Juarez, A., Hughes, C., and Goebel, W. (1982). Cloning of the chromosomal determinants encoding hemolysin production and mannose-resistant hemmaglutination in *Escherichia coli*. *Journal of Bacteriology*, **152**, 1241–1247.

Bindereiff, A., Braun, V., and Hantke, K. (1982). The cloacin receptor of ColV-bearing *Escherichia coli* is part of the Fe^{3+}–aerobactin transport system. *Journal of Bacteriology*, **150**, 1472–1475.

Bindereiff, A., and Neilands, J.B. (1983). Cloning of the aerobactin-mediated iron assimilation system of plasmid ColV. *Journal of Bacteriology*, **153**, 1111–1113.

Binns, M.M., Davies, D.L., and Hardy, K.G. 1979. Cloned fragments of the plasmid ColV, I-K94 specifying virulence and serum resistance. *Nature*, **279**, 778–781.

Bjorn, M.J., Iglewski, B.H., Ives, S.K., Sadoff, J.C., and Vasil, M.L. (1978). Effects of iron on yields of exotoxin A in cultures of *Pseudomonas aeruginosa* PA-103. *Infection and immunity*, **19**, 785–791.

Bjorn, M.J., Sokol, P.A., and Iglewski, B.H. (1979). Influence of iron on yields of extracellular products in *Pseudomonas aeruginosa* cultures. *Journal of Bacteriology*, **138**, 193–200.

Bolivar, F., Rodriguez, R.L., Greene, P.J., Betlach, M.C., Heyneker, H.L., Boyer, H.W., Crosa, J.H., and Falkow, S. (1977). Construction and characterization of new cloning vehicles II. A multipurpose cloning system. *Gene*, **2**, 95–113.

Braun, V. (1981). *Escherichia coli* containing the plasmid ColV produces the iron ionophore aerobactin. *FEMS Microbiology Letters*, **11**, 225–228.

Braun, V., Brazel-Faisst, C., and Schneider, R. (1984). Growth stimulation of *Escherichia coli* in serum by iron (III) aerobactin. Recycling of aerobactin. *FEMS Microbiology Letters*, **21**, 99–103.

Braun, V., and Burkhardt, R. (1982). Regulation of the ColV plasmid-determined iron (III)–aerobactin transport system in *Escherichia coli*. *Journal of Bacteriology*, **152**, 223–231.

Braun, V., Burkhardt, R., Schneider, R., and Zimmerman, L. (1982) Chromosomal genes for ColV plasmid-determined iron (III)–aerobactin transport in *Escherichia coli*. *Journal of Bacteriology*, **151**, 553–559.

Braun, V., Gross, R., Koster, W., and Zimmerman, L. (1983). Plasmid and chromosomal mutants in the iron (III)–aerobactin transport system of *Escherichia coli*. Use of streptonigrin for selection. *Molecular and General Genetics*, **192**, 131–139.

Bullen, J.J. (1981). The significance of iron in infection. *Review of Infectious Diseases*, **3**, 1127–1138.

Bullen, J.J., Rogers, H.J., and Griffiths, E. (1978). Role of iron in bacterial infections. *Current Topics in Microbiology and Immunology*, **80**, 1–35.

Canestrini, G. (1893). La malattia dominante della anguille. *Att dell'Istituto Veneto di Scienze, Lettere ed Arti*, Series 7, 809–814.

Carbonetti, N.H., and Williams, P.H. (1984). A cluster of five genes specifying the aerobactin iron uptake system of plasmid ColV-K30. *Infection and Immunity*, **46**, 7–12.

Cisar, J.O., and Fryer, J.L. (1969). An epizootic of vibriosis in chinook salmon. *Bulletin of the Wildlife Disease Association*, **5**, 73–76.

Clancy, J., and Savage, D.C. (1981). Another colicin V phenotype: *in vitro* adhesion of *Escherichia coli* to mouse intestinal epithelium. *Infection and Immunity*, **32**, 343–352.

Clark-Curtiss, J.E., and Curtiss, III, R. (1983). Analysis of recombinant DNA using *Escherichia coli* minicells. *Methods in Enzymology*, **101**, 347–362.

Costa, J.J., Michel, J.L., Rappuoli, R., and Murphy, J.R. (1981). Restriction map of corynebacteriophages β_c and β_{vir} and physical localization of the diphtheria *tox* operon. *Journal of Bacteriology*, **148**, 124–130.

Crosa, J.H. (1979). *Vibrio anguillarum*: an iron uptake mechanism as a factor of virulence. *Fish Health News*, **8**, 7–9.

Crosa, J.H. (1980) A plasmid associated with virulence in the marine fish pathogen *Vibrio anguillarum* specifies an iron-sequestering system. *Nature*, **284**, 566–568.

Crosa, J.H. (1984). The relationship of plasmid-mediated iron transport and bacterial virulence. *Annual Review of Microbiology*, **38**, 69–89.

Crosa, J.H., Actis, L.A., Mitoma, Y., Perez-Casal, J., and Tolmasky, M.E. (1985). Plasmid-mediated iron sequestering systems in pathogenic strains of *Vibrio anguillarum* and *Escherichia coli*. In *Plasmids in Bacteria* (Eds. D.R. Helinski, S.N. Cohen, D. Clewell, D. Jackson and A. Hollaender). Plenum Publishing Corporation, New York.

Crosa, J.H., and Hodges, L.L. (1981). Outer membrane proteins induced under conditions of iron limitation in the marine fish pathogen *Vibrio anguillarum* 775. *Infection and Immunity*, **31**, 223–227.

Crosa, J.H., Hodges, L.L., and Schiewe, M.H. (1980). Curing of a plasmid is correlated with an attenuation of virulence in the marine fish pathogen *Vibrio anguillarum*. *Infection and Immunity*, **27**, 897–902.

Crosa, J.H., Schiewe, M.H., and Falkow, S. (1977). Evidence for plasmid contribution to the virulence of the fish pathogen *Vibrio anguillarum*. *Infection and Immunity*, **18**, 509–513.

Crosa, J.H., Walter, M.A., and Potter, S.A. (1983a). Iron uptake deficient mutants of *Vibrio anguillarum* 775 generated by insertional inactivation of the virulence plasmid pJM1. In *Microbiology 1983* (Ed. D. Schlessinger) pp. 354–358. American Society for Microbiology, Washington, DC.

Crosa, J.H., Walter, M.A., and Potter, S.A. (1983b). The genetics of plasmid mediated virulence in the marine fish pathogen *V. anguillarum*. In *Bacterial and Viral Diseases of Fish: Molecular Studies* (Ed. J.H. Crosa) pp. 21–30. Washington Sea Grant, Seattle.

Cryz, Jr., S.J., Russell, L.M., and Holmes, R.K. (1983). Regulation of toxinogenesis in *Corynebacterium diphtheriae*: mutations in the bacterial genome that alter the effects of iron on toxin production. *Journal of Bacteriology*, **154**, 245–252.

DeLorenzo, V. and Neilands, J.B. (1986). Characterization of *iuc*A and *iuc*C genes of the aerobactin system of plasmid ColV-K30 in *Escherichia coli. Journal of Bacteriology*, **167**, 350–355.

Ditta, G., Stanfield, S., Corbin, D., and Helinksi, D.R. (1980). Broad host range DNA cloning system for gram-negative bacteria: construction of a gene bank of *Rhizobium meliloti. Proceedings of the National Academy of Sciences* (USA), **77**, 7347–7351.

Dubos, R.G., and Geiger, J. (1946). Preparation and properties of shiga toxin and toxoid. *Journal of Experimental Medicine*, **84**, 143–156.

Eidels, L., Proia, R.L., and Hart, D.A. (1983). Membrane receptors for bacterial toxins. *Microbiological Reviews*, **47**, 596–620.

Elwell, L.P., and Shipley, P.L. (1980). Plasmid-mediated factors associated with virulence of bacteria to animals. *Annual Review of Microbiology*, **34**, 465–496.

Evans, D.G., Silver, R.P., Evans, D.J., Chase, D.G., and Gorbach, S.L. (1975). Plasmid-controlled colonization factor associated with virulence in *Escherichia coli* enterotoxinogenic for humans. *Infection and Immunity*, **12**, 656–667.

Evelyn, T.P.T. (1971). First records of vibriosis in Pacific salmon cultured in Canada and taxonomic status of the responsible bacteria *Vibrio anguillarum. Journal of the Fisheries Research Board of Canada*, **28**, 517–525.

Frederick, P. (1951). Acquisition des proprietes antibiotiques nouvelles par la souche *E. coli* V sous l'action des bacteriophages T.1, T.5 et T.7. *Antonie van Leeuwenhoek Journal of Microbiology and Serology*, **17**, 103–106.

Frederick, P., and Joiris, E. (1950). Distribution des souches productices de colicine V dans les selles normales et pathologiques. *Comptes Rendu de la Societe de Biologie*, **144**, 435–437.

Freeman, V.J. (1951). Studies on the virulence of bacteriophage-infected strains of *Corynebacterium diphtheriae. Journal of Bacteriology*, **61**, 675–688.

Gemski, P., Lazere, J.R., and Casey, T. (1980). Plasmid associated with pathogenicity and calcium dependency of *Yersinia enterocolitica. Infection and Immunity*, **27**, 682–685.

Gibson, F., and McGrath, D.I. (1969). The isolation and characterization of a hydroxamic acid aerobactin formed by *Aerobacter aerogenes* 62–1. *Biochimica et Biophysica Acta*, **192**, 175–184.

Gratia, A. (1925). Sur un remarquable example d'antagonisme entre deux souches de colibacille. *Comptes Rendu de la Societe de Biologie*, **93**, 1040–1041.

Gray, G.L., Smith, D.H., Baldridge, J.S., Harkins, R.N., Vasil, M.L., Chen, E.Y., and Heynecker, H.L. (1984). Cloning, nucleotide sequence, and expression in *Escherichia coli* of the exotoxin A structural gene of *Pseudomonas aeruginosa. Proceedings of the National Academy of Sciences* (USA) **81**, 2645–2649.

Greenfield, L., Bjorn, M.J., Horn, G., Fong, D., Buck, G.A., Collier, J.R., and Kaplan, D.A. (1983). Nucleotide sequence of the structural gene for diphtheria toxin carried by corynebacteriophage β. *Proceedings of the National Academy of Sciences* (USA), **80**, 6853–6857.

Grewal, K.K., Warner, P.J., and Williams, P.H. (1982). An inducible outer membrane protein involved in aerobactin-mediated iron transport by ColV strains of *Escherichia coli. FEBS Letters*, **140**, 27–30.

Griffiths, E. (1983a). Bacterial adaptation to a low-iron environment. In *Microbiology 1983* (Ed. D. Schlessinger), pp. 329–333. American Society for Microbiology, Washington, DC.

Griffiths, E. (1983b). Adaptation and multiplication of bacteria in host tissues. *Philosophical Transactions of the Royal Society of London*, Series B, **303**, 85–96.

Groman, N.B. (1953). Evidence for the induced nature of the change from non-toxigenicity to toxigenicity in *Corynebacterium diphtheriae* as a result of exposure to specific bacteriophage. *Journal of Bacteriology*, **66**, 184–191.

Groman, N.B., and Eaton, M. (1955). Genetic factors in *Corynebacterium diphtheriae* conversion. *Journal of Bacteriology*, **70**, 637–640.

Groman, N.B., Eaton, M., and Booher, Z.K. (1958). Study of mono-and polylysogenic *Corynebacterium diphtheriae. Journal of Bacteriology*, **75**, 320–325.

Gross, R., Engelbrecht, F., and Braun, V. (1984). Genetic and biochemical characterization of the aerobactin synthesis operon on pColV. *Molecular and General Genetics*, **196**, 74–80.

Gross, R., Engelbrecht, F., and Braun, V. (1985). Identification of the genes and their polypeptide products responsible for aerobactin synthesis by pColV plasmids. *Molecular and General Genetics*, **201**, 204–212.

Gyles, C.L., Palchaudhuri, S., and Maas, W.K. (1977). Naturally occurring plasmid carrying genes for enterotoxin production and drug resistance. *Science*, **198**, 198–199.

Gyles, C.L., So, M., and Falkow, S. (1974). The enterotoxin plasmids of *Escherichia coli. Journal of Infectious Diseases*, **130**, 40–49.

Hale, T.L., Sansonetti, P.J., Schad, P.A., Austin, S., and Formal, S.B. (1983). Characterization of virulence plasmids and plasmid-associated outer membrane proteins in *Shigella flexneri*, *Shigella sonnei* and *Escherichia coli. Infection and Immunity*, **40**, 340–350.

Hantke, K. (1981). Regulation of ferric iron transport in *Escherichia coli* K-12: isolation of a constitutive mutant. *Molecular and General Genetics*, **182**, 288–392.

Harbell, S.O., Hodgins, H.O., and Schiewe, M.H. (1979). Studies on the pathology of vibriosis on coho slamon. (*Oncorhynchus kisutch*). *Journal of Fish Diseases*, **2**, 527–535.

Hedges, R.W., and Jacob, A.E. (1974). Transposition of ampicillin resistance from RP4 to other replicon. *Molecular and General Genetics*, **132**, 31–40.

Holmes, R.K., and Barksdale, L. (1969). Genetic analysis of tox^+ and tox^- bacteriophages of *Cornebacterium diphtheriae*. *Journal of Virology*, **3**, 586–598.

Holmes, R.K., and Russell, L.M. (1983). Role of iron in regulating synthesis of bacterial toxins. In *Microbiology 1983* (Ed. D. Schlessinger), pp. 359–362. American Society for Microbiology, Washington, DC.

Iglewski, B.H., and Kabat, D. (1975). NAD-dependent inhibition of protein synthesis by *Pseudomonas aeruginosa* toxin. *Proceedings of the National Academy of Sciences (USA)*, **72**, 2284–2288.

Kaczorec, M., Delpeyroux, F., Chenciner, N., Streeck, R.E., Murphy, J.R., Boquet, P., and Tiollais, P. (1983). Nucleotide sequence and expression of the diphtheria *tox*228 gene in *Escherichia coli. Science*, **221**, 855–858.

Kahn, P.L., and Helinski, D.R. (1964). Relationship between colicinogenic factors E_1 and V and an F factor in *Escherichia coli. Journal of Bacteriology*, **88**, 1573–1579.

Knauff, V., and Nester, E.W. (1982). Wide host range cloning vectors: a cosmid clone bank of an *Agrobacterium* Ti plasmid. *Plasmid*, **8**, 45–54.

Konopka, K., Bindereif, A., and Neilands, J.B. (1982). Aerobactin-mediated utilization of transferrin iron. *Biochemistry*, **21**, 6503–6508.

Kopecko, D.J., Washington, O., and Formal, S.B. (1980). Genetic and physical evidence for plasmid control of *Shigella sonnei* form I cell surface antigen. *Infection and Immunity*, **29**, 207–214.

Krone, W.J.A., Luirink, J., Koningstein, G., Oudega, B., and de Graaf, F.K. (1983a). Subcloning of the cloacin DF 13/aerobactin receptor protein and identification of a pColV-K30-determinant polypeptide involved in ferric-aerobactin uptake. *Journal of Bacteriology*, **156**, 945–948.
Krone, W.J.A., Oudega, B., Stegehuis, F., and de Graaf, F.K. (1983b). Cloning and expression of the cloacin DF13/aerobactin receptor of *Escherichia coli* (ColV-K30). *Journal of Bacteriology*, **153**, 716–721.
Lawlor, K.M., and Payne, S.M. (1984). Aerobactin genes in *Shigella* spp. *Journal of Bacteriology*, **160**, 266–272.
Leong, D., Coleman, K.D., and Murphy, J.R. (1983). Cloned fragment A of diphtheria toxin is expressed and secreted into the periplasmic space of *Escherichia coli* K12. *Science*, **220**, 515–517.
Locke, A., and Main, E.R. (1931). The relation of copper and iron to the production of toxin and enzyme action. *Journal of Infectious Diseases*, **48**, 419–435.
McDougall, S., and Neilands, J.B. (1984). Plasmid- and chromosome-coded aerobactin synthesis in enteric bacteria: insertion sequences flank operon in plasmid-mediated systems. *Journal of Bacteriology*, **159**, 300–305.
Matsuda, M., and Barksdale, L. (1967). System for the investigation of the bacteriophage-directed synthesis of diphtherial toxin. *Journal of Bacteriology*, **93**, 722–730.
Matsuda, M., Kanei, C., and Yoneda, M. (1971). Temperature sensitive mutants of non-lysogenizing corynebacteriophage β_{vir}: their isolation, characterization and relation to toxinogenesis. *Biken Journal*, **14**, 119–130.
Mickelsen, P.A., Blackman, E., and Sparling, P.F. (1982). Ability of *Neisseria gonorrhoeae*, *Neisseria meningitidis* and commensal *Neisseria* species to obtain iron from lactoferrin. *Infection and Immunity*, **35**, 915–920.
Mickelsen, P.A., and Sparling, P.F. (1981). Ability of *Neisseria gonorrhoeae*, *Neisseria meningitidis*, and commensal *Neisseria* species to obtain iron from transferrin and iron compounds. *Infection and Immunity*, **33**, 555–564.
Minshew, B.H., Jorgensen, G., Counts, G.W., and Falkow, S. (1978). Association of hemolysin production, hemmaglutination of human erythrocytes and virulence for chicken embryos of extraintestinal *Escherichia coli* isolates. *Infection and Immunity*, **20**, 50–54.
Mitoma, Y., Aoki, T., and Crosa, J.H. (1984). Phylogenetic relationships among *Vibrio anguillarum* plasmids. *Plasmid*, **12**, 143–148.
Moll, A., Manning, P.A., and Timmis, K.N. (1980). Plasmid-determined resistance to serum bactericidal activity: a major outer membrane protein, the *tra*T gene product, is responsible for plasmid-specified serum resistance in *Escherichia coli*. *Infection and Immunity*, **28**, 359–367.
Moore, D.G., and Earhart, C.F. (1981). Specific inhibition of *Escherichia coli* ferrienterochelin specific immunoglobulin from normal human serum. *Infection and Immunity*, **31**, 631–635.
Mueller, J.H., and Miller, P.A. (1945). Production of tetanal toxin. *Journal of Immunology*, **40**, 21–32.
Murphy, J.R., and Bacha, P. (1979). Regulation of diphtheria toxin production. In *Microbiology 1979* (Ed. D. Schlessinger), pp. 181–186. American Society for Microbiology, Washington, DC.
Murphy, J.R., Michel, J.L. and Teng, M. (1978). Evidence that the regulation of diphtheria toxin production is directed at the level of transcription. *Journal of Bacteriology*, **135**, 511–516.
Murphy, J.R., Pappenheimer, Jr., A.M., and Tayart de Borms, S. (1974). Synthesis of

diphtheria tox gene products in *Escherichia coli* extracts. *Proceedings of National Academy of Sciences* (*USA*), **71**, 11–15.

Nagel de Zwaig, R., and Anton, D. (1964). Interactions between colicinogenic factors and fertility factors. *Biochemical and Biophysical Research Communications*, **17**, 358–362.

Neilands, J.B. (1981) Microbial iron compounds. *Annual Review of Biochemistry*, **50**, 715–731.

Neilands, J.B. (1982). Microbial envelope proteins related to iron. *Annual Review of Microbiology*, **36**, 285–309.

Norrod, P., and Williams, R.P. (1978). Growth of *Neisseria gonorrhoeae* in media deficient in iron without detection of siderophores. *Current Microbiology*, **1**, 281–284.

O'Brien, A.D., Newland, J.W., Miller, S.F., Holmes, R.K., Smith, H.W., and Formal, S.B. (1984). Shiga-like toxin-converting phages from *Escherichia coli* strains that cause haemorrhagic colitis or infantile diarrhoea. *Science*, **226**, 694–696.

Ørskov, I., and Ørskov, F. (1966). Episome-carried surface antigen K88 of *Escherichia coli*. *Journal of Bacteriology*, **91**, 69–75.

Oudega, B., Oldenziel-Werner, W.J.M., Klaasen-Boor, P., Rezee, A., Glas, J., and de Graaf, F.K. (1979). Purification and characterization of cloacin DF13 receptor from *Enterobacter cloacae* and its interation with cloacin DF13 *in vitro*. *Journal of Bacteriology*, **138**, 7–16.

Pappenheimer, Jr., A.M. (1977). Diphtheria toxin. *Annual Review of Biochemistry*, **46**, 69–94.

Pappenheimer, Jr., A.M., and Shaskan, E. (1944). Effect of iron on carbohydrate metabolism of *Clostridium welchii*. *Journal of Biological Chemistry*, **155**, 265–275.

Payne, S.M. (1980). Synthesis and utilization of siderophores by *Shigella flexneri*. *Journal of Bacteriology*, **143**, 1420–1424.

Perez-Casal, J.F., and Crosa, J.H. (1984). Aerobactin iron uptake sequences in plasmid ColV-K30 are flanked by inverted IS*1*-like elements and replication regions. *Journal of Bacteriology*, **160**, 256–265.

Portnoy, D.A., and Falkow, S. (1981). Virulence-associated plasmids from *Yersinia enterocolitica* and *Yersinia pestis*. *Journal of Bacteriology*, **148**, 877–883.

Portnoy, D.A., Moseley, S.L., and Falkow, S. (1981). Characterization of plasmids and plasmid-associated determinants of *Yersinia enterocolitica* pathogenesis. *Infection and Immunity*, **31**, 775–782.

Quackenbusch, R.L., and Falkow, S. (1979). Relationship between colicin V activity and virulence in *Escherichia coli*. *Infection and Immunity*, **24**, 562–564.

Ransom, D.P., Lannan, C.N., Rohovec, J.S., and Fryer, J.L. (1984) Comparison of histopathology caused by *Vibrio anguillarum* and *Vibrio ordalii* in three species of Pacific salmon. *Journal of Fish Diseases*, **7**, 107–115.

Rucker, R.R., Earp, B.J., and Ordal, E.J. (1953). Infectious diseases of Pacific salmon. *Transactions of the American Fisheries Society*, **83**, 297–312.

Russell, L.M., Cryz, Jr., S.J., and Holmes, R.K. (1984). Genetic and biochemical evidence for a siderophore-dependent iron transport system in *Corynebacterium diphtheriae*. *Infection and Immunity*, **45**, 143–149.

Russell, L.M., and Holmes, R.K. (1983). Initial characterization of the ferric iron transport system of *Corynebacterium diphtheriae*. *Journal of Bacteriology*, **155**, 1439–1441.

Russell, L.M. and Holmes, R.K. (1984). Highly toxigenic but avirulent Park-Williams 8 strain of *Corynebacterium diptheriae* does not produce siderophore. *Infection and Immunity*, **47**, 575–578.

Sansonetti, P.J., David, M., and Toucas, M. (1980). Correlation entre la perte d'ADN plasmidique et le passage de la phase I virulence a la phase II avirulence chez *Shigella sonnei*. *Comptes Rendu de l'Academie des Sciences (Paris)*, Series D, **290**, 879–882.

Sansonetti, P.J., d'Hauterille, H., Ecobichon, C., and Pourcel, C. (1983). Molecular comparison of virulence plasmids in *Shigella* and enteroinvasive *Escherichia coli*. *Annales de Microbiologie (Paris)*, **134A**, 295–318.

Sansonetti, P.J., Kopecko, D.J., and Formal, S.B. (1981). *Shigella sonnei* plasmids: evidence that a large plasmid is necessary for virulence. *Infection and Immunity*, **34**, 75–83.

Sansonetti, P.J., Kopecko, D.J., and Formal S.B. (1982). Involvement of a plasmid in the invasive ability of *Shigella flexneri*. *Infection and Immunity*, **35**, 852–860.

Shapiro, J.A. (1983). *Mobile Genetic Elements*. Academic Press, New York.

Singer, K.A. (1973). Temperature-sensitive mutants of toxinogenic corynebacteriophage beta. I. Genetics. *Virology*, **55**, 347–356.

Smith, H.W. (1974). A search for transmissible pathogenic characters in invasive strains of *Escherichia coli*: the discovery of a plasmid-controlled toxin and a plasmid-controlled lethal character associated or identical with colicine V. *Journal of General Microbiology*, **83**, 95–111.

Smith, H.W., and Halls, S. (1967). The transmissible nature of the genetic factor in *Escherichia coli* that controls haemolysin production. *Journal of General Microbiology*, **47**, 153–167.

Smith, H.W., and Halls, S. (1968). The transmissible nature of the genetic factor in *Escherichia coli* that controls enterotoxin production. *Journal of General Microbiology*, **52**, 319–334.

Smith, H.W., and Huggins, M.B. (1976). Further observations on the association of the colicine V plasmid of *Escherichia coli* with pathogenicity and with survival in the alimentary tract. *Journal of General Microbiology*, **92**, 335–350.

Smith, H.W., and Linggood, M.A. (1972). Further observations on *Escherichia coli* enterotoxin with particular regard to those produced by a typical piglet strain and by calf and lamb strains; the transmissible nature of these enterotoxins and of a K antigen possessed by calf and lamb strains. *Journal of Medical Microbiology*, **5**, 243–250.

Smith, W.P., Tai, P.C., Murphy, J.R., and Davis, B.D. (1980). Precursor in cotranslational secretion of diphtheria toxin. *Journal of Bacteriology*, **141**, 184–189.

So M., Crosa, J.H., and Falkow, S. (1975). Polynucleotide sequence relationships among ent plasmids and the relationship between ent and other plasmids. *Journal of Bacteriology*, **121**, 234–238.

Sokol, P.M., Cox, C.D., and Iglewski, B.H. (1982). *Pseudomonas aeruginosa* mutants altered in their sensitivity to the effect of iron on toxin A or elastase yields. *Journal of Bacteriology*, **151**, 783–787.

Stuart, S.J., Greenwood, K.T., and Luke, R.K.J. (1980). Hydroxamate-mediated transport of iron controlled by ColV plasmids. *Journal of Bacteriology*, **143**, 35–42.

Stuart, S.J., Greenwood, K.T., and Luke, R.K.J. (1982). Iron-suppressible production of hydroxamate by *Escherichia coli* isolates. *Infection and Immunity*, **36**, 870–875.

Taylor, P.W., and Hughes, C. (1978). Plasmid carriage and the serum sensitivity of enterobacteria. *Infection and Immunity*, **22**, 10–17.

Tolmasky, M.E., and Crosa, J.H. (1984). Molecular cloning and expression of genetic determinants for the iron uptake system mediated by the *Vibrio anguillarum* plasmid pJMl. *Journal of Bacteriology*, **160**, 860–866.

Toranzo, A.E., Barja, J.L., Potter, S.A., Colwell, R.R., Hetrick, F.M., and Crosa, J.H. (1983). Molecular factors associated with virulence of marine vibrios isolated from striped bass in Chesapeake Bay. *Infection and Immunity*, **39**, 1220–1227.

Uchida, T., Gill, D.M., and Pappenheimer, Jr., A.M. (1971). Mutation in the structural gene for diphtheria toxin carried by temperate phage β. *Nature, New Biology*, **233**, 8–11.

Valvano, M.A., and Crosa, J.H. (1984). Aerobactin iron transport genes commonly encoded by certain ColV plasmids occur in the chromosome of a human invasive strain of *Escherichia coli* K1. *Infection and Immunity*, **46**, 159–167.

van den Bosch, J.F., Postma, P., de Graaff, J., and MacLaren, D.M. (1981). Haemolysis by urinary *Escherichia coli* and virulence in mice. *Journal of Medical Microbiology*, **14**, 321–331.

van Heyningen, W.E., and Gladstone, G.P. (1953). The neurotoxin of *Shigella shigae* 3. The effect of iron on production of the toxin. *British Journal of Experimental Pathology*, **34**, 221–229.

van Tiel-Menkveld, G.J., Mentjox-Vervuurt, J.M., Oudega, B., and de Graaf, F.K. (1982). Siderophore production by *Enterobacter cloacae* and a common receptor protein for the uptake of aerobactin and cloacin DF13. *Journal of Bacteriology*, **150**, 490–497.

van Tiel-Menkveld, G.J., Oudega, B., Kempers, O., and De Graaf, F.K. (1981). Mitomycin C-induced synthesis of cloacin DF13 and lethality in cloacinogenic *Escherichia coli* cells. *FEMS Microbiology Letters*, **12**, 373–380.

Walter, M.A., Bindereif, A., Neilands, J.B., and Crosa, J.H. (1984). Lack of homology between the iron transport regions of two virulence-linked bacterial plasmids. *Infection and Immunity*, **43**, 765–767.

Walter, M.A., Potter, S.A., and Crosa, J.H. (1983). Iron uptake system mediated by *Vibrio anguillarum* plasmid pJMl. *Journal of Bacteriology*, **156**, 880–887.

Warner, P.J., Williams, P.H., Bindereif, A., and Neilands, J.B. (1981). Col V plasmid-specified aerobactin synthesis by invasive strains of *Escherichia coli*. *Infection and Immunity*, **33**, 540–545.

Waters, V. and Crosa, J.H. (1986). DNA environment of the aerobactin iron uptake system genes in prototype ColV plasmids. *Journal of Bacteriology*, **167**, 647–654.

Weinberg, E.D. (1978). Iron and infection. *Microbiological Reviews*, **42**, 45–66.

Welch, R.A., Dellinger, E.P., Minshew, B., and Falkow, S. (1981). Haemolysin contributes to virulence of extra-intestinal *E. coli* infections. *Nature*, **294**, 665–667.

Welkos, S.L., and Holmes, R.K. (1979). Characterization of a screening test for diphtherial toxin antigen produced by individual plaques of corynebacteriophages. *Journal of Clinical Microbiology*, **9**, 693–698.

Welkos, S.L., and Holmes, R.K. (1981a). Regulation of toxinogenesis in *Corynebacterium diphtheriae* I. Mutations in bacteriophage β that alter the effects of iron on toxin production. *Journal of Virology*, **37**, 936–945.

Welkos, S.L., and Holmes, R.K. (1981b). Regulation of toxinogenesis in *Corynebacterium diphtheriae* II. Genetic mapping of a *tox* regulatory mutation in bacteriophage β. *Journal of Virology*, **37**, 946–954.

Williams, P.H. (1979). Novel iron uptake system specified by ColV plasmids: an important component in the virulence of invasive strains of *Escherichia coli*. *Infection and Immunity*, **26**, 925–932.

Williams, P.H., and George, H.K. (1979). ColV plasmid-mediated iron uptake and the enhanced virulence of invasive strains of *Escherichia coli*. In *Plasmids of Medical, Environmental and Commercial Importance*, (Eds. K.N. Timmis and N. Puhler), pp. 161–172. Elsevier–North Holland Biomedical Press, Amsterdam.

Williams, P.H., and Warner, P.J. (1980). ColV plasmid-mediated, Colicin V-independent iron uptake system of invasive strains of *Escherichia coli*. *Infection and Immunity*, **29**, 411–416.

Wolf, M.K. and Crosa, J.H. (1986). Evidence for the role of a siderophore in promoting

Vibrio anguillarum infections, **132**, (in press).
Zink, D.L., Freeley, J.C., Wells, J.G., Vanderzant, C., Vickery, J.C., Roof, W.D., and O'Donovan, G.A. (1980). Plasmid-mediated tissue invasiveness in *Yersinia enterocolitica*. *Nature*, **283**, 224–226.

Iron and Infection
Edited by J.J. Bullen and E. Griffiths

Chapter 5

Iron-binding proteins and host defence

E. GRIFFITHS
National Institute for Biological Standards and Control, Holly Hill, Hampstead, London NW3 6RB, England

J.J. BULLEN
Department of Surgery, University of Miami School of Medicine, Jackson Memorial Medical Center, PO Box 016310, Miami, Florida 33101, USA.

1. INTRODUCTION

The multiplication of bacteria in the largely undefined and changing environment of host tissues is an essential feature of any infection and an ability to interfere with this process plays a major role in host resistance to infection. In this chapter we consider the nature of host antibacterial systems based directly on the iron-binding proteins.

It is now known that the amount of iron that might normally be readily available to bacteria in the tissue fluids of humans and animals is extremely small and that this iron-restricted environment induces phenotypic changes both in the metabolism and in the composition of the outer membranes of bacteria growing *in vivo* (Bullen, 1981; Griffiths, 1983a 1983b, 1985). Body iron is held primarily intracellularly, as ferritin, haemosiderin or haem, and that which is extracellular in serum of other body fluids is attached to the high affinity iron-binding glycoproteins, transferrin and lactoferrin (see Chapters 2 and 3). Growth of bacterial pathogens in the presence of partly saturated iron-binding glycoproteins can lead to the synthesis and secretion of siderophores, to the production of new outer membrane proteins and to changes in transfer RNAs (Griffiths, 1983a, 1983b, 1985; see also Chapters 3 and 4). Such alterations are considered necessary features of cellular economy during the stress of iron-restricted growth, and some phenotypic changes are known to be essential for the acquisition of iron by the bacteria under these environmental conditions. Bacteria which cannot sequester iron *in vivo* are unable to proliferate. However, bacteria which are able to do so, and adapt to and multiply under these iron-restricted growth conditions, sometimes grow more slowly than the iron-replete organisms; the consequences of this are discussed below. Also, it has been found that bacteria which can multiply perfectly well in the presence of an iron-binding glycoprotein *in vitro* are sometimes unable to do so in body fluids such as serum, human milk or bovine colostrum. These body fluids contain not only large amounts of the iron-binding proteins but also other host components such as antibodies and complement factors, and the ability of certain antibodies to inhibit siderophore-mediated iron-uptake systems and to interfere with bacterial iron supply is considered in Section 3. The part played by mechanisms such as these in the ability of human milk to protect neonates against enteric infections is discussed in Section 4.

2. IRON-BINDING PROTEINS ACTING ALONE

2.1 Bacteriostatic effects

There are organisms which, quite simply, are unable to multiply in the presence of partly saturated iron-binding proteins. Such organisms appear to lack a mechanism for removing the iron from transferrin, lactoferrin or ovotransferrin. Some of these bacteria are avirulent strains derived from normally pathogenic organisms such as, for example, strains of *Vibrio anguillarum* which have lost the plasmid pJMl. Highly virulent strains of the fish pathogen *V.anguillarum* carry a 65 kb plasmid designated pJMl which encodes an efficient iron-uptake system that allows the organism to grow in the presence of transferrin (Crosa, 1980; Crosa and Hodges, 1981; see also Chapter 4); on losing this plasmid *V.anguillarum* loses its ability to grow under iron-restricted conditions and also its virulence for fish. Only strains which have the ability to acquire iron *in vivo* are virulent and cause disease. In contrast, *Vibrio vulnificus* is an organism which does not appear to have an efficient high affinity iron-uptake system of its own, although it does possess several other potential virulence factors (Carruthers and Kabat, 1981; Kreger and Lockwood, 1981; Smith and Merkel, 1982). Normally, this organism causes only localized wound

Table 1 Bleomycin-detectable iron in the sera of patients with idiopathic haemochromatosis. Results are the means of duplicate assays on each serum sample

Patient code	Total non-haem iron in serum (μmol/l)	Bleomycin-detectable iron (μmol/l)	Comments
A	115.0	19.4	Newly diagnosed, heavily iron-loaded
B	45.0	1.9	Recently diagnosed, iron-loaded
C	71.0	1.3	Newly diagnosed, iron-loaded
D	43.0	1.3	Previously venesected, reaccumulating iron
D	64.0	4.4	Further iron accumulation (sample taken 3 months later)
E	31.0	0.0	Highly venesected, anaemic
F	38.0	0.0	Hepatoma patient
G	31.0	0.0	Highly venesected
H	51.0	0.7	On maintenance venesection
I	62.0	1.4	On maintenance venesection
Normal controls (6)	24.9±4.4	0.0	—

The presence of 'free' iron is tested for by utilizing the fact that the antibiotic bleomycin requires the presence of iron salts in order to degrade DNA. Suitable calibration of the DNA degradation allows the 'available' iron content of body fluids to be determined. Iron bound to transferrin is unreactive in the bleomycin assay.

From Gutteridge et al. *(1985). Reprinted by permission from The Biochemical Society, London.*

infections in humans and it has been suggested that traces of free haem may serve as a source of iron in this location (Helms, Oliver and Travis, 1984; Chart and Griffiths, 1985). However, in individuals who are suffering from iron-overload diseases, such as haemochromatosis, *V.vulnificus* can cause life-threatening septicaemias which are extremely difficult to control. It has been shown that it is the presence of freely available iron, which is often present in the serum of such individuals (Gutteridge *et al.*, 1985; Table 1), that allows this organism to multiply so rapidly and to cause septicaemia (Chart and Griffiths, 1985); sera from normal individuals do not contain freely available iron.

Figure 1(a) shows how the growth of *V.vulnificus* in broth is inhibited by the presence of ovotransferrin, an effect which is readily reversed by the addition of ferric dicitrate. Figure 1(b) shows how *V.vulnificus* is unable to grow in normal human serum but multiplies rapidly in the sera from patients with

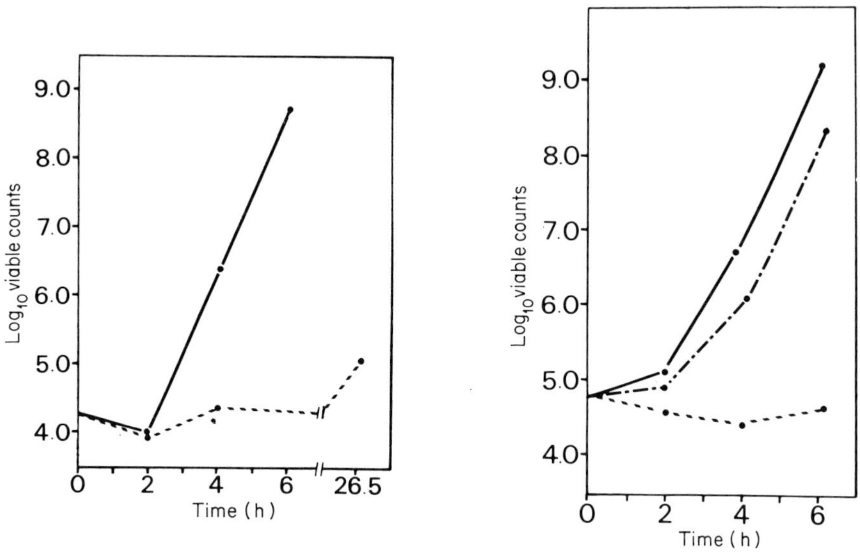

(b)

Figure 1 (a) Graph showing the rapid growth of *V. vulnificus* in trypticase soy broth (——) and the contrasting poor growth in trypticase soy broth containing ovotransferrin (----). The addition of ferric dicitrate (70 μg/ml) to the broth containing ovotransferrin allowed rapid bacterial growth and resulted in a growth curve virtually identical to that obtained with the organism in broth alone (data not shown). (b) Graph showing the ability of *V. vulnificus* to multiply in two 'haemochromatosis' sera (——, —·—) whilst being unable to grow in normal human serum (----). Adding ferric dicitrate to the normal serum resulted in the same rapid growth of the organisms in normal serum as seen in the 'haemochromatosis' serum (data not shown). *From Chart and Griffiths (1985). Reproduced by permission of* FEMS Microbiology Letters

haemochromatosis; adding iron to normal human serum also allows rapid multiplication of the organism. Thus, *V. vulnificus* is an organism that appears to have all the determinants for virulence except the ability to remove iron from unsaturated iron-binding proteins. It therefore cannot grow in the blood and tissues of normal individuals who possess unsaturated transferrin and lactoferrin, although it is resistant to the bactericidal effects of plasma and produces both cytolysin and proteases (Carruthers and Kabat, 1981; Kreger and Lockwood, 1981; Smith and Merkel, 1982). It may be argued, therefore, that the normally partly saturated iron-binding glycoproteins protect the host against potentially lethal infections caused by such organisms. It is very likely, of course, that there are innumerable organisms in the environment which are unable to sequester iron from iron-binding proteins but which pose little threat of infection, even to iron-overloaded individuals, since these organisms also lack other virulence factors.

The various ways in which pathogens remove iron from iron-binding proteins are discussed in Chapter 3. Some are seen to have evolved highly specific iron-uptake systems, capable of removing iron from only certain of the iron-binding proteins and not from all of them. These highly specific iron-uptake systems seem not to involve siderophores but to depend, instead, on a direct contact being made between the organism and the iron-binding protein concerned. For example, all strains of *Neisseria gonorrhoeae* and *N.meningitidis* are able to use the iron in transferrin, whereas most commensal species of *Neisseria* are unable to do so (Mickelsen and Sparling, 1981; Simonson, Brener and DeVoe 1982). Similarly, although all meningococci can obtain iron from lactoferrin, only about 50 per cent of gonococci and 25 per cent of commensal *Neisseria* species can do so (Mickelsen, Blackman and Sparling, 1982). Strains which are unable to remove iron from the iron-binding protein cannot multiply in the presence of that protein. Neither the gonococci nor the meningococci can remove iron from partly saturated ovotransferrin (Archibald and DeVoe, 1979; Mickelsen and Sparling, 1981). *Haemophilus influenzae* type b is another organism which has a very specific iron-uptake system; it is able to remove iron from transferrin but not from human lactoferrin (Herrington and Sparling, 1985). The non-pathogenic microorganism *H.parainfluenzae*, however, is unable to obtain iron from either transferrin or lactoferrin. Whether such specificities play a part in restricting the growth of these organisms to particular ecological niches in the human body remains to be seen, but it is very likely that they do have some influence. It has been suggested that those organisms which cannot ultilize the iron in lactoferrin, but which nevertheless clearly survive on mucosal surfaces, use the haem released by dying cells sloughed from the epithelium as a source of iron (Mickelsen, Blackman and Sparling, 1982).

Although the various high affinity iron-uptake systems used by pathogenic bacteria to acquire iron from iron-binding glycoproteins are often very efficient and allow the organisms to grow well under such conditions, some iron-restricted organisms do, in fact, multiply at a slower rate than the iron-replete cells. For example, certain strains of *Escherichia coli* have a doubling time of about 35 minutes when growing *in vitro* in the presence of an iron-binding protein, but this is reduced to approximately 25 minutes when iron is freely available in the medium (Griffiths and Humphreys, 1978). Similarly, iron-replete *Pseudomonas aeruginosa* grow with a doubling time of about 30 minutes, but in the presence of transferrin or lactoferrin this time is increased to 72 minutes (Bullen, Ward and Wallis 1974). Even a modest reduction in the rate of bacterial growth can make a big difference to the size of a bacterial population over a matter of hours, and this might be crucial in deciding the outcome of an infection. In fact, the growth of many organisms has been shown to be retarded by transferrin or lactoferrin. Reducing the rate of bacterial multiplication gives the host an advantage in that it has time to mount other defensive actions which may be able to control the infection. In contrast, supplying free iron in one form or another will bypass the effects of the iron-binding proteins on the bacteria and will abolish the need for a pathogen to go into what might be termed the iron-stressed state. The organisms will grow faster and will be phenotypically different from the iron-restricted bacteria; no siderophores will be produced, the tRNAs will be unchanged and no new iron-regulated outer membrane proteins will be expressed. Such an increase in the rate of bacterial multiplication may be sufficient to tip the balance in favour of an invading pathogen, other host defences then being unable to contain the infection. This is well illustrated by experimental peritoneal infections with both *Ps.aeruginosa* and *E.coli* (Bullen, Leigh and Rogers, 1968; Bullen, Ward and Wallis, 1974). In both cases, sublethal doses of bacteria grow for a few hours and then decline. In animals injected with ferric ammonium citrate or haematin, however, the same sublethal dose multiplies rapidly and kills the animals. In the case of *Ps.aeruginosa* it was shown that the cellular response was the same with and without iron (see Chapter 6). Experiments such as these show clearly how the outcome of an infection depends on a multiplicity of factors, including the rate of bacterial multiplication and the size of the infective dose, as well as the ability of the host to elicit a polymorph response. Highly virulent organisms which can both multiply successfully under iron restriction and resist other host defences might be expected to be little affected by added iron. It is interesting to note that repeated passage of a strain of *Ps.aeruginosa* made it so virulent for mice that the lethal dose was reduced to approximately ten organisms. In these circumstances the injection of iron had no observable effect, which was not surprising, since it would be difficult to measure a further increase in virulence (Forsberg and Bullen, 1972). However, the point should be made that it is not known whether passage selected a strain of *Ps.aeruginosa* with a more effective iron-uptake system than before or an organism with the same iron-uptake mechanism as the unpassaged bacteria but with greater resistance to other host defences.

2.2 Bactericidal effects

Quite apart from the effects of host iron-binding proteins in simply inhibiting the multiplication of some organisms and retarding the growth of others, there are reports that apolactoferrin has bactericidal activity (Bishop *et al.*, 1976; Arnold, Cole and McGhee, 1977; Arnold *et al.*, 1981, 1982). Arnold and his colleagues (1980–1982) have shown that apolactoferrin, in distilled water, kills a wide range of microorganisms including *E.coli, V.cholerae, Ps.aeruginosa* and streptococci. Figure 2 shows the bactericidal effect of apolactoferrin on *Streptococcus mutans*. However, not all streptococci and *E.coli* are susceptible to killing in this system, and several other organisms, such as *Salmonella newport*,

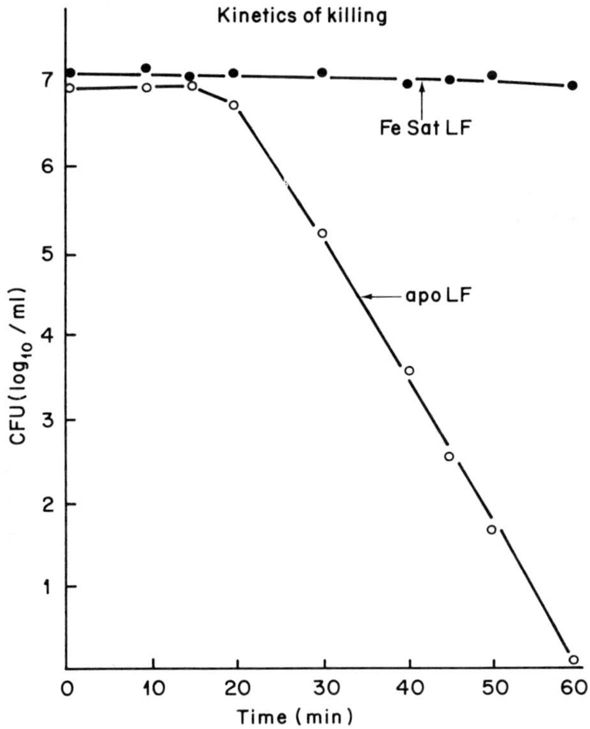

Figure 2 Viability of *S.mutans* harvested in the early exponential phase, incubated at 37°C with apolactoferrin (apoLF;1.2 μ*M*) or with iron-saturated lactoferrin (FesatLF;1.2 μ*M*). *From Arnold* et al. *(1981). Reproduced by permission of the American Society for Microbiology*

Shigella sonnei and staphylococci, are not affected. The bactericidal effect observed with susceptible bacteria is rapid, occurring within about an hour, and it cannot be reversed by iron, although iron-saturated lactoferrin itself has no bactericidal activity. Arnold *et al.* (1981) suggest that the loss of activity seen on saturating the binding capacity of the glycoprotein with iron results from a conformational change in the molecule (Mazurier *et al.*, 1976). Direct contact between the bacterial cell surface and apolactoferrin appears to be essential for killing to take place and death of the organism follows after a lag phase of about 15 minutes (Fig. 2). The process is also energy dependent, no killing taking place at 2°C, and organisms harvested in the exponential phase of growth are markedly more susceptible than those in the stationary phase (Arnold *et al.*, 1981). Furthermore, no bactericidal activity is seen at pH 8, the optimum effect being observed at pH 5.

Detailed studies with *S.mutans* have shown that the killing process involves the inhibition of glucose uptake and metabolism, as well as the inhibition of macromolecular synthesis as determined by the incorporation of ^{14}C-labelled uracil, thymidine and lysine. In this and certain other respects, the bactericidal effect of apolactoferrin on bacteria shows interesting similarities to the bactericidal action of specific antibody, complement and transferrin, acting in concert, on *Pasteurella multocida* and to the action of colicins on susceptible organisms (Griffiths, 1971a, 1971b, 1974b, 1975; Holland, 1975; see also Section 3.2). It is certainly not mediated by simple deprivation of iron. The relevance of the bactericidal effect of apolactoferrin seen *in vitro*, in what might appear to be a rather artificial system, to the various antibacterial systems operating *in vivo* is not clear. Indeed, it has been suggested that the effect might be due to traces of contaminants, such as lactoperoxidase, present in the apolactoferrin preparations used and not to the apolactoferrin itself (Reiter, 1984; Boesman-Finkelstein and Finkelstein, 1985). On the other hand, it is also possible that the bactericidal action of human apolactoferrin does make a direct contribution to the intracellular killing mechanism operating within neutrophils (Bullen and Wallis, 1977; Bullen and Armstrong, 1979; Bullen, 1981; Spitznagel, 1983; see also Chapter 6) and clearly should be investigated further.

3. IRON-BINDING PROTEINS ACTING IN CONJUNCTION WITH OTHER HOST FACTORS

3.1 Bacteriostatic effects

It has been known for many years that certain microorganisms are susceptible to the bactericidal action of fresh serum (Taylor, 1983) and also that many organisms which are not actually killed outright in serum fail to multiply; the bacteriostatic effects of serum can be clearly seen in heat-inactivated serum. Sometimes this inability to multiply in serum may be due simply to the failure of the organism to sequester iron from transferrin, as discussed above. However, in other cases it has been shown that an organism may be capable of removing iron from transferrin and of multiplying well in the presence of an iron-binding protein alone, but is unable to do so in serum (Rogers, 1967, 1973). A smiliar phenomenon is seen in the case of human milk and bovine colostrum, where again an organism capable of multiplying well in the presence of lactoferrin is found to be unable to grow in whole milk or colostrum (Bullen, Rogers and Leigh, 1972; Reiter, Brock and Steel, 1975; Griffiths and Humphreys, 1978; Rogers and Synge, 1978; Spik *et al.*, 1978; Stephens *et al.*, 1980). In each case, serum, milk and colostrum, the bacteriostatic effect can be abolished by adding iron in various forms, strongly suggesting that other components present in these body fluids interfere with some aspects of bacterial iron-uptake mechanisms. For example, serum albumin has been reported to bind the siderophore enterobactin and to decrease its effectiveness in serum and to impede enterobactin-mediated mobilization of iron from transferrin (Konopka and Neilands, 1984; see also Chapter 3). In other cases, antibodies have been shown to be involved in inducing bacteriostasis in the presence of iron-binding proteins (Rogers, 1967, 1976; Bullen, Rogers and Leigh, 1972; Rogers and Synge, 1978; Spik *et al.*, 1978). Of course, the involvement of antibodies introduces a degree of specificity into the system and it is known that a single sample of human milk or bovine colostrum may inhibit one but not another serotype of *E.coli* (Fig. 3) (Griffiths and Humphreys, 1978).

Although it is generally agreed that, in some cases, the presence of both a partly saturated iron-binding protein and an antibody is required to produce bacteriostasis, there is no overall agreement as to the mechanism involved in the inhibitory process. Indeed, it is not always clear with which antigen or antigens such antibodies react. The work of Moore *et al.*(1980) and Moore and Earhart (1981) suggests that normal human serum contains antibodies, apparently IgA, specific for enterobactin which, when acting in concert with transferrin, limit the growth of *E.coli* strains which depend entirely on this iron-sequestering system. These antibodies appear to block enterobactin-mediated iron uptake but not the uptake of iron from ferrichrome or citrate. Since enterobactin is an aromatic molecule it may well adhere to protein, possibly albumin, and act as a hapten for generating antibodies. Another immune mechanism has been described by

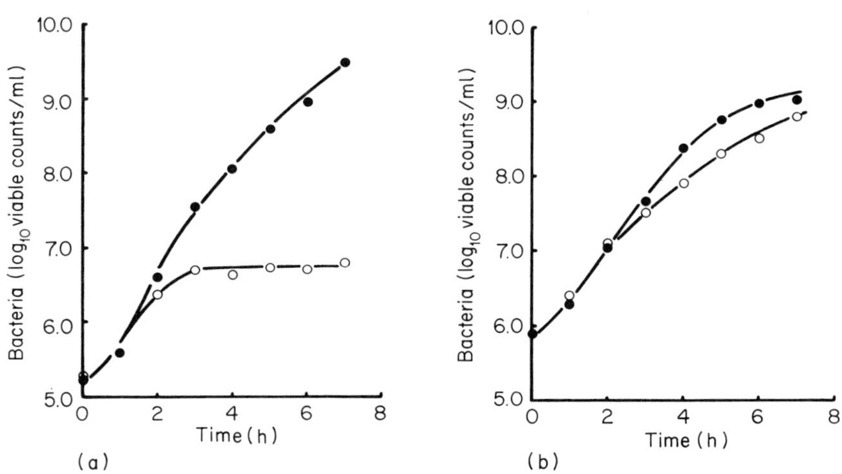

Figure 3 Effect of human milk on the growth of *E.coli*. (a) Bacteriostatic action on *E.coli* 026(○) and its abolition by iron (●). (b) Growth of *E.coli* 0141 in the same batch of human milk used in (a) (○) and in the milk containing added iron (●). In both cases, sufficient iron was added, as ferric dicitrate, to oversaturate the iron-binding capacity of the lactoferrin present in the milk. *From Griffiths and Humphreys (1978). Reproduced by permission of The Federation of European Biochemical Societies*

Fitzgerald and Rogers (1980) who studied serotype specific horse serum antibodies and secretory IgA in human milk. These antibodies, which also act in conjunction with transferrin or lactoferrin to inhibit the multiplication of *E.coli*, appear to interfere with enterobactin synthesis or secretion. It has been suggested that the antibodies involved recognize colitose, which is the terminal sugar of the O-specific side-chain of the lipopolysaccharide of the serotype of *E.coli* used in these experiments, *E.coli*, 0111, and block the production of enterobactin, thus depriving the bacteria of essential iron (Rogers, 1983). Although Brock *et al.* (1983) also concluded that bacteriostasis resulted from the blocking by antibodies of the production or secretion of enterobactin, they found no clear correlation between the bacteriostatic activity and antibodies to the classical O, K and H antigens of *E.coli*. The broader specificity of the antibodies involved in bacteriostasis is also suggested by the work of Dolby and Honour (1979) and by Dolby and Stephens (1983) using human milk, and by that of Reiter (1978b) with bovine colostrum. The results of Dolby and Stephens (1983) suggest that although there are specific anti-O antibodies present in the IgA fraction of human milk, their activity accounts for only a small part of the lactoferrin-dependent bacteriostatic action of whole milk. Clearly, more work is required before all aspects of the growth inhibitory properties of milk are fully understood and it is quite likely that several mechanisms will be found to be acting together. Samson, Mirtle and McClelland (1979) claimed that the addition if IgA to milk 'deficient' in IgA did not enhance its bacteriostatic activity. However, the samples of 'deficient' milk contained approximately 9 mg of IgA per 100 ml. This in itself could be sufficient for bacteriostasis and it is therefore scarcely surprising that the addition of more IgA did not enhance the effect. Recently, antibodies of the IgA class which react with the iron-regulated outer membrane proteins of *E.coli* have been detected in some but not all samples of human milk (Griffiths and Stevenson, unpublished data). Naturally occurring antibodies that react with the iron-regulated outer membrane proteins of *E.coli*, including the siderophore receptors, have also been found in sera from normal healthy human adults as well as in sera from mice, rabbits and guinea-pigs (Griffiths *et al.*, 1985a) (Fig. 4); these particular antibodies were either absent or barely detectable in sera from human infants. The use of murine monoclonal antibodies specific for either IgG or IgM showed that the anti-siderophore receptor antibodies present in human serum, as well as antibodies to the ompA protein, were predominantly of the IgG class. It is not known yet whether such antibodies inhibit siderophore-mediated iron uptake or contribute to the bacteriostatic action of sera and milk. Specific antibodies raised in rabbits to the 78kDa FhuA protein of *E.coli*, which is the receptor for the siderophore ferrichrome as well as for bacteriophage T5, were found only to partially inhibit ferrichrome-promoted iron transport (Coulton, 1982). However, these anti-bodies did block completely the adsorption of the T5 phage on to the 78kDa protein. The results suggest that these antibodies are binding to sites which allow

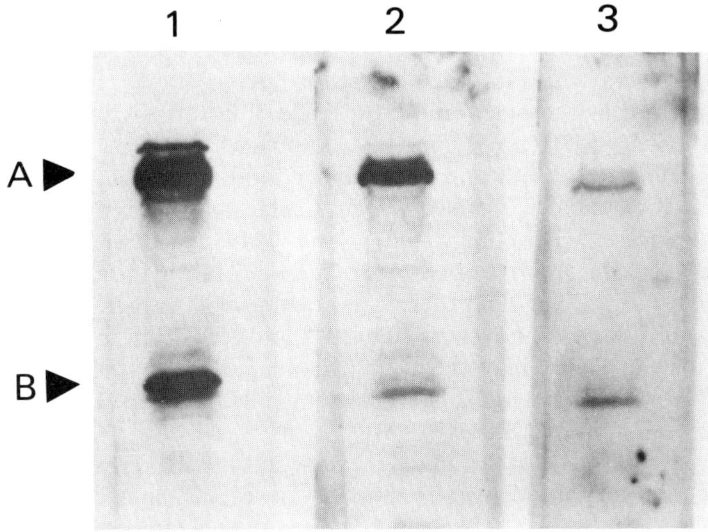

Figure 4 Immunoblots of the separated outer membrane proteins of *E.coli* 0111 reacted with normal human adult serum (100 μl per lane). Bacteria were grown in trypticase soy broth containing ovotransferrin. Serum samples 1, 2 and 3 were from three different individuals. Arrows indicate the approximate positions of the iron regulated membrane proteins (A) and of *omp*A (B). *From Griffiths* et al *(1985a). Reproduced by permission of the American Society for Microbiology*

only partial masking of the domain involved in iron uptake via ferrichrome. Further work is required to see if the same applies to antibodies reacting with the enterobactin receptor.

An interesting aspect of the bacteriostatic effect of milk and colostrum on *E.coli* is the fact that the inhibition of some strains is seen only when bicarbonate is added to the system, whereas other strains are inhibited in the absence of added bicarbonate (Bullen, Rogers and Leigh, 1972; Reiter, Brock and Steel, 1975; Dolby, Stephens and Honour, 1977; Griffiths and Humphreys, 1977; Brock *et al.*, 1983). Human milk and bovine colostrum both contain large amounts of citrate (Peaker and Linzell, 1975; Reiter, Brock and Steel, 1975) and it has been shown that this can make iron available to some strains of *E.coli* (Griffiths and Humphreys, 1977). Citrate-mediated release of the iron bound by transferrin or lactoferrin appears to be blocked by excess bicarbonate and its presence permits the inhibition of bacterial growth to occur. Bicarbonate is known to be essential for the binding of iron by transferrin and lactoferrin, the carbonate/bicarbonate ion forming an integral part of the complex (Aisen *et al.*, 1967; Masson and Heremans, 1968; Schlabach and Bates, 1975; see also Chapter 2). Furthermore, citrate is known to be capable of displacing the bicarbonate from the glycoproteins and to mobilize the iron (Bates, Billups and Saltman, 1967; Aisen and Leibman, 1968; Schlabach and Bates, 1975). Increased bicarbonate levels favour the formation of a stable Fe^{3+}–transferrin–bicarbonate ternary complex in the presence of citrate (Aisen and Leibman, 1968; Schlabach and Bates, 1975). It is not known why the growth of some strains of *E.coli* is inhibited by milk and colostrum in the absence of added bicarbonate, but it is tempting to speculate that these particular strains lack a citrate-mediated iron-uptake system (Rosenberg and Young, 1974; see Chapter 3) and would therefore be unaffected by the presence of ferric–citrate in the medium. It should be mentioned, however, that there is no evidence to suggest that the citrate-mediated mobilization of iron found in milk and colostrum *in vitro* reflects the situation *in vivo*. Citrate may well be absorbed rapidly *in vivo* and it is known that bicarbonate is present in intestinal secretions (Griffiths and Humphreys, 1977; Delachaume-Salem and Sarles, 1970).

Whatever the details of the actual mechanisms involved in the bacteriostatic action of antibodies and iron-binding glycoproteins, it is thought that this process plays an important part in host defences. the bacteriostatic action of IgG and transferrin acting together is considered to operate mainly in serum, and of secretory IgA and lactoferrin together in secretions bathing mucosal surfaces. The combined action of secretory IgA and lactoferrin is also thought to play an important part in breast milk's protective effect against neonatal enteritis caused by *E.coli*; a similar function is attributed to the IgG and lactoferrin present in bovine colostrum. This is discussed in detail in Section 4. The presence of freely available iron *in vivo* would negate all such defences including those resulting from the action of iron-binding proteins acting alone (Section 2), and it is well known that animals injected with iron in various forms are much more susceptible to various bacterial infections than the untreated control animals (Bullen, 1981; Griffiths, 1983b; see also Chapter 1).

3.2 Bactericidal effects

Although the enhancement of experimental bacterial infections in animals by iron compounds appears in many cases to be due to iron acting as a nutrient, there is evidence which suggests that iron may also sometimes interfere with the activities of other antibacterial systems (Griffiths, 1975; Kochan, Wasynczuk and McCabe, 1978; Kochan, Wagner, and Wasynczuk, 1984). It has been suggested that a distinction should be made between the role of iron compounds in providing an essential growth factor and their ability to abolish the bactericidal action of certain sera (Griffiths, 1975). Specific antibody, transferrin and a heat labile factor in fresh serum, which appears to be complement, have been implicated in the bactericidal action of sera on *Pasteurella multocida* (originally known as *Pasteurella septica*); this antibacterial effect can be abolished by adding

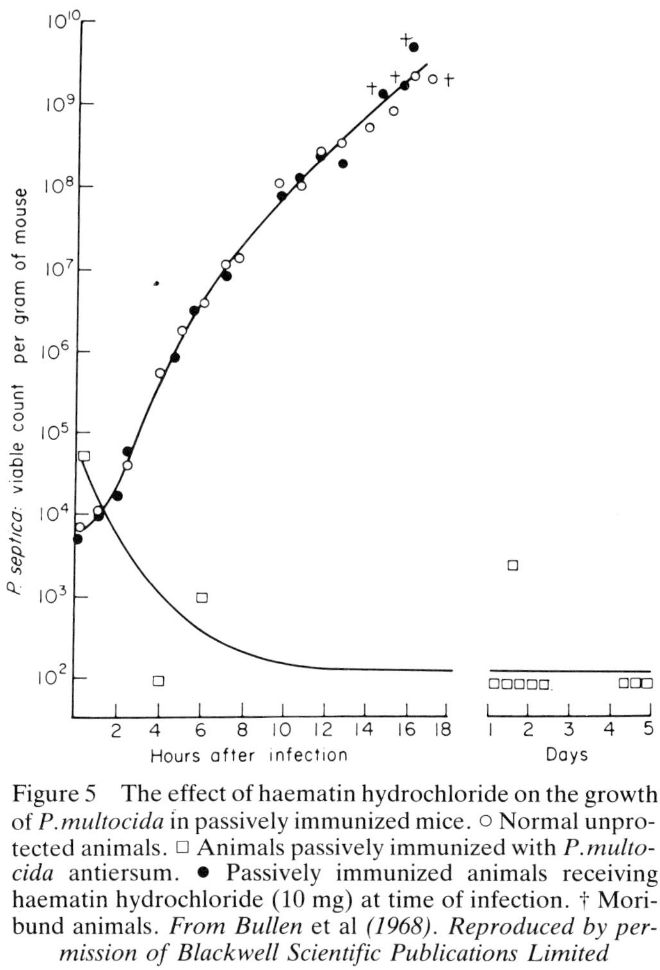

Figure 5 The effect of haematin hydrochloride on the growth of *P.multocida* in passively immunized mice. ○ Normal unprotected animals. □ Animals passively immunized with *P.multocida* antiersum. ● Passively immunized animals receiving haematin hydrochloride (10 mg) at time of infection. † Moribund animals. *From Bullen* et al *(1968). Reproduced by permission of Blackwell Scientific Publications Limited*

iron compounds. *Pasteurella multocida* is an organism which can be highly virulent for mice with a lethal dose of <10 organisms. In normal animals, the bacteria grow rapidly with viable counts rising from 10^4/g tissue to 10^9/g in 16 hours. Specific antibody is highly protective and the viable counts in protected animals decline rapidly, although the bacteria do persist in low numbers for several days (Fig. 5). The protective effect of specific antibody can be completely reversed by injecting haematin hydrochloride along with the bacteria (Fig. 5). Ferric ammonium citrate (5 mg Fe/kg) has a similar though less well-marked effect. The striking feature of the experiments involving haematin is that the bacteria grow at the same rate as in normal unprotected animals, in spite of the presence of a normally protective dose of *P.multocida* antiserum (Bullen *et al.*,

1968). The effects of iron on *P.multocida in vivo* are closely paralleled *in vitro* where it has been shown that specific antibody, complement and partly saturated transferrin are all essential for the bactericidal effect seen in normal serum to which has been added a small amount of *P.multocida* antiserum. Experiments involving radioactive labels have shown that the inhibitory process

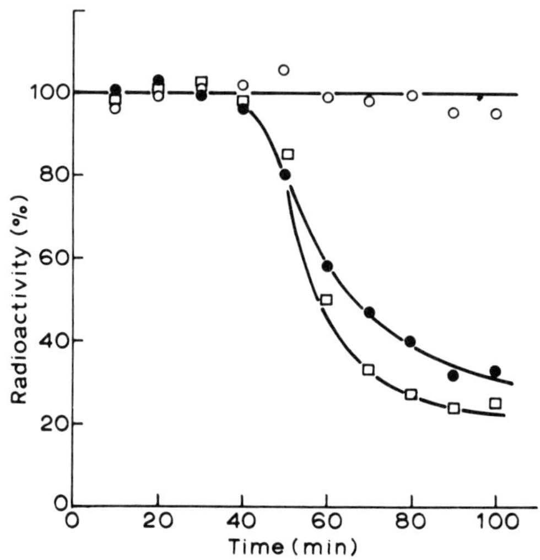

Figure 6 The effect of 2,4-dinitrophenol on antiserum-induced RNA breakdown in *P.multocida*. Specific antiserum was added at time 0 to bacteria prelabelled with ^{14}C-uracil growing in normal horse serum under controlled conditions. □ Antiserum alone added; note the delay of about 40 minutes before degradation of RNA commences; 100% = 4,000 c.p.m. ○ Dinitrophenol added 5 minutes after antiserum; 100% = 3,900 c.p.m. ● Dinitrophenol added 35 minutes after antiserum but before RNA degradation had started; 100% = 3,950 c.p.m. Final dinitrophenol concentration in the serum was $4 \times 10^{-3} M$ in each case. Adding dinitrophenol 5 minutes after adding antiserum also abolished the bactericidal effect of the antiserum, although the growth of the organisms was inhibited. Adding dinitrophenol 35 minutes after antiserum but before the onset of cell death had no effect on the subsequent bactericidal event (data not shown). *From Griffiths (1974b), Reproduced by permission of Elsevier Biomedical Press B.V.*

operates by interfering with the metabolism of the bacterial cell (Griffiths, 1971a, 1971b). Net synthesis of RNA is depressed within 20 minutes of adding specific antiserum to the bacteria growing in fresh normal horse serum and is blocked completely after 40–50 minutes. Protein accumulation proceeds normally for over 40 minutes after the addition of antiserum but stops at about the fiftieth minute. Little loss of label occurs from this fraction, showing that the rapid death which follows the cessation of cell division at 35–40 minutes is not due to gross lysis of the bacterial cell. DNA accumulation continues for up to 90–100 minutes before stopping. Adding iron or haematin reverses these events, with the resumption of net macromolecular synthesis following the same sequence as its initial inhibition.

An interesting feature of this bactericidal effect is the 40 minute delay which elapses between the time of addition of antiserum and the onset of RNA degradation and cell death which occurs soon after the cessation of multiplication at 35–40 minutes (Fig. 6) (Griffiths, 1974a, 1974b). Griffiths (1974b) showed that some metabolic event had to occur before RNA breakdown and killing could be initiated and that this was dependent on bacterial oxidative metabolism (Fig. 6). Thus, the bactericidal effect could be prevented by inhibiting bacterial aerobic metabolism with cyanide or anaerobiosis, or by uncoupling oxidative phosphorylation with 2,4-dinitrophenol or carbonyl cyanide *m*-chlorophenylhydrazone. In this and certain other respects, the bactericidal action of antiserum on *P. multocida* shows interesting similarities to the action of colicins on bacteria (Griffiths, 1974b; Holland, 1975) and to the bactericidal effects of lactoferrin acting alone, as described in Section 2.2. Another antibacterial system which is abolished by adding iron or haematin and also profoundly affected by various respiratory inhibitors, or by agents altering cellular energetics, is the bactericidal action of the cationic proteins from rabbit polymorphonuclear leukocytes on staphylococci (Gladstone and Walton, 1971; Walton and Gladstone, 1976).

The antibacterial action of antiserum on *P. multocida* is also sensitive to small changes in pH. Both the bactericidal effect and the degradation of RNA are abolished when the pH is lowered from 7.4 to 6.8 (Bullen, Rogers and Lewin, 1971; Griffiths, 1974a, 1975). This pH effect resembles the action of haem compounds in that the killing is abolished immediately (Griffiths, 1971b, 1975). This is in contrast to the effect of added ferric iron which does not prevent antiserum from initiating the inhibitory process but does reverse the effects after a delay of 2–3 hours (Griffiths, 1971a, b). It was originally assumed that haem compounds abolished the bactericidal action of antiserum, providing *P. multocida* with a source of available iron or haem (Bullen, Rogers and Lewin, 1971). If this was so, and if depletion of iron or haem from a critical cellular role was the only factor involved in the inhibitory process, then *P. multocida* growing in antiserum in the presence of haem should have behaved like the organisms growing in normal serum. Experiments showed that this was not the case

(Griffiths, 1975). The addition of certain antibiotics to *P.multocida* growing apparently normally in antiserum containing haem compounds led to a rapid killing of the bacteria and to the degradation of their RNA. The same happened when these antibiotics were added to the organisms growing in antiserum at pH 6.8. When the same antibiotics were added to *P.multocida* growing in normal serum, however, only a bacteriostatic effect was seen and no degradation of RNA was observed.

It must be concluded, therefore, that although iron compounds undoubtedly interfere with the bactericidal action of antiserum on *P.multocida*, an explanation of the antibacterial action of antiserum based on an interference by antibody and complement with bacterial iron supply is not sufficient. The process is more complex and must involve other factors (Griffiths, 1975). However, the mechanism whereby surface-bound antibody and complement induce RNA breakdown and cell death in *P.multocida* and the way in which iron compounds counteract these effects is still not clear. What is clear is that the energy-dependent nature of the serum bactericidal reaction is not peculiar to *P.multocida*. Taylor and Kroll (1983) have found that an inhibitor (cyanide) and an uncoupler (2,4-dinitrophenol) of oxidative phosphorylation will inhibit completely the bactericidal action of serum on *E.coli*. Furthermore, *E.coli*, as in *P.multocida*, exposure to serum results in the inhibition of macromolecular synthesis (Melching and Vas, 1971; Martinez and Carroll, 1980; Taylor and Kroll, 1983). Details of the bactericidal and bacteriolytic activity of serum against Gram-negative bacteria and of the possible mechanisms involved have been extensively reviewed by Taylor (1983, 1985).

4. THE PROTECTIVE EFFECT OF MILK

The ability of iron compounds to overcome the antibacterial effects of body fluids *in vitro* is, as discussed above, now well established and correlates with the vastly enhanced susceptibility of iron-treated animals to infection (Bullen, 1981; Griffiths, 1983b; see Chapter 1). Sometimes iron acts as a nutrient and promotes bacterial multiplication and sometimes it may interfere with host antibacterial systems. Since an increased availability or iron exerts such a marked effect on experimental bacterial infections in animals, it might be expected that similar alterations in the availability of iron might lead to reduced resistance to infection in humans. Generally, only freely available iron or haem compounds would be expected to have such an effect, although it is fair to say that little detailed work has been done to examine the influence of increasing the percentage saturation of the iron-binding proteins on various infections. It is important to note that not all iron compounds donate iron equally well to iron-binding proteins and some caution should be exercised when interpreting data from experimental studies in which these have been used. In some cases, it is likely that the available iron comes not from highly saturated transferrin, for example, but from iron complexes bound non-specifically to various plasma proteins (Hegenauer and Saltman, 1975).

Clinical enchancement of infection must arise either by liberation of haem compounds or by increased availability of iron, and this is discussed in detail in Chapter 7. Generally, increasing the availability of iron does predispose humans, like other animals, to infection and this shows how essential it is to restrict the availability of the metal *in vivo*. The key to the importance of iron lies in the fact that it is not normally readily available to invading organisms and that host defences normally operate against an iron-restricted background. Milk and colostrum, like serum, also inhibit the growth of certain organisms and this bacteriostatic effect is overcome by iron. It is pertinent therefore to ask if this inhibitory system operates *in vivo*. Bishop *et al.* (1976) have suggested that lactoferrin is one of the factors which contributes to the protection of the bovine mammary gland itself. The lactoferrin concentration of the exosecretions of the cow's udder varies with the functional state of the gland (Schanbacher & Smith, 1975). In bovine colostrum the concentration of lactoferrin is 2–5 mg/ml and in cow's milk 0.1–0.3 mg/ml. During involution of the gland, the concentration of lactoferrin increases dramatically, attaining levels of 20–30 mg/ml. The lactoferrin concentration also increases significantly during mammary infections (Harmon *et al.*, 1975, 1976). Furthermore, Reiter and Bramley (1975) have shown that the involuted gland is more resistant than the lactating gland to infection with *E.coli*. However, more work is needed in order to evaluate fully the function of the very high levels of lactoferrin seen in the involuted bovine mammary gland. In this section we consider the role of milk in protecting the newborn against infections and, in particular, the part played by the bacteriostatic action of iron-binding proteins and antibodies.

It has long been recognized that human milk has a protective effect against various infections in infants, especially enteric infections. In 1922 Woodbury made an extensive survey of the morbidity and mortality among 22,422 infants born in eight American cities. The feeding regimes were exclusively breast, exclusively artificial and partly breast and artificial. During the first year of life the mortality among the artifically fed infants was nearly four times that of breast-fed infants, while deaths from gastroenteritis were nearly eight times as high. The higher levels of mortality appeared in all ethnic groups and at all levels of family income. The mortality among those partly breast fed was midway between the other two groups. Similar results have been obtained by Robinson (1951). Again, Alexander (1948) recorded a death rate of 4.8 per cent among 456 infants with enteritis, all of whom had been artificially fed. Few breast-fed infants were admitted to hospital with enteritis and with these all that was usually required for their recovery was the maintenance or reestablishment of breast feeding. Giles, Sangster and Smith (1949) described a disastrous outbreak of gastroenteritis involving 207 cases with a mortality of over 50 per cent; of these only four infants had been entirely breast fed. With all of the rest breast feeding had been replaced or supplemented with artifical feeding for at least a week before the onset of symptoms. The significantly lower ($P < 0.01$) incidence of gastroenteritis in breast-fed children in the United States of America has also been noted by Larsen and Homer (1978). A study of Guatemalan Indians living under primitive conditions also showed the benefits of breast feeding: breast-fed infants were better protected against a variety of infections and particularly against enteric diseases caused by *E.coli* and *Shigella* (Mata and Urrutia, 1971). An important finding of this study was that there was a marked increase in the incidence of infection after weaning.

Some workers have shown that fresh human milk can be used to control outbreaks of enteritis caused by *E.coli* even when all other means of control have failed. Svirsky-Gross (1958) found that feeding human milk brought to an end an outbreak of enteritis in premature infants after two years of failure of other forms of treatment, including the use of antibiotics. Tassovatz and Kotsitch (1961) successfully treated a previously uncontrollable epidemic of enteritis in newly born infants caused by the enteropathogen *E.coli* 0111 by feeding unheated human milk; heated milk had no effect.

Clearly, there is a wealth of evidence showing the beneficial and protective effects of breast milk against bacterial infections. More recent studies and reviews have been assembled by Feachem and Koblinsky (1984). However, it is worth emphasizing the fact that primates have the advantage over many other mammals in that transmission of IgG to the young is largely prenatal (Brambell, 1958, 1970). This is vital for preventing systemic bacterial infections. In contrast, animals with epitheliochorial placentation, like the pig and calf, almost invariably die of infections, both systemic and enteric, if deprived of colostrum since they need to absorb protective IgG from the colostrum during the first few hours of life (Porter and Allen, 1978; Morris and Sojka, 1985; Porter *et al.*, 1985). Human babies deprived of colostrum or milk are clearly not so susceptible to such septicaemias, but the evidence suggests that they may lack protective factors in the gut which are provided by milk and they can suffer diarrhoeas that are sometimes fatal. It has been suggested that the protective effects of breast feeding against enteric infections can be best demonstrated in high risk populations subject to considerable environmental contamination such as the lower socioeconomic population of the underdeveloped countries (Chandra, 1977). However, careful studies also show the protective effect of breast feeding for infants in families in high socioeconomic status in developed countries, such as Canada, England, Finland, New Zealand and the United States (Feachem and Koblinsky, 1984).

4.1 The composition of human and bovine milk

Only those aspects of human milk that are involved in resistance to infection are considered here. However, it is important to compare some aspects of human

Table 2 Approximate composition of human and bovine milk

Content/100g	Human milk	Cow's milk
Total proteins (g)	1.3	3.3
Total fats (g)	4.1	3.8
Lactose (g)	7.2	4.7
Calcium (mg)	34	120
Magnesium (mg)	3	12
Sodium (mg)	14	50
Potassium (mg)	58	150
Iron (mg)	0.07	0.05
Zinc (mg)	0.28	0.35
Phosphorus (mg)	14	95
Chlorine (mg)	42	95
Caseins (g)	0.4	2.8
IgA (mg)	100	10
IgG (mg)	4	45
IgM (mg)	10	8
Lactoferrin (mg)	100–300	2–30
Transferrin (mg)	1–2	2–30

Data from Masson and Heremans (1971), Schanbacher and Smith (1975), Ribadeau-Dumas (1983).

milk with cow's milk since most artificial feeds for babies are based on cow's milk. Both milks have a similar content of water and total solids but cow's milk contains about three times the total protein of human milk and the bulk of this difference is due to casein (Table 2). Cow's milk also contains about seven times as much phosphorus and the casein and phosphorus together give it a relatively high buffering capacity. Thus to reduce the pH of cow's milk from 7 to 5 requires three times as much acid as that required for human milk (C.L. Bullen and Willis, 1971). Human milk contains more lactose and a little more fat than Cow's milk (Table 2).

The proportions of immunoglobulins in the two milks are also quite different. The most abundant immunoglobulin in cow's milk is IgG. In bovine colostrum its concentration can be as high as 6g per 100 ml although this value drops rapidly to that of mature milk. In human milk the most abundant immunoglobulin is secretory IgA; in human colostrum its concentration is about 1–2 g per 100 ml and in milk about 0.1 g per 100 ml. Mature human milk contains only small amounts of IgG and IgM; in contrast cow's milk contains small amounts of IgA and IgM (Table 2). In addition human and cow's milk differ greatly in their content of iron-binding protein. Human colostrum can contain as much as 600 mg of lactoferrin per 100 ml, but this falls to 100–300 mg per 100 ml within a few days but remains at this level in mature milk for some time (Masson and

Heremans, 1971). Human milk also contains 1–2 mg of transferrin per 100 ml. Mature cow's milk contains only relatively small amounts of lactoferrin and transferrin, in equal proportion (Table 2). These major differences in both the type and quantity of antibodies and iron-binding proteins present in human and cow's milk are considered to be partly responsible for the important differences seen in the ability of these fluids to control bacterial multiplication. Cow's milk also contains 2–8 times as much citrate as human milk (Jenness, 1974; Peaker and Linzell, 1975).

4.2 The inhibition of bacterial proliferation in the small intestine

Although it is easy to demonstrate the difference between the bacteriostatic activity of human and cow's milk *in vitro*, it is not so easy to show that this property plays a part in protecting the infant against infection. In so complex a matter it is likely that many different factors will be operating. Furthermore, before considering whether or not suppression of bacterial growth by milk components does occur in the small intestine, it must be shown that the potential antibacterial agents present in human milk, such as antibodies and lactoferrin, survive the detrimental effects of low pH in the stomach and also resist proteolytic digestion. As far as the detrimental effect of low pH and digestion in the stomach is concerned, Mason (1962) observed that the pH of the stomach contents of breast-fed infants remained relatively high (pH 6–6.5) for about one hour after feeding. Also, 90 minutes after feeding no hydrolysed

Table 3 Groups of *Escherichia coli* causing diarrhoeal disease: virulence properties

Group	Sero groups	Adhesive factors	Toxins	Genetic control
Enterotoxigenic *E.coli* (ETEC)	Wide variety	Animal:K88, K99, 987P, F41 Human: CFA/I, CFAII(CS1, CS2,CS3)	Heat-labile toxin (LT) Heat-stable toxin (ST)	Mostly plasmid mediated
Enteropathogenic *E.col* (EPEC)	Restricted range, e.g. 0111, 055	Details unknown	Possibly shiga-like toxin	Possibly plasmid mediated
Enteroinvasive *E.coli* (EIEC)	Restricted range e.g. 0164 0124	Properties similar to *Shigella*		Plasmid and chromosomal

protein could be detected in eight specimens of gastric contents. Mason (1962) concluded that in newborn infants the major part of the feed leaves the stomach without any digestion having occurred. It is also known that antibodies present in human milk survive passage through the intestinal canal of newborn infants (Kenny, Boesman and Michaels, 1967; Gindrat *et al.*, 1972) and that IgA is quite resistant to proteolysis by gastrointestinal juice (Brown, Newcomb and Ishizaka, 1970). Some of the lactoferrin in human milk is bound to secretory IgA (Watanabe *et al.*, 1984) and both apolactoferrin and lactoferrin saturated with iron are highly resistant to digestion by proteolytic enzymes (Brines and Brock, 1983). In addition, both human and cow's milk contain protease inhibitors which are effective against trypsin, chymotrypsin and elastase (Lindberg, 1979). Thus, the evidence strongly points to the fact that both the antibodies and lactoferrin in human milk can pass through the stomach undamaged, can survive proteolytic digestion and can function in the upper part of the small intestines of infants.

Epidemiological observations over many years have led to the identification of *E.coli* as a major cause of enteric infections in infants and young children, and it is the way breast feeding controls such infections that is mainly considered here. In recent years it has become clear that three groups of organisms play important roles in the etiology of acute diarrhoea: enterotoxigenic *E.coli* (ETEC), enteropathogenic *E.coli* (EPEC) and enteroinvasive *E.coli* (EIEC) (Rowe, 1979; WHO Scientific Working Group, 1980) (Table 3). It is now recognized that ETEC are an important cause of diarrhoea, including infantile enteritis, in many parts of the world, but more especially in tropical and developing countries. ETEC produce one or both of two well-characterized enterotoxins: a heat-labile enterotoxin (LT) that is immunologically related to cholera toxin and a low molecular weight heat-stable non-antigenic toxin (ST). They also possess filamentous protein appendages on their surfaces called colonization or adhesive factors; these are the pili or fimbriae and enable the organisms to adhere to the mucosal surfaces of the epithelial cells and initiate colonization (Levine, 1981; Klemm, 1985; Parry and Rooke, 1985). For example, the presence of the K88, K99 or 987P fimbriae confers specific adhesive properties on *E.coli* with regard to piglet intestinal epithelium. The K99 antigen together with another fimbrial antigen called F41 enable ETEC to adhere to bovine intestinal epithelium. In human strains of ETEC, the colonization factors are known as CFA1 and CFA2 (CS1, CS2 and CS3). The genes coding for the various toxins and colonization factors found in ETEC are often found on plasmids (Smith, Scotland and Rowe, 1985). Although the ETEC belong to a wide variety of O:K:H serotypes, certain associations between serotypes and specific fimbriation can in fact be identified (Smith, Scotland and Rowe, 1985; Klemm, 1985). Generally, the EPEC belong to a restricted range of serotypes which differ from those to which ETEC and EIEC strains belong; the prototype strains are *E.coli* 0111 B4 and *E.coli* 055 B5. The EPEC group of pathogens are the classical strains shown to be responsible for outbreaks of enteritis in infants in both developing and developed countries. They have been recognized by epidemiological studies combined with serology. Unlike the ETEC, EPEC do not produce the now well-characterized enterotoxins, LT and ST, although it seems that another toxin may be involved in pathogenesis (Edelman and Levine, 1983). The ability of EPEC to colonize the epithelial mucosa of the upper intestines is also important in pathogenesis but, in contrast to ETEC, the mechanisms of adhesion are not known and no well-defined colonization factors similar to those in ETEC have been found (Levine *et al.*, 1985). Since 1960 there has been a noticeable decrease in the incidence of epidemic diarrhoea due to EPEC in developed countries, but the reason for this marked decrease is not known. The third group of pathogenic *E.coli* are the EIEC which produce diarrhoeal disease resembling bacillary dysentry, and these have been shown to be responsible for occasional outbreaks of infantile enteritis. EIEC strains are often atypical biochemically and non-motile, and they resemble *Shigella* (Rowe, 1979; WHO Scientific Working Group 1980; Griffiths *et al.*, 1985b; Smith, Scotland and Rowe, 1985). The best-known serotype is 0164. Like *Shigella*, the EIEC cause dysentry-like disease by invading the epithelium of the large bowel, producing inflammation and ulceration of the mucosa.

Given the evidence that human milk protects against enteritis caused by *E.coli* and that IgA and lactoferrin can survive in the digestive tract, the relevant question becomes one of mechanisms: exactly how does protection occur in the newborn human infant? An obstacle to answering this directly is that samples of intestinal material are not easily obtainable from living infants. Although examination of faeces can give much useful information about conditions in the lower part of the gut, little reliable information can be obtained about conditions in the small intestines. However, there is no reason to suppose that the essential features of protection against enteric infection in babies are any different from those in the young of other mammals. There may, of course, be differences in detail between species, but the fundamental need of maternal milk to suppress unwanted bacterial growth might be expected to be the same for all. In order to cause enteritis pathogenic *E.coli* must establish itself and multiply to large numbers in the small intestine (Rutter *et al.*, 1975; Smith, 1976; Smith and Huggins, 1978; Levine, 1981). Protection by milk or colostrum might, therefore, be expected to operate by preventing the initial adherence of the pathogen or by inhibiting subsequent bacterial multiplication or both.

Kohler (1974) has shown that a very large difference does exist, up to 6×10^6 times, between the viable counts in the small intestines of piglets dying from *E.coli* infections and those protected by colostrum from immunized sows. Similarly, Smith (1972) showed that the viable count of pathogenic *E.coli* in the small intestines of pigs protected by antiserum could be 1000–10,000 times less than in the unprotected controls.

The protective effect of antibodies directed against specific colonization factors has been extensively studied. Anti-fimbrial antibodies have been detected in breast milk (Svanborg-Eden *et al.*, 1979) and several purified fimbrial vaccines prepared from enterotoxigenic *E.coli* have been evaluated in farm animals, including the K88, K99 and 987P antigens (WHO Scientific Working Group, 1980; Beachey, 1981; Levine, 1981; Porter *et al.*, 1985). For example, the purified fimbrial vaccines have been administered to pregnant sows and cows in order to see if the offspring would be protected against diarrhoea. In many cases, protection was indeed seen to correlate with the presence of specific anticolonization factor in the colostrum and with impaired colinization of the ileum by ETEC. Piglets suckling sows parenterally vaccinated with partially purfied K88 fimbriae, which are important in the colonization of piglet small intestine by certain ETEC (Parry and Rooke, 1985), were protected against diarrhoeal disease caused by oral challenge with a $K88^+$ ETEC. Such specific antibodies do not of course protect against challenge with ETEC bearing heterologous fimbriae such as K99 or 987P (WHO Scientific Working Group, 1980; Porter *et al.*, 1985). However, although data obtained from veterinary studies suggest that anti-adhesive antibodies in milk or colostrum may protect the offspring, there are clearly other antibodies present which also contribute to protection. Indeed, work with the K88 antigen in pigs has shown that, in spite of the fact that colonization factor (K88)-mediated adhesion is essential for establishing infection by some strains of ETEC, antibodies that specifically block adhesion are not essential for maintaining protection of the host. Thus, although the K88 antigen is common to many O-serotypes that are pathogenic for piglets, the presence of anti-K88 antibodies in colostrum and milk are not always the essential protective factor in this particular species (Porter and Linggood, 1983; Porter *et al.*, 1985). Observations by Porter and his colleagues on the natural passage of infection from sow to piglet emphasize the importance of carefully considering the route of immunization for inducing passive antibodies. These workers suggest that a capacity for 'curing' pathogenic *E.coli* of the K88 plasmid, i.e. the deletion of the plasmid by means of mucosal antibodies in the gut of the sow and subsequently by milk antibodies in the gut of the offspring is a feature of the protection observed; neither anti-K88 antibodies nor O-antigen-specific antibodies seem to be involved in this process.

As far as the human infant is concerned, it should be recalled that the classical enteropathogenic strains (EPEC) do not have well-defined fimbrial adhesive factors similar to those of ETEC, although adhesion is involved in pathogenesis and breast milk clearly protects (Tassovatz and Kotsitch, 1961). It is possible that different mechanisms operate with different types of pathogenic *E.coli*, the ETEC, EPEC and EIEC, and it is likely that the bacteriostatic action of antibodies acting in conjunction with lactoferrin also plays a significant part in protection. If the bacteriostatic action of antibodies and lactoferrin contributes to protection against *E.coli* in the gut of the newborn, then it would be expected that the effect could be reversed by feeding iron, just as the presence of free iron abolishes the bacteriostatic effect of milk and colostrum *in vitro*. Experiments using guinea-pigs suggested that iron compounds could indeed reverse the protective effect of milk *in vivo*. Suckling guines-pigs can be considered as a reasonable substitute for human babies since guinea-pig's milk contains large amounts of iron-binding proteins, both transferrin and lactoferrin, and like man, transfer of passive immunity to the young is largely prenatal (Brambell, 1958). Bullen, Rogers and Leigh (1972) carried out experiments in which newborn suckling guinea-pigs were dosed orally with approximately 10^6 cells of *E.coli* 0111 and kept with their mothers. At intervals the animals were killed and viable counts made of the numbers of *E.coli* 0111 in the small and large intestines; similar counts were made of the lactobacilli. Results showed that the viable count of *E.coli* declined rapidly in both the small and large intestines and that these organisms were rapidly replaced by a predominant flora of lactobacilli. When the newborn guinea-pigs were separated from their mothers and fed on an artificial diet, the *E.coli* 0111 reached far higher numbers in the intestines, both large and small, compared with suckled animals and the lactobacilli were also far slower in establishing themselves. When suckling newborn animals were dosed orally with 10^6 cells of *E.coli* 0111 together with 50 mg of haematin, then a very large number of *E.coli* 0111 was found in the small intestine, about 10,000-fold more than in animals given *E.coli* 0111 alone. Similarly, the number of *E.coli* 0111 in the large intestines of haematin-treated animals was about 100-fold greater than in the controls (Bullen, Rogers and Leigh, 1972) (Fig. 7). These results have been taken to indicate that the iron-binding proteins present in milk do play a vital role in suppressing the growth of *E.coli* in the gut, especially in the small intestines. However, these experiments need to be repeated, perhaps in other animals, before a protective role for iron-binding protein in the small intestine can be definitely established.

The iron content of human milk is low (Table 2) and it has been suggested that this concentration may not maintain an adequate iron supply for infants, especially when breast feeding continues for more than six months (Saarinen, 1978; Siimes, Vuori and Kuitinen, 1979). Therefore, it has been proposed that breast fed infants be supplemented with iron (Formon *et al.*, 1979). Others have argued that supplementation with large amounts of iron might be deleterious (Addy, 1976; Bullen, Rogers and Griffiths, 1978) and may compromise the antibacterial action of milk in a way similar to the effect of iron compounds *in vitro*. This argument has not yet been resolved but Lonnerdal *et al.* (1980) consider that, ideally, iron supplementation should be carried out without interfering with the bacteriostatic properties of human milk. In this respect it is important to bear in mind the way supplementation might be achieved and that not all iron compounds donate iron equally well to iron-binding proteins (Hegenauer and Saltman, 1975). Supplementation with small amounts of an iron compound which donated its iron poorly to lactoferrin would still leave an undersaturated iron-binding protein but would possibly provide a pool of available iron. Maternal dietary supplementation with iron appears to have no

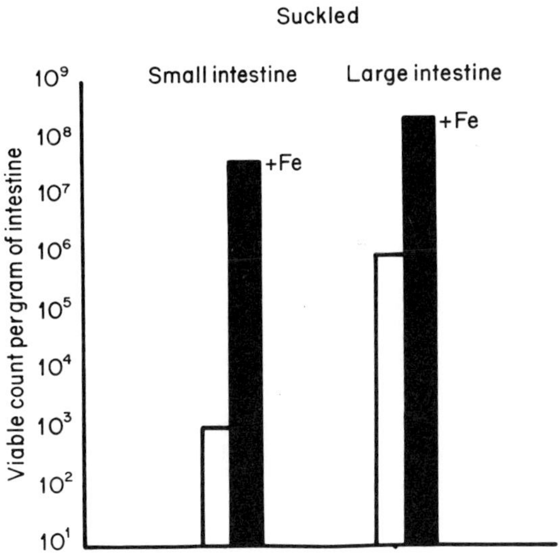

Figure 7 Effect of feeding haematin to suckled guinea-pigs dosed with approximately 1×10^6 *E.coli* 0111 at birth. □ No haematin. ■ Haematin twice daily. Viable counts taken three days after birth. *From Bullen, Rogers and Leigh (1972) Reproduced by permission of the British Medical Association*

effect on the iron content nor the degree of saturation of lactoferrin in breast milk (Reddy *et al.*, 1977; Murray *et al.*, 1978).

Human milk also contains some cells (about 4×10^5/ml). These consist of polymorphs, macrophages, lymphocytes and eosinophils (Robinson, Harvey and Soothill, 1978). It has been shown that these cells can phagocytose and kill *E.coli*, as well as *Staphylococcus aureus*, *in vitro*, and they could undoubtedly have an antibacterial effect in the mammary gland. However, whether they contribute to resistance of the infant is uncertain. Antibody-forming cells have also been detected in human colostrum after oral immunization (Goldblum *et al.*, 1975) and studies show a close relationship between antigenic sensitization by way of the gastrointestinal tract and the development of secretory IgA-producing cells in the milk. Milk and colostrum also contain other antibacterial proteins, such as lysozyme, and it has been suggested that a lactoperoxidase system may play a protective role in the calf (Reiter, 1984) but its role in human milk is unknown (Gothefors and Marklund, 1975; Reiter, 1978a, 1978b, 1984; Reiter and Harnulv, 1984). Of course, milk and colostrum protect against many different organisms and it is unwise to assume that the various antibacterial mechanisms operating in these fluids always operate in the same way against all organisms.

Recent evidence has added to the list of protective properties of milk (Table 4). Murray, Murray and Murray (1980) have shown that drinking bovine milk

Table 4 Possible antibacterial properties and components of human milk operating in the gut

Antitoxin antibodies
Antiadhesive antibodies
Bacteriostatic action of lactoferrin and IgA
Lysozyme
Lactoperoxide
Non-immunoglobulin substances which prevent bacterial adhesion
Non-immunoglobulin substances which prevent action of certain toxins
Factors encouraging growth of *Bifidobacteria*

protects the Masai tribesman in Africa against amoebiasis and that this is linked to the low levels of iron in milk. In a controlled experiment inolving 76 Masai free of *Entamoeba histolytica* infestation and whose diet was largely milk, 35 were given 300 mg of ferrous sulphate twice weekly for a year. Giving iron led to a statistically significant increase in amoebiasis, suggesting that the dietary iron acted to promote infestation directly in the gut. It has been shown that the intestinal protozoan *Giardia lamblia*, which is a major cause of waterborne enteritis in the United States, is rapidly killed by human milk, although the mechanisms involved are not known (Gillin, Reiner and Wang, 1983). In the case of *Vibrio cholerae* infections, Glass *et al.* (1983) have shown that human milk protects against clinical disease but not against colonization with the organisms. Here there was a direct relationship between the level of IgA to *V.cholerae* and protection. Children receiving milk containing high titres of secretory IgA which reacted with cholera toxin or with the lipopolysaccharide of *V.cholerae* developed clinical cholera with significantly lower frequency than those receiving breast milk with lower specific secretory IgA antibody titres, but no less total secretory IgA. Neutralizing antibodies directed against the heat-labile enterotoxin of *E.coli* have also been found in breast milk (Holmgren *et al.*, 1976; Stoliar *et al.*, 1976). However, although some milks contain antibodies which prevent the binding of both cholera and *E.coli* enterotoxins to the receptor ganglioside GM1, there are present non-immunoglobulin substances which also interfere with these binding reactions, at least *in vitro* (Holmgren *et al.*, 1981). In addition, the non-immunoglobulin substances in milk can inhibit haemaglutination mediated by the colonization factors of ETEC, CFA I, CFA II and the K88 antigen, as well as inhibit the action of non-immunogenic low molecular weight heat-stable (ST) enterotoxin of *E.coli* (Holmgren, Svennerholm and Ahren, 1981; Cleary, Chambers and Pickering, 1983). Clearly with such a galaxy of potential protective mechanisms it is difficult to decide which particular mechanism operates in any one case. Of course, it is very likely that more than one mechanism would be operating. In fact, a well-designed protective system might be expected to counteract all three of the crucial steps in the infection process, attachment, multiplication and toxin production.

4.3 The protective effect of the normal gut flora

It is now well appreciated that the protective mechanisms of breast feeding are complex. In addition to the protection afforded by the immunological and direct antimicrobial properties of breast milk, the nature of the intestinal flora established during breast feeding is very different to that found under artificial feeding schemes. This difference, sometimes referred to as the 'Bifidus factor' (Feachem and Koblinsky, 1984), is also considered to play a part in inhibiting the colonization of the gut by Gram-negative species, such as *E.coli*, and is likely to be important mainly in the large intestine.

Breast-fed infants have faeces which are yellowish green in colour, of small bulk, a watery curdled consistency and a 'cheesy' odour. In contrast, bottle fed infants have faeces of large bulk, a firm putty-like consistency and a putrid odour. These differences are fundamental and reflect the composition of the feed and the nature of the bacterial flora in the large intestine. The flora depends upon the substrate provided by the babies' food and it has been found that all artificial feeds produce a gut flora which is profoundly different from that provided by maternal milk (Beerens, Romond and Neut, 1980; C.L. Bullen, 1980). The flora of the premature neonate separated at birth from the mother, housed in a humidicrib and treated from birth with parenteral antibiotics differs from that of both breast-fed and artificially fed healthy full-term babies (Blakey *et al.*, 1982).

Human milk has a relatively high content of lactose, a low level of protein, a low level of phosphate and a poor buffering capacity compared to cow's milk (Table 2; C.L. Bullen and Willis, 1971). Studies by C.L. Bullen and colleagues (C.L. Bullen and Willis, 1971; C.L. Bullen, Tearle and Willis, 1976) showed that the faeces of breast-fed infants had a predominant flora of *Bifidobacteria*, which are Gram-positive anaerobic organisms, with counts in the region of 10^9–10^{11}/g. *E.coli* and *Streptococcus faecium* were present in approximately equal numbers of about 10^7–10^8/g, and *Bacteroides* species and *Clostridia* species at about 10^3–10^6/g. Comparatively few other organisms were encountered. Mata and Urrutia (1971), working with a population exposed to relatively unhygenic conditions, obtained similar but not identical bacteriological results. Overall, the viable counts in the faeces of breast-fed infants were somewhat higher. However, *Bifidobacteria* (10^{11}–10^{12}/g) outnumbered all other bacteria during the first sixteen weeks of life while *E.coli* had average counts of about 10^8/g during the same period. *Bacteroides* species were present at about 10^{10}/g while *Veillanellae* species were present at 10^8–10^{11}/g. Streptococci varied from 10^8 to 10^{11}/g and *Clostridia* species were in the range 10^6–10^{11}/g.

The relatively high level of lactose in human milk, which, incidentally, can be detected in the infant's faeces (C.L. Bullen and Willis, 1971), is believed to be a key factor in the establishment of the characteristic flora (Willis *et al.*, 1973). It is postulated that lactose-fermenting organisms like *E.coli* and *S.faecium* cause a rapid fall in the pH and *Eh* of the gut contents. This is helped by the low buffering capacity of breast milk. A low pH and anaerobic conditions provide ideal conditions for the growth of *Bifidobacteria* and it should be emphasized that the counts of this organism are 10–1,000 times greater than all other bacteria present (Mata and Urrutia, 1971; C.L. Bullen, Tearle and Willis, 1976; C.L. Bullen, 1980). The consequence of very high counts of *Bifidobacteria* is the production of large amounts of acetic acid and the presence of an acetic acid buffer in more than 60 per cent of breast-fed infants during the first week of life (C.L. Bullen, 1980). The pH of the faeces of breast-fed infants between the ages of 7 days and 7 weeks varied from 5.0 to 5.7 (C.L. Bullen and Willis, 1971; C.L. Bullen, Tearle and Willis, 1976; C.L. Bullen, 1980). Within this pH range an acetate buffer either causes bacteriostasis or has a lethal effect on a number of enteric organisms. Bergheim (1940) showed that an acetate buffered medium was lethal to *E.coli* at pH 6.0, whereas the organism grew rapidly in medium without acetate until a pH of 4.5 was reached. Levison (1973) found that *Pseudomonas aeruginosa* was more sensitive to the inhibitory effect of propionic, isobutyric, butyric, acetic and formic acids than *E.coli, K.pneumoniae* or *P.mirabilis*. This was true of all fatty acid concentrations within the pH range 5.5 to 6.5. C.L. Bullen and Tearle (1975) found that an acetate buffered medium (0.2 *M*) was bactericidal at pH 5.0 or below to *E.coli*, *Bacillus fragilis, Ps.aeruginosa, Salmonella typhimurium, Shigella sonnei* and *V.cholerae* El Tor. Between pH 5.0 and 5.8 the medium was strongly bacteriostatic for 24 hours, although slow growth of some organisms did eventually take place. The growth of *B.fragilis* was the least effected while the most sensitive organism was *V.cholerae* which showed no growth at any time. In the absence of acetate buffer, there was no bacteriostatic effect on *E.coli* above pH 4.6. *Bifidobacteria* and *S.faecium* were largely unaffected by the acetate buffer and grew well at pH 4.6 and 5.4 respectively. There is, therefore, good evidence that fatty acids can have a marked bactericidal and bacteriostatic effect on many enteric bacteria within the pH range found in the large intestine of the breast-fed infant. The ability of *Bifidobacteria* to tolerate acetate buffer at low pH may be one reason why this organism has such a dominant position in the large intestine of the breast-fed infant and is able to suppress the growth Gram-negative pathogens which are unable to survive the low pH and presence of acetate. It has also been suggested that the *Bifidobacteria* in large numbers in the intestines of breast-fed infants decreases further the availability of iron for other organisms (Bezkorovainy, 1984; Bezkorovainy, Topouzian and Miller-Catchpole, 1986). In baby guinea-pigs and piglets there is also a large population of lactobacilli in the small intestine (Smith and Jones, 1963; Bullen, Rogers and Leigh, 1972). It is possible that in these animals their presence in the small intestines is important. There are no quantitative data on the bacterial flora of the human infant's small intestine.

The substitution of artificial feeds based on cow's milk for maternal milk means the introduction of a high protein, high phosphorus substrate which has a high buffering capacity; there will also be less lactose supplied. Together these changes encourage the maintenance of a high pH (8–9) which discourages the growth of *Bifidobacteria* and prevents the production of the acetate buffer (C.L. Bullen, 1980). The faeces of bottle-fed infants have relatively high counts of *E.coli, S.faecium, Bacteoides* species, *Clostridia* species, *Proteus* species, *Klebsiella* species and *Ps.aeruginosa*. This putrefactive flora contains relatively low numbers of *Bifidobacteria*, which eventually disappear altogether (C.L. Bullen, Tearle and Willis, 1976). The presence of large numbers of putrefactive organisms, some of which are potential pathogens, could certainly be a disadvantage and may be responsible for the initiation of serious infection. Mata *et al.* (1976) pointed out that infections in breast-fed infants increased with the onset of weaning, together with a change in the faecal flora from the 'breast-fed' to the 'adult' type. If a decline in the intake of breast milk is a disadvantage at weaning it must, clearly, be a greater loss in the artificially fed newborn who is deprived of this asset from birth.

It is also important to remember that supplementary feeding of artificial feeds to breast-fed babies interferes with the establishment of a fermentative flora in the large intestine and seriously delays the appearance of the acetate buffer (C.L. Bullen, 1980). What effect supplementary feeds have on protective mechanisms in the small intestine is unknown. Babies receiving mixed feeds of breast milk and artificial food have a higher mortality and morbidity than those entirely breast fed (see above) and, therefore, every effort should be made to ensure that, where possible, newly born infants receive breast milk alone. The case for natural feeding of infants is also made by Reiter (1978a), Welsh and May (1979), Hanson (1982) and Ribadeau-Dumas (1983).

4.4 The problem of necrotizing enterocolitis in infants

The aetiology of necrotizing enterocolitis in infants has not yet been fully explained but there is enough evidence to suggest that it is closely connected with abnormal bacterial growth in the small intestine. It is primarily a disease of small infants weighing less than 1,500 g (Editorial, 1978) and is characterized by necrosis of the intestinal mucosa, particularly in the ileo-caecal region (Editorial, 1977). It occurs only in those infants who have received food (Editorial, 1978; Goldman, 1980), and the bacterial flora of the small intestine is grossly abnormal (Kliegman, 1979; Lawrence, Bates and Gaul, 1982).

It is surprising that more attention has not been paid to the fact that the great majority of cases occur in artificially fed babies. The protective effect of breast feeding against infection is well established, and as pointed out already protection may be associated with several factors, among them being the bacteriostatic properties of milk itself and the development of a characteristic bacterial flora in the large intestine. It should be emphasized that supplementary feeding interferes with the establishment of the characteristic flora and nullifies the beneficial effect of exclusive breast feeding (C.L. Bullen, 1980). This could account for several reported instances of enterocolitis in breast-fed infants where supplementary feeding had been given. For example, Guinan *et al.* (1979) state that of 39 infants developing enterocolitis only one was exclusively breast fed. Seven infants given breast milk developed the disease but all had received supplementary feeding. Kosloske (1979) quotes two sources (Denes *et al.*, 1970; Stein, 1977) where enterocolitis is alleged to have occurred in breast-fed infants, but in neither communication is there any reference to this, and in fact Stein (1977) states that the low incidence of enterocolitis reported could well have been due to the protective effect of breast milk.

Barlow *et al.* (1974) have provided good evidence that maternal milk protects against experimental enterocolitis. Lesions resembling enterocolitis were induced by subjecting newly born rats to hypoxia. After this treatment, with or without oral doses of *E.coli* or *Klebsiella pneumoniae*, the animals developed enterocolitis if fed artificially, but had no lesions if fed on maternal milk. Similarly, de Lemos, Rogers and McLaughlin (1974) produced mucosal necrosis in newborn goats by feeding hypertonic maternal milk. Animals fed unmodified maternal milk remained normal. All those deprived of maternal milk died of sepsis, which was scarcely surprising since this procedure deprives the young of maternal IgG antibodies normally absorbed from the intestines in the first few hours of life.

Of course, the results of Barlow *et al.* (1974) and de Lemos, Rogers and McLaughlin (1974) do not explain the pathogenesis of enterocolitis, but they reinforce the view that maternal milk is highly beneficial to the newly born. However, there is, as yet, no indication as to which of the antibacterial properties of milk (Table 3) may be important for protecting against enterocolitis. The harmful effects of artificial feeding in relation to gastroenteritis have been discussed already, and there is some circumstantial evidence to show that artificial feeding predisposes to necrotizing enterocolitis (Krouskip, Brown and Sweet, 1974). In addition, Goldman (1980) found that there was a significant correlation between the yearly incidence of enterocolitis and the percentage of infants who had received large increases of artificial food.

Enterocolitis of infants bears a strong resemblance to other infections of the ileum which result from massive bacterial growth associated with overfeeding or the feeding of abnormal diets. In enterotoxaemia of sheep, for example, an essential feature is a sudden change of diet followed by overeating. The bacteria responsible, *Clostridium perfringens* type D, are part of the normal intestinal flora. When the diet is changed, and overeating occurs, large amounts of undigested food in the small intestine provide the substrate for rapid bacterial multiplication. Death is due to toxaemia (Bullen and Scarisbrick, 1957). Similar conditions in man associated with overeating include enteritis necroticans caused by *Cl.perfringens* type C (Murrell *et al.*, 1966; Lawrence and Walker, 1976) and *Cl.per-*

fringens type F (Zeissler and Rassfeld-Sternberg, 1949). Volstead Pedersen *et al.* (1976) suggested that necrotic enterocolitis might be a form of gas gangrene of the bowel. There are indeed many similarities to clostridial myonecrosis, including the production of gas, extensive tissue necrosis and sometimes the presence of large numbers of *Cl.perfringens* type A. However, little is known about the quantitative aspects of the bacteriology of this disease, and it is difficult to decide which bacteria are primarily responsible until these data are available.

REFERENCES

Addy, D.P. (1976). Infant feeding: a current view. *British Medical Journal*, **1**, 1268–1271.

Aisen, P., Aasa, R., Malmstrom, B.G., and Vanngard, T. (1967). Bicarbonate and the binding of iron to transferrin. *Journal of Biological Chemistry*, **242**, 2484–2490.

Aisen, P., and Leibman, A. (1968). Citrate-mediated exchange of Fe^{3+} among transferrin molecules. *Biochemical and Biophysical Research Communications*, **32**, 220–226.

Alexander, M.B. (1948). Infantile diarrhoea and vomiting: a review of 456 infants treated in a hospital for enteritis. *British Medical Journal*, **2**, 973–978.

Archibald, F.S., and DeVoe, I.W. (1979). Removal of iron from human transferrin by *Neisseria meningitidis*. *FEMS Microbiology Letters*, **6**, 159–162.

Arnold, R.R., Cole, M.F., and McGhee, J.R. (1977). A bactericidal effect for human lactoferrin. *Science*, **197**, 263–265.

Arnold, R.R., Russell, J.E., Champion, W.J., and Gauthier, J.J. (1981). Bactericidal activity of human lactoferrin: influence of physical conditions and metabolic state of the target microorganism. *Infection and Immunity*, **32**, 655–660.

Arnold, R.R., Russell, J.E., Champion, W.J., Brewer, M., and Gauthier, J.J. (1982). Bactericidal activity of human lactoferrin: differentiation from the stasis of iron deprivation. *Infection and Immunity*, **35**, 792–799.

Barlow, B., Santulli, T.V., Heira, W.C., Pitt, J., Blanc, W.A., and Schullinger, J.N. (1974). An experimental study of acute neonatal enterocolitis; the importance of breast milk. *Journal of Pediatric Surgery*, **9**, 587–594.

Bates, G.W., Billups, C., and Saltman, P. (1967). The kinetics and mechanisms of iron (III) exchange between chelates and transferrin I. The complexes of citrate and nitrilotriacetic acid. *Journal of Biological Chemistry*, **242**, 2810–2815.

Beachey, E.H. (1981). Bacterial adherence; adhesin-receptor interactions mediating the attachment of bacteria to mucosal surfaces. *Journal of Infectious Diseases*, **143**, 325–345.

Beerens, H., Romond, C., and Neut, C. (1980). Influences of breast feeding on the bifid flora of the newborn intestine. *American Journal of Clinical Nutrition*, **33**, 2434–2439.

Bergheim, O. (1940). Toxicity of intestinal volatile fatty acids for yeast and *Escherichia coli*. *Journal of Infectious Diseases*, **66**, 222–234.

Bezkorovainy, A. (1984). Iron uptake by the microaerophilic anaerobe *Bifidobacterium bifidum var Pennsylvanicus*. *Clinical and Physiological Biochemistry*, **2**, 291–297.

Bezkorovainy, A., Topouzian, N., and Miller-Catchpole, R. (1986). Mechanisms of ferric and ferrous iron uptake by *Bifidobacterium bifidum var Pennsylvanicus*. *Clinical Physiology and Biochemistry* (in press).

Bishop, J.G., Schanbacher, F.L., Ferguson, L.C., and Smith, K.L. (1976). *In vitro* growth inhibition of mastitis–causing coliform bacteria by bovine apolactoferrin and reversal of inhibition by citrate and high concentrations of apolactoferrin. *Infection and Immunity*, **14**, 911–918.

Blakey, J.L., Lubitz, L., Barnes, G.L., Bishop, R.F., Campbell, N.T., and Gillam, G.L. (1982). Development of gut colonization in pre-term neonates. *Journal of Medical Microbiology*, **15**, 519–529.

Boesman-Finkelstein, M., and Finkelstein, R.A. (1985). Antimicrobial effects of human milk: inhibitory activity on enteric pathogens. *FEMS Microbiology Letters*, **27**, 167–174.

Brambell, F.W.R. (1958). The passive immunity of the young mammal. *Biological Reviews*, **33**, 488–531.

Brambell, F.W.R. (1970). The transmission of passive immunity from mother to young. In *Frontiers of Biology* (Eds. A. Neuberger and L. Tatum), Vol. 18. North Holland, Amsterdam.

Brines, R.O., and Brock, J.H. (1983). The effect of trypsin and chymotrypsin on the *in vitro* antimicrobial and iron-binding properties of lactoferrin in human and bovine colostrum. *Biochimica et Biophysica Acta*, **759**, 229–235.

Brock, J.H., Pickering, M.G., McDowall, M.C., and Deacon, A.G. (1983). Role of antibody and enterobactin in controlling growth of *Escherichia coli* in human milk and acquisition of lactoferrin- and transferrin-bound iron by *Escherichia coli*. *Infection and Immunity*, **40**, 453–459.

Brown, W.R., Newcomb, R.W., and Ishizaka, K. (1970). Proteolytic degradation of exocrine and serum immunoglobulins. *Journal of Clinical Investigation*, **49**, 1374–1380.

Bullen, C.L. (1980). Infant feeding and faecal flora. In *The Immunology of Infant Feeding*, 13th Course of the International School of Medical Sciences, Sicily, Italy, pp. 41–53. Plenum Press, New York.

Bullen, C.L., and Tearle, P.V. (1975). Bifidobacteria in the intestinal tract of infants: an *in vitro* study. *Journal of Medical Microbiology*, **9**, 335–344.

Bullen, C.L., Tearle, P.V., and Willis, A.T. (1976). Bifidobacteria in the intestinal tract of infants: an *in vivo* study. *Journal of Medical Microbiology*, **9**, 325–333.

Bullen, C.L., and Willis, A.T. (1971). Resistance of the breast-fed infant to gastroenteritis. *British Medical Journal*, **3**, 338–343.

Bullen, J.J. (1981). The significance of iron in infection. *Reviews of Infectious Diseases*, **3**, 1127–1138.

Bullen, J.J., and Armstrong, J.A. (1979). The role of lactoferrin in the bactericidal function of polymorphonuclear leukocytes. *Immunology*, **36**, 781–791.

Bullen, J.J., Leigh, L.C., and Rogers, H.J. (1968). The effect of iron compounds on the virulence of *Escherichia coli* for guinea pigs. *Immunology*, **15**, 581–588.

Bullen, J.J., Rogers, H.J., and Lewin, J.E. (1971). The bacteriostatic effect of serum on *Pasteurella septica* and its abolition by iron compounds. *Immunology*, **20**, 391–406.

Bullen, J.J., Rogers, H.J., and Leigh, L. (1972). Iron-binding proteins in milk and resistance to *Escherichia coli* infections in infants. *British Medical Journal*, **1**, 69–75.

Bullen, J.J., Rogers, H.J., and Griffiths, E. (1978). Nutrient deficiencies in breast fed infants. *New England Journal of Medicine*, **299**, 1471.

Bullen, J.J. and Scaribrick, R. (1957). Enterotoxaemia of sheep. Experimental reproduction of the disease. *Journal of Pathology and Bacteriology*, **73**, 495–509.

Bullen, J.J., and Wallis, S.N. (1977). Reversal of the bactericidal effect of polymorphs by a ferritin–antibody complex. *FEMS Microbiology Letters*, **1**, 117–120.

Bullen, J.J., Ward, C.G., and Wallis, S.N. (1974). Virulence and the role of iron in *Pseudomonas aeruginosa* infection. *Infection and Immunity*, **10**, 443–450.

Bullen, J.J., Wilson, A.B., Cushnie, G.H., and Rogers, H.J. (1968). The abolition of the protective effect of *Pasteurella septica* antiserum by iron compounds. *Immunology*, **14**, 889–898.

Carruthers, M.M., and Kabat, W.J. (1981). *Vibrio vulnificus* (lactose-positive vibrio) and *Vibrio parahaemolyticus* differ in their susceptibility to human serum. *Infection and Immunity*, **32**, 964–966.

Chandra, R.K. (1977). Iron status, immune response and susceptibility to infection. Ciba Foundation, *Symposium*, **51**, 249–262.

Chart, H., and Griffiths, E. (1985). The availability of iron and the growth of *Vibrio vulnificus* in sera from patients with haemochromatosis. *FEMS Microbiology Letters*, **26**, 227–231.

Cleary, T.G., Chambers, J.P., and Pickering, L.K. (1983). Protection of suckling mice from the heat-stable enterotoxin of *Escherichia coli* by human milk. *Journal of Infectious Diseases*, **148**, 1114–1119.

Coulton, J.W. (1982). The ferrichrome-iron receptor of *Escherichia coli* K12: antigeneticity of the fhuA protein. *Biochimica et Biophysica Acta*, **717**, 154–162.

Crosa, J.H. (1980). A plasmid associated with virulence in the marine fish pathogen *Vibrio anguillarum* specifies an iron sequestering system. *Nature*, **284**, 556–568.

Crosa, J.H., and Hodges, L.L. (1981). Outer membrane proteins induced under conditions of iron limitation in the marine fish pathogen *Vibrio anguillarum*. *Infection and Immunity*, **31**, 223–227.

Delachaume-Salem, E. and Sarles, H. (1970). Evolution en fonction de l'age de la secretion pancreatique humaine normale. Biologie et Gastroenterologie, **2**, 135–146.

Denes, J., Gergely, K., Wolmuth, G., and Leb, J. (1970). Necrotizing enterocolitis in premature infants. *Surgery*, **68**, 558–561.

Dolby, J.M., and Honour, P. (1979). Bacteriostasis of *Escherichia coli* by milk IV. The bacteriostatic antibody of human milk. *Journal of Hygiene*, **83**, 255–265.

Dolby, J.M., and Stephens, S. (1983). Antibodies to *Escherichai coli* O antigens and the *in vitro* bacteriostatic properties of human milk and its IgA. *Acta Paediatrica Scandinavica*, **72**, 577–582.

Dolby, J.M., Stephens, S., and Honour, P. (1977). Bacteriostasis of *Escherichia coli* by milk II. Effect of bicarbonate and transferrin on the activity of infant feeds. *Journal of Hygiene*, **78**, 235–242.

Edelman, R., and Levine, M.M. (1983). Summary of a workshop of enteropathogenic *Escherichia coli*. *Journal of Infectious Diseases*, **147**, 1108–1118.

Editorial (1977). Necrotizing enterocolitis. *Lancet*, **1**, 459–460.

Editorial (1978). Necrotizing enterocolitis. *British Medical Journal*, **1**, 132.

Feachem, R.G., and Koblinsky, M.A. (1984). Interventions for the control of diarrhoeal diseases among young children: promotion of breast-feeding. *Bulletin of the World Health Organization*, **62**, (2), 271–291.

Fitzgerald, S.P., and Rogers, H.J. (1980). Bacteriostatic effect of serum: role of antibody to lipopolysaccharide. *Infection and Immunity*, **27**, 302–308.

Formon, S.J., Filer, L.J., Anderson, T.A., and Ziegler, E.E. (1979). Recommendations for feeding normal infants. *Pediatrics*, **63**, 52–59.

Forsberg, C.M., and Bullen, J.J. (1972). The effect of passage and iron on the virulence of *Pseudomonas aeruginosa*. *Journal of Clinical Pathology*, **25**, 65–68.

Giles, C., Sangster, G., and Smith, J. (1949). Epidemic gastro-enteritis of infants in Aberdeen during 1947. *Archives of Diseases in Childhood*, **24**, 45–53.

Gillin, F.D., Reiner, D.S., and Wang, C.S. (1983). Human milk kills parasitic intestinal protozoan. *Science*, **221**, 1290–1292.

Gindrat, J.J., Gothefors, L., Hanson, L.A., and Winberg, J. (1972). Antibodies in human milk against *E.coli* of the serogroups most commonly found in neonatal infections. *Acta Paediatrica Scandinavica*, **61**, 587–590.

Gladstone, G.P., and Walton, E. (1971). The effect of iron and haematin on the killing of staphylococci by rabbit polymorphs. *British Journal of Experimental Pathology*, **52**, 452–464.

Glass, R.I., Svennerholm, A.M., Stoll, B.J., Khan, M.R., Hossain, K.M.B., Huq, M.I., and Holmgren, J. (1983). Protection against cholera in breast fed children by antibodies in breast milk. *New England Journal of Medicine*, **308**, 1389–1392.

Goldblum, R.M., Ahlstedt, S, Carlsson, B., Hanson, L.A., Jodal, U., Lindin-Janson, G., and Sohl-Akerlund, A. (1975). Antibody-forming cells in human colostrum after oral immunization, *Nature*, **257**, 797–798.

Goldman, H.I. (1980). Feeding and necrotizing enterocolitis. *American Journal of Diseases of Children*, **134**, 553–555.

Gothefors, L., and Marklund, S. (1975). Lactoperoxidase activity in human milk and in saliva of newborn infants. *Infection and Immunity*, **11**, 1210–1215.

Griffiths, E., (1971a). Selective inhibition of macromolecular synthesis in *Pasteurella septica* by antiserum and its reversal by iron. *Nature (New Biology)*, **232**, 89–90.

Griffiths, E. (1971b). Mechanism of action of specific antiserum on *Pasteurella septica*: selective inhibition of net macromolecular synthesis and its reversal by iron compounds. *European Journal of Biochemistry*, **23**, 69–76.

Griffiths, E. (1974a). Rapid degradation of ribosomal RNA in *Pasteurella septica* induced by specific antiserum. *Biochimica et Biophysica Acta*, **340**, 400–412.

Griffiths, E. (1974b). Metabolically controlled killing of *Pasteurella septica* by antibody and complement. *Biochimica et Biophysica Acta*, **362**, 598–602.

Griffiths, E. (1975). Effect of pH and haem compounds on the killing of *Pasteurella septica* by specific antiserum. *Journal of General Microbiology*, **88**, 345–354.

Griffiths, E. (1983a). Adaptation and multiplication of bacteria in host tissues. *Philosophical Transactions of the Royal Society, London*, Series B, **303**, 85–96.

Griffiths, E. (1983b). Availability of iron and survival of bacteria in infection, In *Medical Microbiology* (Eds. C.S.F. Easmon, M. Brown and P. Lambert), Vol. 3, pp. 153–177. Academic Press, London.

Griffiths, E. (1985). Candidate virulence markers. In *The Virulence of Escherichia coli* (Ed. M. Sussman), Society for General Microbiology Special Publication No. 13, pp. 193–226. Academic Press, London.

Griffiths, E., and Humphreys, J. (1977). Bacteriostatic effect of human milk and bovine colostrum on *Escherichia coli*: importance of bicarbonate. *Infection and Immunity*, **15**, 396–401.

Griffiths, E., and Humphreys, J. (1978). Alterations in tRNAs containing 2-methylthio-N^6-($\triangle^2$-isopentenyl)-adenosine during growth of enteropathogenic *Escherichia coli* in the presence of iron-binding proteins. *European Journal of Biochemistry*, **82**, 503–513.

Griffiths, E., Stevenson, P., Thorpe, R., and Chart, H. (1985a). Naturally occurring antibodies in human sera that react with the iron-regulated outer membrane proteins of *Escherichia coli*. *Infection and Immunity*, **47**, 808–813.

Griffiths, E., Stevenson, P., Hale, T.L., and Formal, S.B. (1985b). The synthesis of aerobactin and a 76000 dalton iron-regulated outer membrane protein by *Escherichia coli* K12-*Shigella* hybrids and by enteroinvasive strains of *Escherichia coli*. *Infection and Immunity*, **49**, 67–71.

Guinan, M., Schaberg, D., Bruhn, F.W., Richardson, C.J. and Fox, W.W. (1979). Epidemic occurrence of neonatal necrotizing enterocilitis. *American Journal of Diseases of Children*, **133**, 594–597.

Gutteridge, J.M.C., Rowley, D.A., Griffiths, E., and Halliwell, B. (1985). Low-molecular-weight iron complexes and oxygen radical reactions in idiopathic haemochromatosis. *Clinical Science*, **68**, 463–467.

Hanson, L.A. (1982). The mammary gland as an immunological organ. *Immunology Today*, **3**, 168–172.

Harmon, R.J., Schanbacher, F.L., Ferguson, L.C., and Smith, K.L. (1975). Concentration of lactoferrin in milk of normal lactating cows and changes occurring during mastitis. *American Journal of Veterinary Research*, **36**, 1001–1007.

Harmon, R.J., Schanbacher, F.L., Ferguson, L.C., and Smith, L.C. (1976). Changes in lactoferrin, immunoglobulin G, bovine serum albumin and α-lactalbumin during acute experimental and natural coliform mastitis in cows. *Infection and Immunity*, **13**, 533–542.

Hegenauer, J., and Saltman, P. (1975). Iron and susceptibility to infectious diseases. *Science*, **188**, 1038–1039.

Helms, S.D., Oliver, J.D., and Travis, J.C. (1984). Role of heme compounds and haptoglobin in *Vibrio vulnificus* pathogenicity. *Infection and Immunity*, **45**, 345–349.

Herrington, D.A., and Sparling, P.F. (1985). *Haemophilus influenzae* can use human transferrin as a sole source of required iron. *Infection and Immunity*, **48**, 248–251.

Holland, I.B. (1975). Physiology of colicin action. *Advances in Microbial Physiology*, **12**, 55–139.

Holmgren, J., Hanson, L.A., Carlsson, B., Lindblad, B.S., and Rahintoola, J. (1976). Neutralizing antibodies against *Escherichia coli* and *Vibrio cholerae* enterotoxins in human milk from a developing country. *Scandinavian Journal of Immunology*, **5**, 867–871.

Holmgren, J., Svennerholm, A.M., and Ahren, C. (1981). Non-immunoglobulin fraction of human milk inhibits bacterial adhesion (hemagglutination) and enterotoxin binding of *Escherichia coli* and *Vibrio cholerae*. *Infection and Immunity*, **33**, 136–141.

Jenness, R. (1974). Composition of milk. In *Lactation* (Eds. B.L. Larsen and V.R. Smith), Vol. III. pp. 3–107. Academic Press, New York.

Kenny, J.F., Boesman, M.T., and Michaels, R.H. (1967). Bacterial and viral coproantibodies in breast-fed infants. *Pediatrics*, **39**, 202–213.

Klemm P. (1985). Fimbrial adhesins of *Escherichia coli*. *Reviews of Infectious Diseases*, **7**, 321–340.

Kliegman, R.M. (1979). Neonatal necrotizing enterocolitis: implications for an infectious disease. *Pediatrics Clinics of North America*, **26**, 327–344.

Kochan, I., Wagner, S.K., and Wasynczuk, J. (1984). Effect of iron on antibacterial immunity in vaccinated mice. *Infection and Immunity*, **43**, 543–548.

Kochan, I., Wasynczuk, J., and McCabe, M.A. (1978). Effects of injected iron and siderophores on infections in normal and immune mice. *Infection and Immunity*, **22**, 560–567.

Kohler, E.M. (1974). Protection of pigs against neonatal enteric colibacillosis with colostrum and milk from orally vaccinated sows. *American Journal of Veterinary Research*, **35**, 331–338.

Konopka, K., and Neilands, J.B. (1984). Effect of serum albumin on siderophore-mediated utilization of transferrin iron. *Biochemistry*, **23**, 2122–2127.

Kosloske, A.M. (1979). Necrotizing enterocolitis in the neonate. *Surgery, Gynecology and Obstetrics*, **148**, 259–269.

Kreger, A., and Lockwood, D. (1981). Detection of extra-cellular toxin(s) produced by *Vibrio vulnificus*. *Infection and Immunity*, **33**, 583–590.

Krouskop, R.W., Brown, E.G., and Sweet, A.Y. (1974). The relationship of feeding to necrotizing enterocolitis. *Pediatric Research*, **8**, 383.

Larsen, S.A., and Homer, D.R. (1978). Relation of breast feeding to hospitalization in a middle-class U.S. population. *Journal of Pediatrics*, **92**, 417–418.

Lawrence, G., Bates, J., and Gaul, A. (1982). Pathogenesis of neonatal necrotizing enterocolitis. *Lancet*, **1**, 137–139.

Lawrence, G. and Walker, P.D. (1976). Pathogenesis of enteritis necroticans in Papua New Guinea. *Lancet*, **1**, 125–126.

Levine, M.M. (1981). Adhesion of enterotoxigenic *Escherichia coli* in humans and animals. In *Adhesion and Microorganism Pathogenicity*, Ciba Foundation Symposium No. 80, pp. 142–160.

Levine, M.M., Nataro, J.P., Karch, H., Baldini, M.M., Kaper, J.B., Black, R.E., Clements, M.L., and O'Brien, A.D. (1985). The diarrhoeal response of humans to some classic serotypes of enteropathogenic *Escherichia coli* is dependent on a plasmid encoding an enteroadhesiveness factor. *Journal of Infectious Diseases*, **152**, 550–559.

Levison, M.E. (1973). Effect of colon flora and short chain fatty acids on growth *in vitro* of *Pseudomonas aeruginosa* and enterobacteriaceae. *Infection and Immunity*, **8**, 30–35.

Lindberg, T. (1979). Protease inhibitors in human milk. *Pediatric Research*, **13**, 969–972.

Lonnerdal, B., Keen, C.L., Fransson, G.B., Hambraeeus, L., and Hurley, L.S. (1980). New perspectives on iron supplementation of milk. *The Journal of Paediatrics*, **96**, 242.

Martinez, R.J., and Carroll, S.F. (1980). Sequential metabolic expressions of the lethal process in human serum-treated *Escherichia coli*: role of lysozyme. *Infection and Immunity*, **28**, 735–745.

Mason, S. (1962). Some aspects of gastric function in the new born. *Archives of Diseases in Childhood*, **37**, 387–391.

Masson, P.L., and Heremans, J.F. (1968). Metal-combining properties of human lactoferrin (red milk protein) I. The involvement of bicarbonate in the reaction. *European Journal of Biochemistry*, **6**, 579–584.

Masson, P.L., and Heremans, J.F. (1971). Lactoferrin in milk from different species. *Comparative Biochemistry and Physiology*, **39B**, 119–129.

Mata, L.J., Kronmel, R.A., Garcia, B., Butler, W., Urrutia, J.J., and Murillo, S. (1976). Breast feeding, weaning and the diarrhoeal syndrome in a Guatemalan Indian village. In *Acute Diarrhoea in Childhood*, Ciba Symposium No. 42, pp. 45–46. Elsevier, Amsterdam.

Mata, L.J., and Urrutia, J.J. (1971). Intestinal colonization of breast fed children in a rural area of low socioeconomic level. *Annals of the New York Academy of Sciences*, **176**, 93–109.

Mazurier, J., Aubert, J.P., Loucheux-Lefevre, M.H., and Spik, G. (1976). Comparative circular dichroism studies of iron-free and iron-saturated forms of human serotransferrin and lactoferrin. *FEBS Letters*, **66**, 238–242.

Melching, L., and Vas, I. (1971). Effects of serum components on Gram-negative bacteria during bactericidal reactions. *Infection and Immunity*, **3**, 107–115.

Mickelsen, P.A., Blackman, E., and Sparling, P.F. (1982). Ability of *Neisseria gonorrhoeae*, *Neisseria meningitidis* and commensal *Neisseria* species to obtain iron from lactoferrin. *Infection and Immunity*, **35**, 915–920.

Mickelsen, P.A., and Sparling, P.F. (1981). Ability of *Neisseria gonorrhoeae*, *Neisseria meningitidis* and commensal *Neisseria* species to obtain iron from transferrin and iron compounds. *Infection and Immunity*, **33**, 555–564.

Moore, D.G., and Earhart, C.F. (1981). Specific inhibition of *Escherichia coli* ferrienterochelin uptake by a normal human serum immunoglobulin. *Infection and Immunity*, **31**, 631–635.

Moore, D.G., Yancey, R.J., Lankford, C.E., and Earhart, C.F. (1980). Bacteriostatic enterochelin-specific immunoglobulin from normal human serum. *Infection and Immunity*, **27**, 418–423.

Morris, J.A., and Sojka, W.J. (1985). *Escherichia coli* as a pathogen in animals. In *The Virulence of Escherichia coli* (Ed. M. Sussman), Special Publications of the Society for General Microbiology No. 13, pp. 47–77. Academic Press, London.

Murray, M.J., Murray, A., and Murray, C.J. (1980). The salutary effect of milk on amoebiasis and its reversal by iron. *British Medical Journal*, **1**, 1351–1352.

Murray, M.J., Murray, A.B., Murray, C.J., and Murray, M.B. (1978). The effect of iron status of Nigerian mothers on that of their infants at birth and 6 months, and on the concentration of Fe in breast milk. *British Journal of Nutrition*, **39**. 624–630.

Murrell, G.C., Roth, L., Egerton, J., Samels, J. and Walker, P.D. (1966). Pig-Bel; enteritis necroticons. *Lancet*, 217–222.

Parry, S.H., and Rooke, D.M. (1985). Adhesins and colonization factors. In *The Virulence of Escherichia coli* (Ed. M. Sussman), Special Publications of the Society for General Microbiology No. 13, pp. 79–155. Academic Press, London.

Peaker, M., and Linzell, J.L. (1975). Citrate in milk: a harbinger of lactogenesis. *Nature* **253**, 464.

Porter, P., and Allen, W.D. (1978). Antibody response in pigs and calves to antigens from the intestinal lumen and the efficacy of oral immunoprophylaxis against post-weaning enteric infection. In *Antigen Absorption by the Gut* (Ed. W.A. Hemmings), pp. 81–92. MTP Press, Lancaster.

Porter, P., and Linggood, M.A. (1983). Development of oral vaccines for preventing diarrhoea caused by enteropathogenic *Escherichia coli*. *Journal of Infection*, **6**, 111–121.

Porter, P., Powell, J.R., Allen, W.D., and Linggood, M.A. (1985). The immune response to *Escherichia coli*. In *The Virulence of Escherichia coli* (Ed. M. Sussman), Special Publications of the Society for General Microbiology No. 13, pp. 271–283. Academic Press, London.

Reddy, V., Bhaskaram, C., Raghuramulu, N., and Jagadeesan, V. (1977). Antimicrobial factors in human milk. *Acta Paediatrica Scandinavica*, **66**, 229–232.

Reiter, B. (1978a). Review of the progress of dairy science: antimicrobial systems in milk. *Journal of Dairy Research*, **45**, 131–147.

Reiter, B. (1978b). Review of non-specific antimicrobial factors in colostrum. *Annales de Recherches Veterinaires*,**9**, 205–224.

Reiter, B. (1984). Role of non-antibody proteins in milk in the protection of the newborn. In *Human Milk Banking* (Eds. A.F. Williams and J.D. Baum), pp. 29–53. Nestle Nutrition, Vevey/Raven Press, New York.

Reiter, B., and Bramley, A.J. (1975). Defense mechanisms of the udder and their relevance to mastitis control. In *Proceedings of Seminar on Mastitis Control—1975* (Eds. F.H. Dodd, T.K. Griffin and R.G. Kingwill), pp. 210–222. International Dairy Federation, Brussels.

Reiter, B., Brock, J.H., and Steel, E.D. (1975). Inhibition of *Escherichia coli* by bovine colostrum and post-colostral milk II. The bacteriostatic effect of lactoferrin on a serum susceptible and serum resistant strain of *E.coli*. *Immunology*, **28**, 83–95.

Reiter, B., and Harnulv, G. (1984). Lactoperoxidase antibacterial system: natural occurrence, biological functions and practical applications. *Journal of Food Protection*, **47**, 724–732.

Ribadeau-Dumas, B. (1983). Human milk. *Endeavour (New Series)*, **7**, 80–87.

Robinson, J.E., Harvey, B.A.M., and Soothill, J.F. (1978). Phagocytosis and killing of bacteria and yeast by human milk cells after opsonization in aqueous phase of milk. *British Medical Journal*, **1**, 1443–1445.

Robinson, M. (1951). Infant morbidity and mortality: a study of 3266 infants. *Lancet*. **1**, 788–794.

Rogers, H.J. (1967). Bacteriostatic effects of horse sera and serum fractions on *Clostridium welchii* type A, and the abolition of bacteriostasis by iron salts. *Immunology*, **12**, 285–301.

Rogers, H.J. (1973). Iron-binding catechols and virulence in *Escherichia coli*. *Infection and Immunity*, **7**, 445–456.

Rogers, H.J. (1976). Ferric iron and the antibacterial effects of horse 7S antibodies to *Escherichia coli* 0111. *Immunology*, **30**, 425–433.

Rogers, H.J. (1983). Role of iron chelators, antibodies and iron-binding proteins in infection. In *Microbiology—1983*, pp. 334–337. American Society for Microbiology.

Rogers, H.J., and Synge, C. (1978). Bacteriostatic effect of human milk on *Escherichia coli*: the role of IgA. *Immunology*, **34**, 19–28.

Rosenberg, H., and Young, I.G. (1974). Iron transport in the enteric bacteria. In *Microbial Iron Metabolism* (Ed. J.B. Neilands), pp. 67–82. Academic Press, New York.

Rowe, B. (1979). The role of *Escherichia coli* in gastroenteritis. *Clinics in Gastroenterology*, **8**, 625–644.

Rutter, J.M., Burrows, M.R., Sellwood, R., and Gibbons, R.A. (1975). A genetic basis for resistance to enteric disease caused by *E. coli*. *Nature*, **257**, 135–136.

Saarinen, U.M. (1978). Need for iron supplementation in infants on prolonged breast feeding. *Journal of Pediatrics*, **93**, 177–180.

Samson, R.R., Mirtle, C., and McClelland, D.B.L. (1979). Secretory IgA does not enhance the bacteriostatic effects of iron-binding or vitamin B12 binding proteins in human colostrum. *Immunology*, **38**, 367–373.

Schanbacher, F.L., and Smith, L.K. (1975). Formation and role of unusual whey proteins and enzymes: relation to mammary function. *Journal of Dairy Science*, **58**, 1048–1062.

Schlabach, M.R., and Bates, G.W. (1975). The synergistic binding of anions and Fe^{3+} by transferrin; implications for the interlocking site hypothesis. *Journal of Biological Chemistry*, **250**, 2182–2188.

Siimes,,M.A., Vuori, E., and Kuitinen, P. (1979). Breast milk iron—a declining concentration during the course of lactation. *Acta Paediatrica Scandinavica*, **68**, 29–31.

Simonson, C., Brener, D., and DeVoe, I.W. (1982). Expression of a high-affinity mechanism for acquisition for transferrin iron by *Neisseria meningitidis*. *Infection and Immunity*, **36**, 107–113.

Smith, G.C., and Merkel, J.R. (1982). Collagenolytic activity of *Vibrio vulnificus*: potential contribution to its invasiveness. *Infection and Immunity*, **35**, 1155–1156.

Smith, H.R., Scotland, S.M., and Rowe, B. (1985). Genetics of *Escherichia coli* virulence. In *The Virulence of Escherichia coli* (Ed. M. Sussman), Special Publications of the Society for General Microbiology No. 13, pp. 227–269. Academic Press, London.

Smith, H.W. (1972). The nature of the protective effect of antisera against *Escherichia coli* diarrhoea in piglets. *Journal of Medical Microbiology*, **5**, 345–353.

Smith, H.W. (1976). Neonatal *Escherichia coli* infections in domestic mammals: transmissibility of pathogenic characteristics. In *Acute Diarrhoea in Childhood*, Ciba Symposium No. 42, pp. 45–64.

Smith, H.W., and Huggins, M.B. (1978). The influence of plasmid determined and other characteristics of enteropathogenic *Escherichia coli* on their ability to proliferate in the alimentary tract of piglets, calves and lambs. *Journal of Medical Microbiology*, **11**, 471–492.

Smith, H.W., and Jones, J.E.T. (1963). Observations on the alimentary tract and its bacterial flora in healthy and diseased pigs. *Journal of Pathology and Bacteriology*, **86**. 387–412.

Spik, G., Cheran, A., Montreuil, J., and Dolby, J.M. (1978). Bacteriostasis of a milk-sensitive strain of *Escherichia coli* by immunoglobulins and iron-binding proteins in association. *Immunology*, **35**, 663–671.

Spitznagel, J.K. (1983). Microbial interactions with neutrophils. *Reviews of Infectious Diseases*, **5**, S806–S822.

Stein, H. (1977). Necrotizing enterocolitis in black neonates. *South African Medical Journal*, **51**, 199–200.

Stephens, S., Dolby, J.M., Montreuil, J., and Spik, G. (1980). Differences in inhibition of the growth of commensal and enteropathogenic strains of *Escherichia coli* by lactotransferrin and secretory immunoglobulin A isolated from human milk. *Immunology*, **41**, 597–603.

Stoliar, O.R., Pelley, R.P., Kaniecki-Green, E., Klaus, M.H., and Carpenter, C.C.J. (1976). Secretory IgA against enterotoxins in breast milk. *Lancet*, **1**, 1258–1261.

Svanborg Eden, C., Carlsson, B., Hanson, L.A., Jann, K., Korhonen, T.K., and Wadstrom, T. (1979). Anti-pili antibodies in breast milk. *Lancet*, **2**, 1235.

Svirsky-Gross, S. (1958). Pathogenic strains of coli (0111) among prematures and the use of human milk in controlling the outbreak of diarrhoea. *Annals Paediatrici*, **190**, 100–115.

Sweeny, M.J., de Lemos, R.A., Rogers, J.H., and McLaughlin, G.W. (1974). Experimental production of necrotizing enterocolitis in new-born goats. *Pediatric Research*, **8**, 380.

Tassovatz, B., and Kotsitch, A. (1961). Le lait de femme et son action de protection contre les infections intestinales chez le nouveau-ne. *Annales de Pediatrie*, **8**, 285–290.

Taylor, P.W. (1983). Bactericidal and bacteriolytic activity of serum against Gram-negative bacteria. *Microbiological Reviews*, **47**, 46–83.

Taylor, P.W. (1985). Measurement of the bactericidal activity of serum. In *The Virulence of Escherichia coli* (Ed. M. Sussman), Special Publications of the Society for General Microbiology No. 13, pp. 445–456. Academic Press, London.

Taylor, P.W., and Kroll, H.P. (1983). Killing of an encapsulated strain of *Escherichia coli* by human serum. *Infection and Immunity*, **39**. 122–131.

Volstead Pederson, P., Hart Hansen, F., Halveg, A.B., Christiansen, E.D., Justesen, T., and Hogh, P. (1976). Necrotizing enterocolitis of the newborn—is it gas-gangrene of the bowel? *Lancet*, **2**, 715–716.

Walton, E., and Gladstone, G.P. (1976). Factors affecting the susceptibility of staphylococci to killing by the cationic proteins from rabbit polymorphonuclear leucocytes, the effects of alteration of cellular energetics and of various iron compounds. *British Journal of Experimental Pathology*, **57**, 560–570.

Watanabe, T., Nagura, H., Watanabe, K. and Brown, W.R. (1984). The binding of human milk lactoferrin to immunoglobulin A. *FEBS Letters*, **168**, 203–207.

Welsh, J.K., and May, J.T. (1979). Anti-infective properties of breast milk. *Journal of Pediatrics*, **94**, 1–9.

WHO Scientific Working Group (1980). *Escherichia coli* diarrhoea. *Bulletin of the World Health Organization*, **58**, 23–36.

Willis, A.T., Bullen, C.L., Williams, K., Fagg, C.G., Bourne, A., and Vignon, M. (1973). Breast milk substitute: a bacteriological study. *British Medical Journal*, **4**, 67–72.

Woodbury, R.M. (1922). The relation between breast and artificial feeding and infant mortality. *American Journal of Hygiene*, **2**, 668–687.

Zeissler, J. and Rassfeld-Sternberg, L., (1949). Enteritis necroticans due to *Clostridium welchii* Type F. *British Medical Journal*, I, 267–269.

Iron and Infection
Edited by J.J. Bullen and E. Griffiths

Chapter 6

Iron and the antibacterial function of polymorphonuclear leucocytes

J.J. BULLEN
Department of Surgery,
University of Miami School of Medicine,
Jackson Memorial Medical Center,
PO Box 016310, Miami,
Florida 33101, USA

1. THE INFLUENCE OF IRON-BINDING PROTEINS ON PHAGOCYTOSIS

Much has been written about the antibacterial mechanisms of polymorphonuclear leucocytes and there are several excellent reviews on this topic (Root and Cohen, 1981; Ryter and de Chastellier, 1983; Spitznagel, 1983). However, comparatively few studies have been made on the quantitative relationships between phagocytic cells and bacteria which ultimately decide the outcome of any infection. For example, if the number of polymorphs is fixed and the bacteria continue to multiply in the extracellular fluid, then the task of the polymorph in controlling the infection becomes progressively more difficult. Exactly the opposite applies if the plasma is bactericidal. These relationships, which are often of fundamental importance, are best studied *in vivo* where all the circumstances of an infection come into play. Studies *in vitro* may be essential for a particular purpose, but in the end it is their relevance to conditions *in vivo* that really matters.

In vivo, the effectiveness of phagocytosis depends essentially on the following: the ratio of bacteria to phagocytic cells, the rate of ingestion of the bacteria, the rate of destruction or growth of the intracellular bacteria and the rate of destruction or growth of the extracellular bacteria. The medium in which

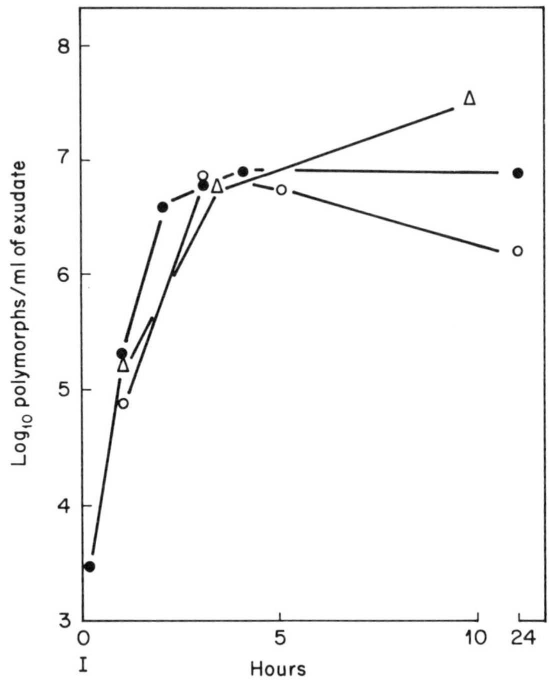

Figure 1 Counts of polymorphonuclear leucocytes in the peritoneal cavity of rabbits infected with *Pseudomonas aeruginosa*. ○ Sublethal infection. ● Lethal infection. △ Lethal infection (with haematin). *From Bullen, Ward and Wallis (1974). Reproduced by permission of the American Society for Microbiology*

polymorphs function consists of plasma or inflamatory exudate. Both contain unsaturated iron-binding proteins, which, depending on individual circumstances, consist of transferrin, lactoferrin or a mixture of both. The influence of these proteins, in combination with other antibacterial factors, such as specific antibacterial antibody, complement and lysozyme, can be of decisive importance. This is illustrated by the fate of *Pseudomonas aeruginosa* in experimental intraperitoneal infections in rabbits (Bullen, Ward and Wallis, 1974; Bullen, Wallis and Griffiths, 1976).

In these experiments animals were equipped with permanent cannulae so that samples could be removed without damaging the peritoneal lining. The introduction of *Ps aeruginosa* produced a massive exudate of polymorphs. The response was the same in both lethal and non-lethal infections, with or without the addition of iron compounds (Fig. 1) and in all cases there was comparatively little change in the mononuclear cell population (Bullen, Ward and Wallis,

Table 1 Iron-binding capacities of plasma and peritoneal fluid of rabbits infected with *Pseudomonas aeruginosa*. (Data calculated for samples adjusted to same protein concentration, 10 mg/ml.) SIBC = saturated iron-binding capacity, UIBC = unsaturated iron-binding capacity, TIBC = total iron-binding capacity

			Plasma and peritoneal fluid			
Infection	Sample	Hours after infection	SIBC	UIBC (10^{-6} *M* Fe)	TIBC	Satuaration with Fe (%)
Sublethal	Plasma	0	5.0	2.0	7.0	71
		7	5.9	4.9	10.8	55
	Peritoneal fluid	0	11.6	12.5	24.1	48
		7	9.1	23.7	32.8	28
Lethal	Plasma	0	13.1	2.9	16.0	82
		7	3.9	6.0	9.9	39
	Peritoneal fluid	0	19.3	8.6	27.9	69
		7	5.2	11.0	16.2	32
Protected with antibody	Plasma	0	9.7	2.4	12.1	80
		7	9.7	2.7	12.4	78
	Peritoneal fluid	0	10.3	17.3	27.6	37
		7	8.7	14.4	23.1	38

From Bullen, Ward and Wallace (1974). Reproduced by permission of the American Society for Microbiology.

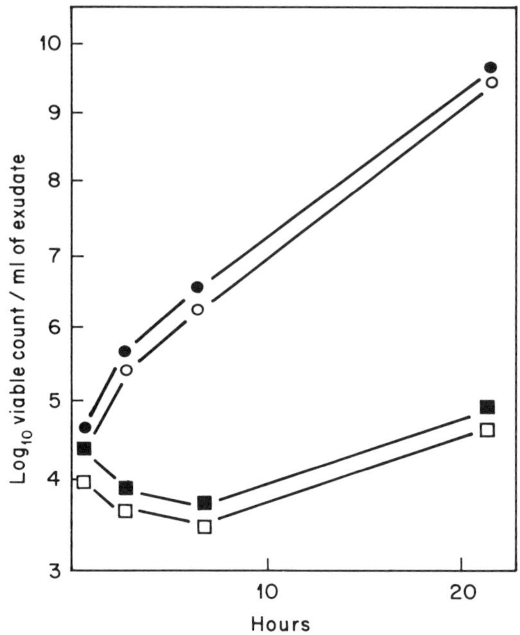

Figure 2 Viable counts of *Pseudomonas aeruginosa* in sublethal and lethal infections in the peritoneal cavity of rabbits. ■ Sublethal total count. □ Sublethal extracellular count. ● Lethal total count (+ 5 mg of Fe/per kg live weight). ○ Lethal extracellular count. *From Bullen, Ward and Wallis (1974). Reproduced by permission of the American Society for Microbiology*

1974). In normal rabbits the plasma transferrin was relatively highly saturated (71–80 per cent), but the peritoneal fluid was less so (37–69 per cent) (Table 1). Why this should be is not known at present. Infection produced a sharp fall in the percentage saturation of both the plasma and the peritoneal fluid (Table 1).

In both lethal and non-lethal infections the majority of the viable bacteria were extracellular (Fig. 2) which suggested that the internal bactericidal mechanisms of the polymorphs were highly efficient (Bullen, Ward and Wallis, 1974). This was confirmed by experiments with ^{32}P-and ^{14}C-labelled bacteria where only a small percentage of intracellular organisms was viable (Table 2) (Bullen, Wallis and Griffiths, 1976). Since the number of polymorphs was the same in both lethal and non-lethal infections, it was clear that the rate of extracellular growth and the rate of phagocytosis decided the outcome of the infection.

In non-lethal infections the rate of phagocytosis was high with 55–87 per cent (mean 73 per cent) of labelled bacteria being ingested at 5 and 20 hours after

Table 2 Percentage of labelled intracellular bacteria and viable intracellular bacteria in the peritoneal exudate of rabbits infected with *Pseudomonas aeruginosa*. (Bacteria labelled with ^{32}P and ^{14}C)

Infection	Time after infection (hours)	Time after labelled bacteria added (minutes)	Intracellular viable bacteria (%)	Intracellular labelled bacteria (%)
	5	10	7	80
		60	40	82
Non-lethal	20	10	0	87
		60	0	84
	20	10	0	55
		60	23	78
Lethal	1	10	10	37
		60	11	38
	1	10	0	33
		60	12	46
Protected with antibody	1	10	48	57
		60	56	88
	1.5	10	88	66
		60	96	80

From Bullen, Wallis and Griffiths (1976). Reproduced by permission of Blackwell Scientific Publications Limited.

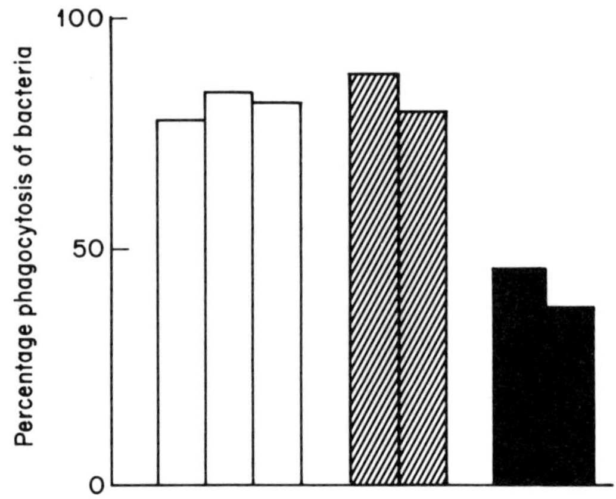

Figure 3 Percentage phagocytosis of *Pseudomonas aeruginosa* in the peritoneal cavity of rabbits. □ Non-lethal infection. ■ Lethal infection. ▨ Protected with specific antibody. Measurements made 60 minutes after introduction of bacteria labelled with ^{32}P or ^{14}C. *From Bullen, Wallis and Griffiths (1976). Reproduced by permission of Blackwell Scientific Publications Limited*

infection (Table 2; Fig. 3) *In vitro*, *Ps aeruginosa* grew slowly in pertioneal fluid with a generation time of 72 minutes (Table 3). In the peritoneal cavity the bacteria were apparently incapable of growing fast enough to replace those destroyed by the polymorphs, and the infection slowly declined, although the rate of multiplication was sufficient to allow the bacteria to persist for several days (Figs. 2 and 4). This might have been due partly to the fall in the percentage of polymorphs in the peritoneal exudate that occurred after 24 hours (Fig. 4).

In lethal infections, without added iron, using large inocula of 10^7–10^9 bacteria, the total viable count rose steadily (Bullen, Ward and Wallis, 1974; Bullen, Wallis and Griffiths, 1976). The failure to control the infection was not due to a lack of polymorphs (Fig. 1). Nor was it due to inefficient killing of ingested bacteria since the number of viable intracellular bacteria was small (0–12 per cent, Table 2). However, the overall rate of phagocytosis was low, as shown by the small percentage of labelled bacteria ingested by the polymorphs (mean 39 per cent, Table 2 and Fig. 3). This was probably due to the high ratio of bacteria to polymorphs, and this inability to ingest a large proportion of the bacteria present appeared to be decisive. Even with a comparatively slow generation time of 72 minutes (Table 3) extracellular growth continued until death occurred from septicaemia (Bullen, Ward and Wallis, 1974).

Specific antibacterial antibody gave complete protection against a normally lethal dose of *Ps aeruginosa* and it was interesting that the rate of phagocytosis was greatly improved and almost equalled that seen in non-lethal infections

Table 3 Effect of added iron on the rate of growth of *Pseudomonas aeruginosa* in peritoneal fluid or in 199 medium plus transferrin

Culture fluid	Saturation with Fe (%)	*Ps aeruginosa* generation time (minutes)
Rabbit peritoneal fluid	34	72
Rabbit peritoneal fluid + Fe	100	34
Human transferrin in 199 medium	46	72
Human transferrin in 199 medium + Fe	100	34
Bacteriological broth	—	29

From Bullen, Ward and Wallis (1974). Reproduced by permission of the American Society for Microbiology.

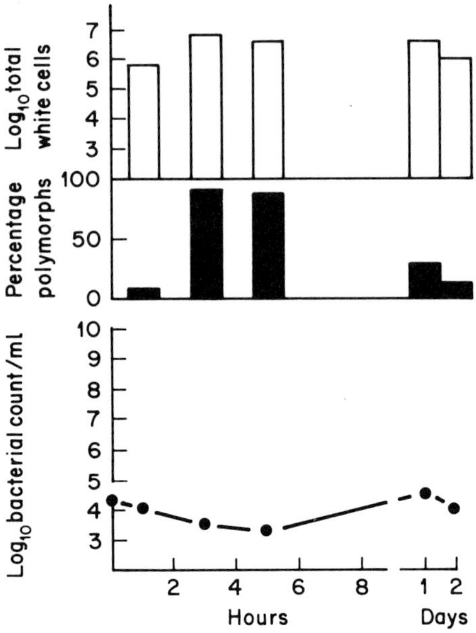

Figure 4 Non-lethal infection with *Pseudomonas aeruginosa* in the peritoneal cavity of a rabbit. Total white cells, percentage of polymorphs and viable bacterial counts. *From Bullen, Wallis and Griffiths (1976). Reproduced by permission of Blackwell Scientific Publications Limited*

(Table 2). Equally interesting was the fact that several hours after infection passively immunized animals showed no fall in the percentage saturation of the plasma or peritoneal iron-binding proteins (Table 1). This was in sharp contrast to the situation in unimmunized animals (see above and Table 1). The reason for this is uncertain, but it presumably means that the specific antibody interferes in some way with the mechanism responsible for hypoferraemia. It could be related to the neutralization of endotoxin and the failure to release lactoferrin from polymorphonuclear leucocytes (see Chapter 7).

In non-lethal infections all the evidence suggests that the unsaturated iron-binding proteins made a large contribution to resistance. When enough Fe^{3+} was injected to saturate the serum transferrin or when haem compounds (which are not bound by transferrin) were injected with the bacteria a normally non-lethal infection became a lethal one. Instead of declining in numbers the extracellular bacteria increased rapidly until death occurred (Fig. 2). *In vitro*, it was found that saturation of the iron-binding capacity of the peritoneal fluid allowed the bacteria to grow twice as quickly as before with a generation time of 34 minutes (Table 3). Assuming that this also occurred *in vivo* the increase in the speed of extracellular growth appeared to be crucial and was sufficient to overwhelm the polymorphs. The importance of iron-binding proteins in resistance to *Ps aeruginosa* is also shown by the increase in susceptibility that occurs when the iron-binding capacity of the plasma transferrin is saturated. In rabbits the lethal dose was reduced by 100-fold (Bullen, Ward and Wallis, 1974) and in mice the LD 50 by 1,000-fold (Forsberg and Bullen, 1972).

In a different context, the work of Eaton *et al.* (1982) showed that the binding of haemoglobin by haptoglobin rendered the iron in haemoglobin unavailable to *E. coli* and that haptoglobin could have a protective effect. This is discussed in Chapter 7, but it raises the question as to whether the degree of saturation of serum proteins that bind haemoglobin or haem can affect phagocytic efficiency.

Experiments with human polymorphs cannot be done *in vivo*, but Ward, Hammond and Bullen (1986) investigated this problem by using polymorphs from normal individuals incorporated in a clot of autologous plasma. This technique was a modification of the method originally described by Gladstone and Walton (1971) and Bullen and Joyce (1982), and was used to mimic conditions *in vivo* as closely as possible. Working with *Klebsiella pneumoniae* it

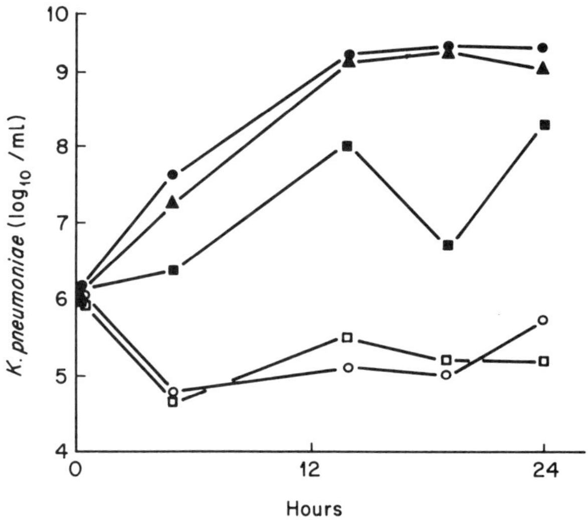

Figure 5 Effect of hematin on growth of *K. pneumoniae* in plasma clots with polymorphs (2.5×10^7/ml). Symbols: ○, control; □, 5% saturation of plasma albumin with hematin; ■, 10% saturation; ▲, 50% saturation; ●, 100% saturation. *Reproduced by permission of the American Society for Microbiology*

was found that normal human plasma (without polymorphs) was bactericidal for small numbers (10^3/ml or less) of bacteria and slowed down the growth of larger numbers (ca.10^6/ml). When polymorphs (2.5×10^7/ml) were added to the plasma, control of bacterial growth was much more effective. With an inoculum of 10^6 bacteria/ml there was an initial fall in numbers followed by a prolonged bacteriostatic effect which lasted for at least 24 hours (Fig. 5). This was in contrast to the slow but persistent growth that occurred in plasma alone.

In plasma clots with polymorphs experiments were made on the effect of varying levels of saturation of the plasma proteins binding iron or iron compounds. With haptoglobin, 100 per cent saturation of its haemoglobin binding capacity abolished the bacteriostatic effect, but 50 per cent saturation did not, suggesting that *K. pneumoniae* could utilize the iron in free haemoglobin but not when it was bound to haptoglobin. With albumin, 50 per cent saturation of its haem-binding capacity (which would also saturate the haem-binding capacity of haemopexin) abolished the bacteriostatic effect and even 10 per cent saturation gave a significant increase in bacterial growth (Fig. 5). This suggested that the organism could utilize the iron in haem bound to albumin. With transferrin a 100 per cent saturation with Fe^{3+} led to rapid growth and even 60 per cent saturation led to rapid growth after a delay of 19 hours. In all cases where rapid growth occurred the majority of the bacteria appeared to be extracellular.

These experiments provide additional evidence that an increase in the availability of iron, which destroys the bactericidal or bacteriostatic properties of plasma, has a very adverse effect on phagocytic efficiency, and can lead to the polymorphs being overwhelmed by the bacteria. As far as local conditions are concerned, additional iron-binding capacity could be provided by the release of lactoferrin following degranulation of polymorphs on contact with immune complexes (Leffell and Spitznagel, 1975) or Interleukin-1 (Klempner, Dinarello and Gallin, 1978, and Chapter 7). Up to 40 per cent of the lactoferrin in polymorphs can degranulate and of this about 90 per cent may leave the cell (Leffell and Spitznagel, 1975); indeed, it has been found that a whole range of granular enzymes may be released in a similar fashion (Wright and Malawista, 1972).

However, while there is no doubt that some lactoferrin may leave the cell on contact with immune complexes it is by no means certain that this always happens. Leffell and Spitznagel (1975) used latex beads coated with immune complexes which may have provided an exceptional stimulus for degranulation. Bullen and Armstrong (1979) found no detectable fall in the total iron-binding capacity (TIBC) of polymorph extracts after the cells had been exposed to *Ps. aeruginosa* treated with specific antibacterial antibody (Table 4). It is interesting that it is precisely this combination of *Ps. aeruginosa* and specific antibody that failed to cause hypoferraemia in the intact animal (Bullen, Ward and Wallis, 1974, and Table 1). It could be that this was due to the failure to release any lactoferrin from the polymorphs (see Chapter 7).

There is evidence that the concentration of extracellular lactoferrin is increased in some clinical conditions and that the lactoferrin is derived from the polymorphs. Gutteberg, Haneberg and Jorgensen (1984a) reported that the concentration of lactoferrin in serum was significantly increased in all but one of eleven children suffering from meningococcal septicaemia who had been ill for less than 18 hours. In this respect lactoferrin acted like an acute phase protein. The authors gave an upper limit (mean + 2 SD) for healthy infants of approximately 11 mg of lactoferrin per litre of serum. In infected patients the level varied from approximately 15 mg/litre to over 200 mg/litre. Gutteberg, Haneberg and Jorgensen (1984b) also found raised levels of lactoferrin in the serum of 22 out of 49 newborn infants with suspected or known bacterial or viral infections.

Wolach *et al.* (1984) gave figures of 1.5 ± 1.8 mg/litre for plasma lactoferrin in normal male controls, and found that patients with more than a 30 per cent burn had levels of 10–40 mg/litre. Furthermore, there was some correlation between the extent of the burn and the level of lactoferrin on the first day after injury. There was also a correlation with the degree of leukocytosis. In addition there was a significant increase in lactoferrin in those burned patients that developed pneumonia compared with those that did not.

Venge *et al.* (1978) give the concentration of lactoferrin in normal human polymorphs as 4.3 ± 1.2 mg/10^9 cells. They found that in 10 out of 12 cases of bacterial infection there was a fall in intracellular lactoferrin (below–2 SD). This was reflected by an increase in the concentration of lactoferrin in the plasma.

There is no doubt that iron-binding proteins can have a powerful influence on extracellular bacterial growth (see above). In local infections lactoferrin could act as a bacteriostatic agent by itself, or it could have a bacteriostatic effect in conjunction with specific antibacterial antibody (see Chapter 5). It might have an important effect by binding iron in an area of low pH. A fall in pH is not uncommon in local infections (Stoner and Green, 1948; Bullen, Cushnie and Stoner, 1966). The bacteriostatic properties of serum which involves unsaturated transferrin, specific antibody, and complement, disappear at pH 6.8 or below, at least in the case of *Pasteurella multocida* (Bullen, Rogers and Lewin, 1971). This deficiency might be made up by lactoferrin which can have a powerful bacteriostatic effect at pH 6.8 if no citrate is present (Griffiths and Humphreys, 1977). In local infections lactoferrin may be partly responsible for the inhibition of staphylococci, streptococci, *Klebsiella* species and *E. coli* in the bovine mammary gland (Harmon *et al.*, 1975; Bishop *et al.*, 1976; and see Chapter 5). With protozoan infections the presence of lactoferrin appears to encourage the phagocytosis and killing of *Trypanosoma cruzi* (Lima and Kierszenbaum, 1985). However, much more needs to be known about the antibacterial or antiprotozoal role of extracellular lactoferrin.

Indirectly, lactoferrin probably contributes to the control of infection by altering the surface charge on polymorphs and increasing their adhesive properties. Polymorphs normally have a negative surface charge which helps to keep them in suspension (Gallin, 1980). Lactoferrin causes aggregation of polymorphs in a dose-dependent manner (Oseas *et al.*, 1981) and reduces their surface charge which leads to an increase in adhesiveness (Boxer *et al.*, 1982c). In particular, lactoferrin appears to encourage the adherence of polmorphs to the endothelial cells of blood vessels (Boxer *et al.*, 1982a). This must occur before the polymorphs can migrate through the wall of the blood vessel towards the site of infection.

2. THE ROLE OF LACTOFERRIN IN THE BACTERICIDAL MECHANISMS OF POLYMORPHS

Masson, Heremans and Schonne (1969) were the first to discover the presence of lactoferrin in human and guinea-pig polymorphonuclear leukocytes. The protein is located in the specific granules (Leffell and Spitznagel, 1972; Briggs, Montiel and Wojtkowiak, 1983) and is present in fairly large amounts. Masson Heremans and Schonne (1969) and van Snick, Masson and Heremans (1974) found 3 mg/10^9 human polymorphs and Venge *et al.* (1978) 4.3 ± 1.2 mg/10^9 of the same cells.

The lactoferrin is relatively unsaturated with iron. Van Snick, Masson and Heremans (1974) gave a figure of 8 per cent saturation. This was measured by the binding of ^{59}Fe by extracts of polymorphs in 1 *M* saline after the cells had been disrupted by freezing and thawing. Bullen and Wallis (1977) found that lysosomal extracts from rabbit polymorphs with a total iron-binding capacity (TIBC) of 2.43×10^{-5} *M* Fe were approximately 31 per cent saturated, while a sonnicated extract of rabbit polymorphs with a TIBC of 3.9×10^{-5} *M* Fe was approximately 15 per cent saturated. Bullen and Armstrong (1979) using sonicated extracts of rabbit polymorphs with TIBCs of $4.47\text{–}5.7 \times 10^{-5}$ *M* Fe found a 14–40 per cent saturation with Fe (Table 4).

When bacteria are phagocytosed by polymorphs the cytoplasmic granules are discharged into the phagocytic vacuole. The specific granules are discharged first (Bainton, 1973). In the rabbit these contain lactoferrin, collagenase, alkaline phosphatase and lysozyme. The azurophil granules which follow contain myeloperoxidase, cationic proteins, lysozyme and hydrolases (Bainton, 1975).

Much attention has been paid to the activity of the large number of different enzymes involved in the bactericidal system within the phagocytic vacuole (Jensen and Bainton, 1973; Root and Cohen, 1981). However, there is plenty of evidence to show that while some bactericidal agents may be important in the polymorphs of some species they have no relevance in others. For example, myeloperoxidase may be essential for the proper function of human polymorphs (Root and Cohen, 1981; Spitznagel, 1983). However, it is not present in chicken heterophile leukocytes which have powerful bactericidal effects against several

Table 4 Iron-binding capacities of extracts of peritoneal exudate cells after exposure to: (1) *Pseudomonas aeruginosa* plus specific antibody, (2) an apoferritin–antiferritin complex, (3 and 4) a ferritin–antiferritin complex. SIBC = saturated iron-binding capacity, UIBC = unsaturated iron-binding capacity, TIBC = total iron-binding capacity

	Experiment	Polymorphs (%)	Cell extracts			Saturation with Fe (%)
			SIBC	UIBC (10^{-5} *M* Fe)	TIBC	
1.	Cells alone (control)	84	2.0	3.0	5.0	40
	Cells + *Ps aeruginosa* + *Ps auruginosa* antibody		2.23	3.27	5.5	40
2.	Cells alone (control)	76	1.45	4.3	5.75	25
	Cells + apoferritin complex		1.0	3.3	4.3	23
3.	Cells alone (control)	80	1.4	4.7	6.1	23
	Cells + ferritin complex		2.2	0	2.2	100
4.	Cells alone (control)	98	0.634	3.84	4.47	14
	Cells + ferritin complex		0.89	0	0.89	100

From Bullen and Armstrong (1979). Reproduced by permission of Blackwell Scientific Publications Limited.

bacteria and fungi (Brune, Leffell and Spitznagel, 1972). Again, bovine leukocytes do not contain lysozyme yet can kill *Salmonella typhimurium* and other bacteria (Padgett and Hirsch, 1967).

The question is whether lactoferrin is essential for the bactericidal function of polymorphs that contain it, and as far as we know there are no examples of its absence, at least in normal cells. There is no doubt that lactoferrin itself can act as an antibacterial agent (see Chapter 5) but in many cases it acts in conjunction with other components of the immune system, such as Ig A, for example, in human milk (see Chapter 5). It seems perfectly possible that the iron-binding capacity of lactoferrin, and especially its ability to bind iron at a low pH, could be essential for many bactericidal mechanisms that operate within the phagocytic vacuole.

The fact that some bactericidal mechanisms can operate *in vitro* (Root and Cohen, 1981; Spitznagel, 1983) without the presence of unsaturated iron-binding proteins does not exclude the possibility that lactoferrin could be important *in vivo*. At present, there is no way of imitating exactly the conditions inside the intact cell where all the bactericidal systems operate simultaneously in a controlled environment.

To explore the role of lactoferrin it was essential to find some way of saturating its iron-binding capacity inside polymorphs. Some of the first experiments on the effects of iron compounds on polymorphs were done by Gladstone and Walton (1971), and although no attempt was made to measure the saturation of intracellular lactoferrin the results suggested that iron could be important inside the cell. The iron compounds used were $FeSO_4$ and soluble haematin. Whether these compounds can enter the cell is not know but 1.84 m*M* Fe^{2+} had a sparing effect on the destruction of staphylococci by rabbit polymorphs suspended in an amino acid–glucose medium containing 20 per cent rabbit serum. In other experiments the polymorphs were suspended in a plasma clot. Here, both Fe^{2+} (= 1.84 m*M* Fe) and haematin (= 0.23 m*M* Fe) appeared to stimulate extracellular and intracellular growth, although the haematin was much more effective than the Fe^{2+}

Working with *Ps aeruginosa* sensitized with *Ps aeruginosa* antibody, Bullen and Wallis (1977) found that neither ferric ammonium citrate (= 2.2 m*M* Fe) nor ferritin (= 3.3 m*M* Fe) could prevent the bactericidal effect of rabbit polymorphs suspended in rabbit serum. The failure of the ferric ammonium citrate to stimulate extracellular growth as described previously was probably due to the rapid phagocytosis of the bacteria in the presence of specific antibody (see above and Bullen and Armstrong, 1979). However, a ferritin–antiferritin complex appeared to reverse the bactericidal effect and stimulate intracellular growth while an apoferritin–antibody complex did not.

Further work by Bullen and Armstrong (1979) with *Ps aeruginosa* (3.6×10^7/ml) sensitized with *Ps aeruginosa* antibody and suspended in autologous serum with 1×10^7 cells/ml (80–90 per cent polymorphs, the rest being macrophages and a few lymphocytes) showed that there was a rapid fall in the

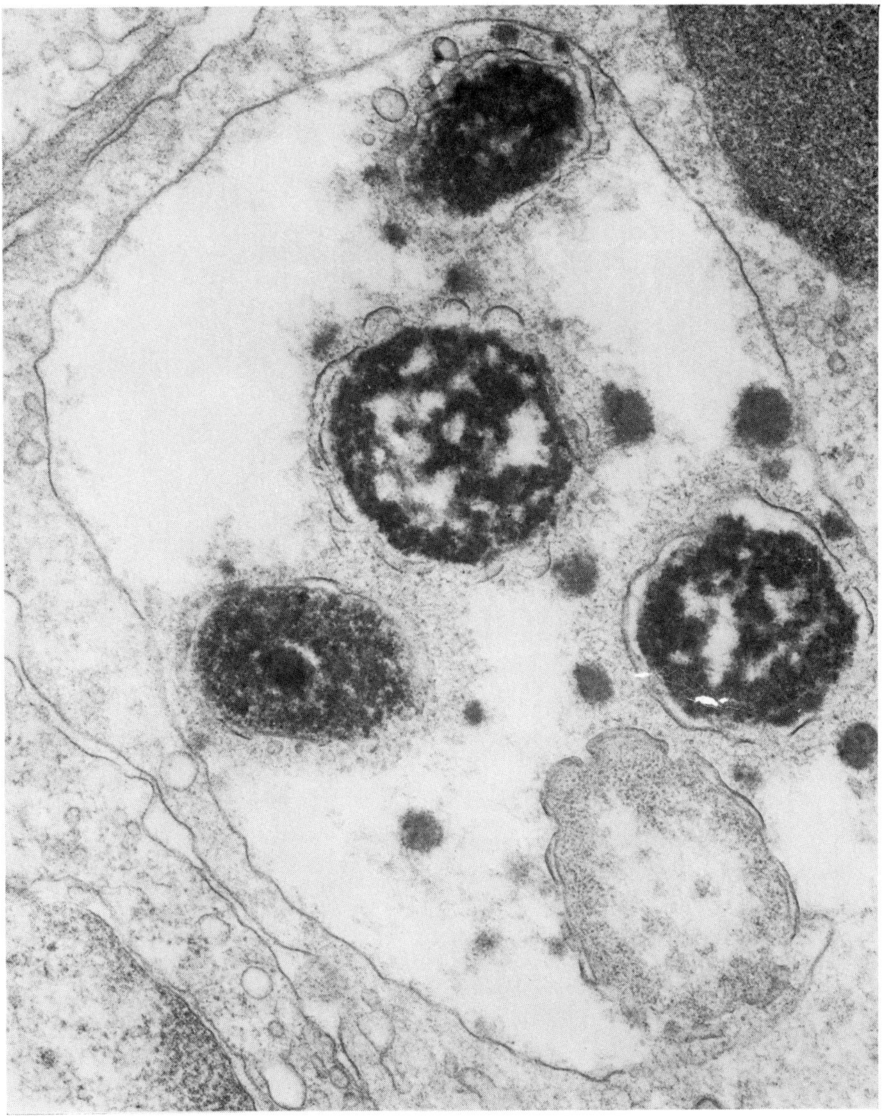

Figure 6 Phagocytosis of *Pseudomonas aeruginosa* by rabbit polymorph. Typical phagolysosome containing five structurally degraded bacteria. Dense bodies between bacteria are products of degranulation (× 37,600). *From Bullen and Armstrong (1979). Reproduced by permission of Blackwell Scientific Publications Limited*

viable count over a period of 6 hours. Electron micrographs after 2.75 hours showed widespread phagocytosis with phagolysosomes containing structurally degraded bacteria (Fig. 6). Extensive degranulation had occurred and many of the polymorph granules had fused with the phagosomes (Fig. 6). Measurement

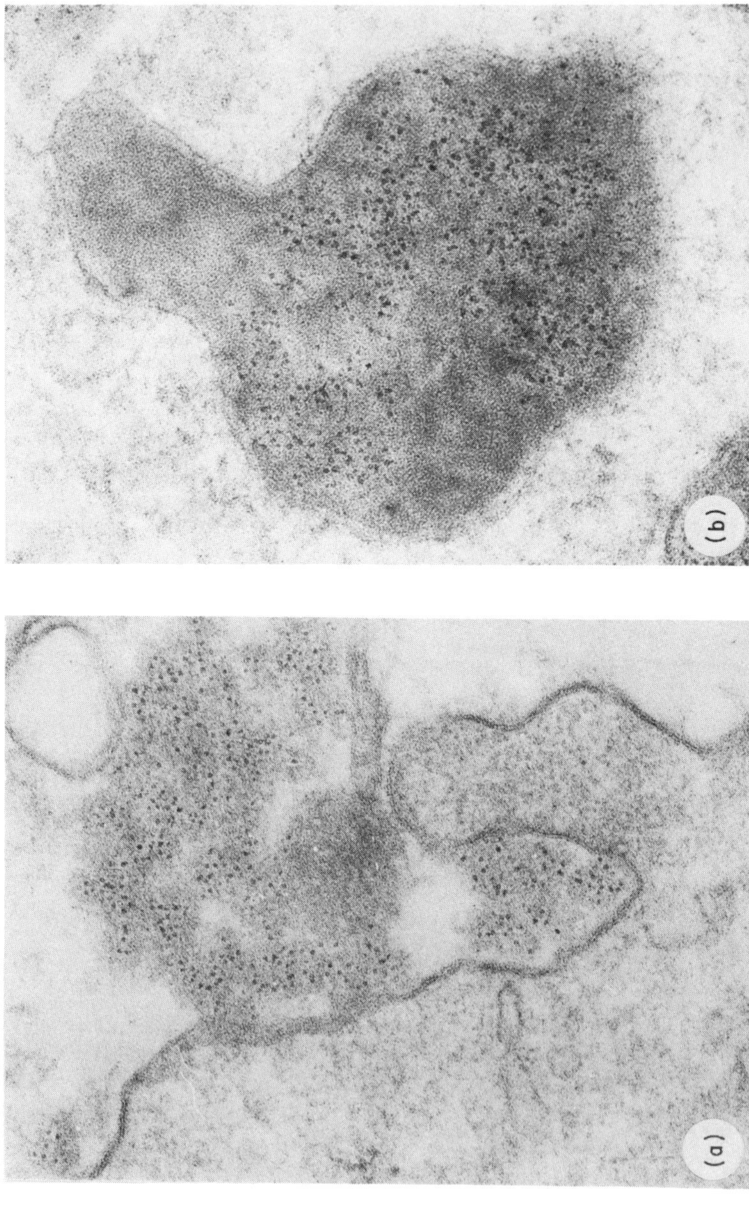

Figure 7 (a) Entry and (b) localization of ferritin–antiferritin complex in polymorph. Shows restriction of ferritin to vacuolar and granular systems of cell (× 110,000). *From Bullen and Armstrong (1979). Reproduced by permission of Blackwell Scientific Publications Limited.*

of the iron-binding capacity of sonicated extracts of the polymorphs after two hours showed no fall in TIBC (Table 4). This is consistent with the absence of any degranulation to the exterior of the cell, and, as mentioned before, is also consistent with the absence of hypoferraemia in the intact animal (Table 1). It seems likely that *Ps aeruginosa* sensitized with specific antibody does not provide enough stimulus to the polymorph to cause extracellular degranulation of the specific granules, although there was well-marked degranulation into the phagosomes (Fig. 6). A rough calculation suggested that the bacteria themselves could not supply enough iron to upset the iron-binding capacity of the cell, even if all the iron in the bacteria was liberated into the phagolysosomes. This is based on the figure of 0.1 mg of iron per gram dry weight of bacteria (Stephenson, 1949).

When ferritin–antiferritin complexes were added (1.0×10^7 cells: 90 per cent polymorphs, 3.6×10^7 bacteria and the complex = to 0.014 mg of ferritin/ml) considerable amounts of the complex were ingested by endocytosis after 2.75 hours (Fig. 7a). The complex appeared as flocculent material of only moderate density within which the characteristic dense cores of ferritin were scattered uniformly but with much wider spacing then seen with purified specimens of ferritin alone (Fig. 7a). It was detectable in numerous small endocytic vesicles and channels near the cell surface and also within the polymorph granules (Fig. 7b).

Ingested bacteria were numerous in both polymorphs and macrophages and hardly any were found extracellularly at 2.75 hours. Extensive fusion of the granules with phagosomes containing bacteria had occurred. The ferritin complex was found adjacent to the bacteria in the phagolysosomes, and sometimes the complex was seen in the process of being transferred from the granule into the phagosome by fusion, together with normal lysosomal dense material from the granule (Fig. 8). The great majority of intracellular bacteria showed obvious signs of structural degradation and had presumably been killed, but here and there bacilli were found which, though located in typical fused phagolysosomes, appeared to be completely intact, and could have been viable (Fig. 9). It should be emphasized that the small percentage of apparently 'spared' organisms did nevertheless seem to have been exposed to the same granule fusion products as all the other intracellular bacilli and there was no obvious morphological explanation of their survival. In phagosomes containing more than one bacterium the different types were never mixed but always 'intact' or 'degraded'. This might indicate that the composition of the granule contents, rather than any inherent bacterial resistance, determined the outcome in the first few hours after infection.

This picture was consistent with the viable counts where there was considerable destruction of the bacteria during the first few hours. Later, at 5.75 hours, the picture changed dramatically, in keeping with a rapid increase in the viable bacterial count. Almost all the polymorphs and a high proportion of macro-

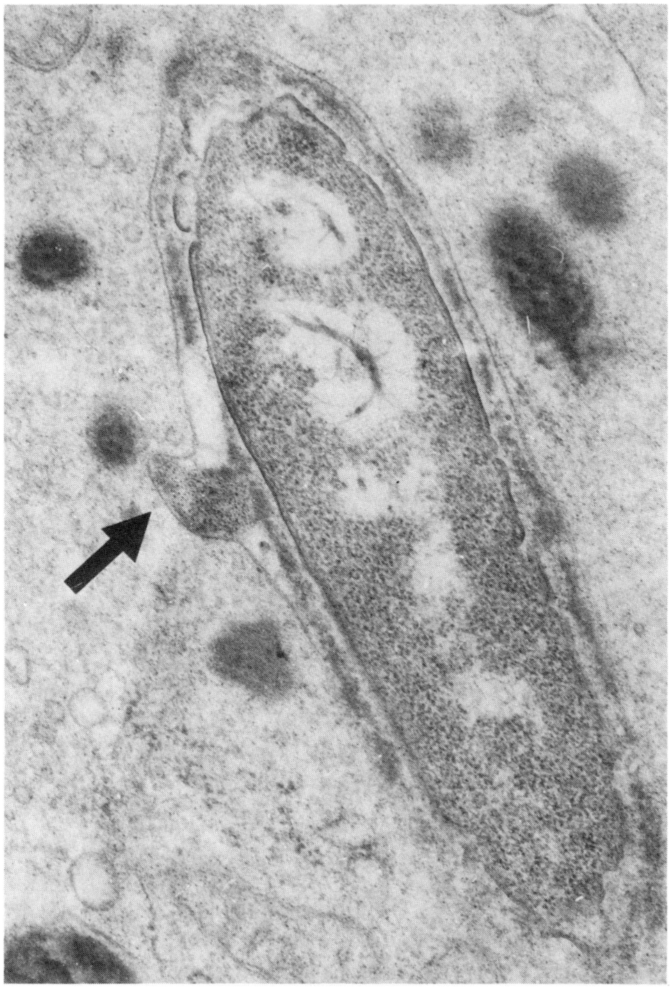

Figure 8 Section of polymorph exposed to *Pseudomonas aeruginosa* and ferritin–antiferritin complex. Fusion of ferritin-containing cytoplasmic granule (arrowed) with phagosome containing the organism (× 60,000). *From Bullen and Armstrong (1979). Reproduced by permission of Blackwell Scientific Publications Limited*

phages showed obvious cytolytic changes, with masses of cell fragments intermingled with multiplying *Ps. aeruginosa* (Fig. 10). Thus the ferritin–antibody complex eventually destroyed the bactericidal power of the cells. In addition, it completely saturated the iron-binding capacity of the polymorph extracts (Table 4). This is consistent with the entry of the ferritin–antiferritin complex into the cell and the transfer of Fe from the ferritin to the lactoferrin

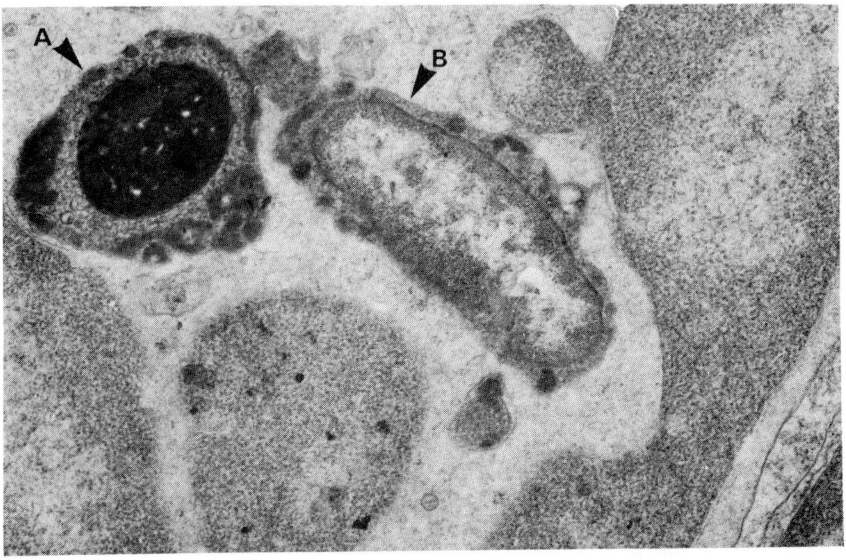

Figure 9 Section of polymorph plus *Pseudomonas aeruginosa* and the ferritin–antiferritin complex. Two phagolysosomes contain bacteria. (A) Degranulation results in destruction of the organism. (B) Organism intact despite degranulation (× 24,800). *From Bullen and Armstrong (1979). Reproduced by permission of Blackwell Scientific Publications Limited*

derived from the specific granules. It strongly suggests that the unsaturated iron-binding capacity of the intracellular lactoferrin is essential for the bactericidal properties of the polymorphs against *Ps aeruginosa*.

The apoferritin–antiferritin complex was a useful control since the polymorphs were exposed to identical amounts of antigenic material as in the experiments with the ferritin–antiferritin complex but no iron was present. Since there were no iron cores in the apoferritin it was more difficult to identify it in the electron micrographs, but flocculent masses of moderately electron dense material were seen within the polymorphs and macrophages, both in the granule contents and in the larger endocytic vacuoles. The apoferritin compex failed to interfere with the killing of *Ps aeruginosa* by the polymorphs and the electron micrographs showing destruction of the bacteria were very similar to those of the control with cells and bacteria alone (Fig. 11). The apoferritin complex had no effect on the percentage saturation of the lactoferrin in the cell (Table 4). This was expected, but it did cause some loss of total iron-binding capacity which was consistent with an escape of lactoferrin during phagocytosis of an immune complex (Leffell and Spitznagel, 1975).

The evidence that the iron-binding capacity of lactoferrin in polymorphs may be essential for the cell's bactericidal power, at least with some bacteria, made it all the more important to see if similar results could be obtained *in vivo*. Bullen and Joyce (1982) produced evidence that with *K. pneumoniae* and *E.coli*

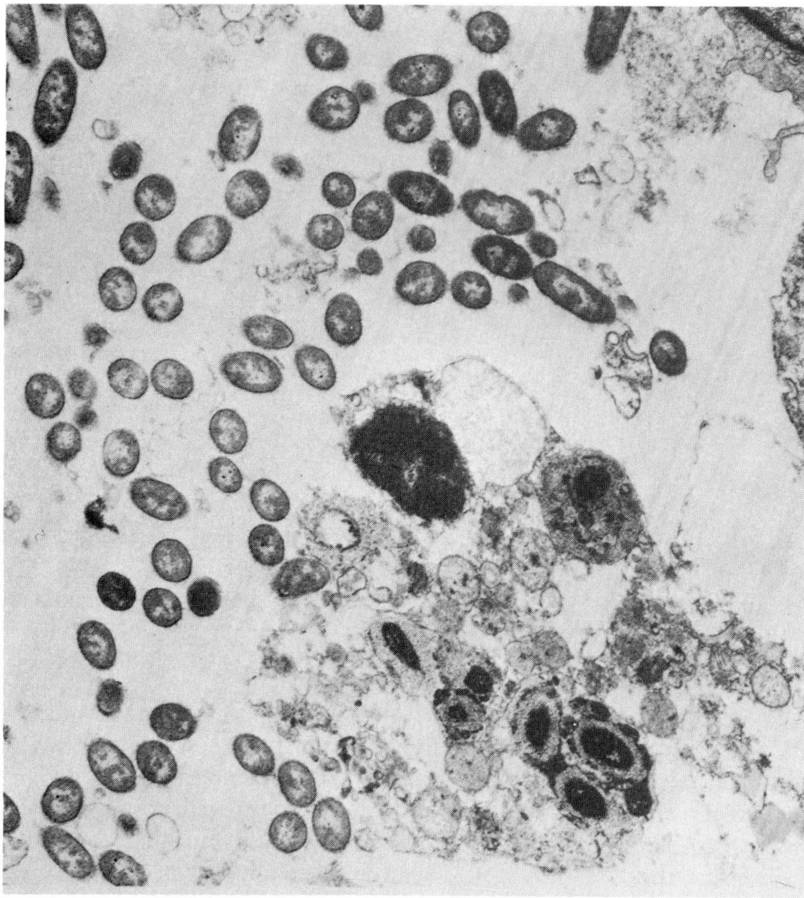

Figure 10 Destruction of polymorph by growth of *Pseudomonas aeruginosa* following exposure to bacteria and the ferritin–antiferritin complex. Cell remnants surrounded by growing organisms. Some bacteria emerging from cell (× 5,120). *From Bullen and Armstrong (1979). Reproduced by permission of Blackwell Scientific Publications Limited*

infections the ingestion of ferritin complexes by polymorphs can lead to intracellular bacterial growth instead of destruction of the bacteria. This results in rapidly fatal infections. Table 5 shows that the injection of 0.1 mg of Fe as a ferritin–antiferritin complex in passively immunized animals which are normally protected against *K. pneumoniae* gave a high death rate. Ferritin alone without the antiferritin antibody had little effect. The apoferritin–antiferritin complex had no effect.

Similar, but not identical, results were obtained with *E.coli* (Table 6). In this

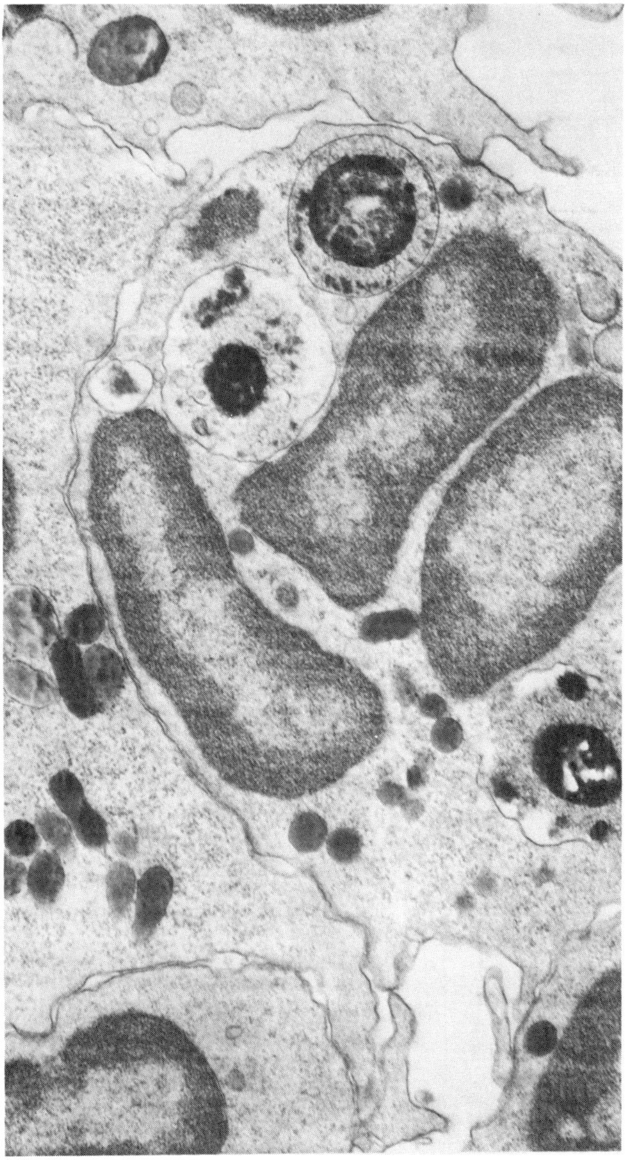

Figure 11 Section of polymorph exposed to *Pseudomonas aeruginosa* and apoferritin–antiferritin complex. Destruction of bacteria in the vacuoles (× 14,000). *From Bullen and Armstrong (1979). Reproduced by permission of Blackwell Scientific Publications Limited*

Table 5 Reduction of the protective effect of *K.pneumoniae* antibody in mice by injection of a ferritin–antiferritin complex.

	Infection	Death rate	Deaths (%)
1.	*K.pneumoniae*	24/24	100
2.	*K.pneumoniae* plus protective antibody	0/23	0
3.	*K.pneumoniae* plus protective antibody plus apoferritin–antiferritin complex	0/46	0
4.	*K.pneumoniae* plus protective antibody plus ferritin–antiferritin complex	41/46	89
5.	*K.pneumoniae* plus ferritin	1/15	7

From Bullen and Joyce (1982). Reproduced by permission of Blackwell Scientific Publications Limited.

Table 6 Enhancement of the lethal effect of *E.coli* in mice by injection of a ferritin–antiferritin complex (Ferritin alone also has some effect)

	Infection	Death rate	Deaths (%)
1.	*E.coli*	3/46	6.5
2.	*E.coli* plus apoferritin–antiferritin complex	1/68	1.5
3.	*E.coli* plus ferritin–antiferritin complex	60/68	88
4.	*E.coli* plus Ferritin	10/27	37

From Bullen and Joyce (1982). Reproduced by permission of Blackwell Scientific Publications Limited.

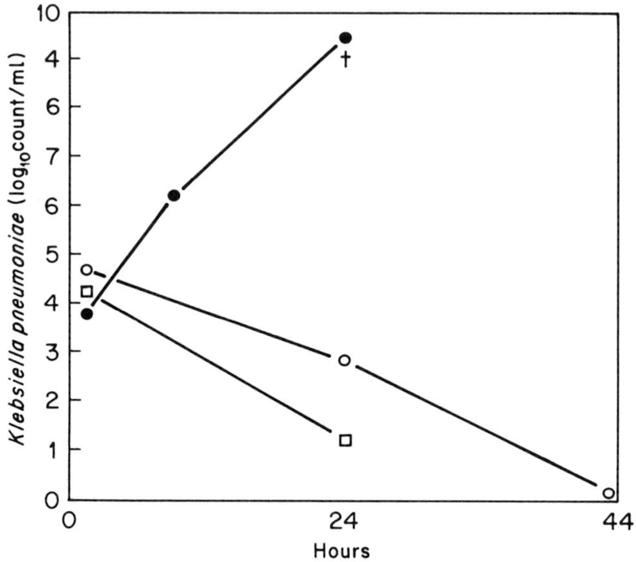

Figure 12 *Klebsiella pneumoniae* in the peritoneal cavity of passively immunized mice. □ Control. ○ Plus an apoferritin–antiferritin complex. ● Plus a ferritin–antiferritin complex. † Dying animal. *From Bullen and Joyce (1982). Reproduced by permission of Blackwell Scientific Publications Limited*

case no protective antibody was used and there was a small number of deaths in the controls. The ferritin-antiferritin complex (= 0.1 mg Fe) gave nearly 90 per cent deaths while the apoferritin–antiferritin complex gave only 1.5 per cent. Ferritin alone, however, gave 37 per cent deaths, suggesting that in this case the iron in the ferritin was enough to tip the balance towards a fatal infection, even without the antiferritin antibody.

With both *E.coli* and *K.pneumoniae* infections the apoferritin–antiferritin complex did produce slightly higher bacterial counts *in vivo* than the controls, but the ferritin–antiferritin complex stimulated bacterial growth to a far greater extent (Figs. 12 and 13). With *E.coli* infections it was possible to see intracellular bacterial multiplication in the polymorphs of animals receiving the ferritin–antiferritin complex (Fig. 14). The apoferritin complex showed relatively few bacteria and the great majority of these were extracellular (Fig. 14).

These experiments, both *in vitro* and *in vivo*, strongly suggested that the iron-binding capacity of lactoferrin within polymorphs could indeed be important for its bactericidal function. However, one has to remember that the role of iron-binding proteins in controlling extracellular bacterial growth, which has been discussed already, may be equally important, and the possibility that both mechanisms could operate simultaneously must be borne in mind.

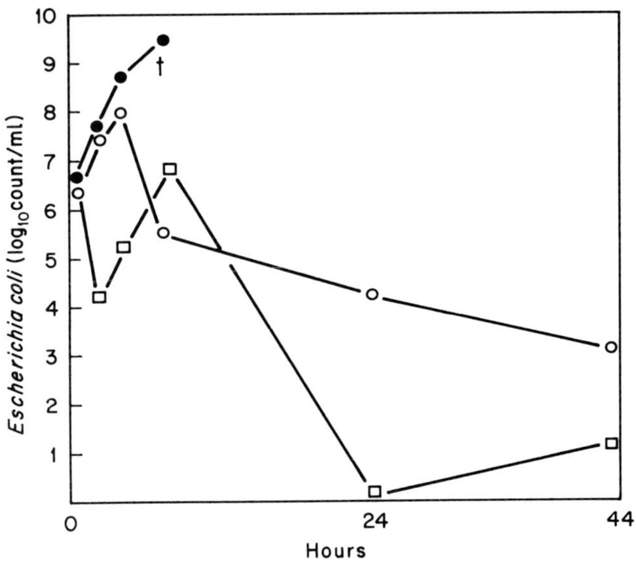

Figure 13 *Escherichia coli* in the peritoneal cavity of mice. □ Control. ○ Plus an apoferritin–antiferritin complex. ● Plus a ferritin–antiferritin complex, † Dying animal. *From Bullen and Joyce (1982). Reproduced by permission of Blackwell Scientific Publications Limited*

There is some clinical evidence that lactoferrin deficiency in polymorphs is associated with increased susceptibility to infection. Boxer *et al.* (1982b) describe a patient in which the lactoferrin content of the specific granules (0.24 ± 0.01 mg/10^9 cells) was approximately 3.4 per cent of the normal value (7.0 ± 1.5 mg/10^9 cells). The patient was reported to suffer from repeated deep-seated abscesses and there was some evidence of reduced bactericidal activity of the polymorphs. The authors also suggested that a relative deficiency of lactoferrin could contribute to the patient's cells showing poor adhesiveness and aggregation, and that this could contribute to lack of effectiveness in dealing with infections. Breton-Gorius *et al.* (1980) described the case of a boy suffering from repeated infections where the specific granules in the polymorphs were absent. They found that the bactericidal activity of the polymorphs against a strain of *Serratia marscescens* and *Staphylococcus aureus* was 'normal', but the *in vitro* tests were of very short duration (90 minutes) and the cells were suspended in Hanks solution containing 20 per cent of serum from normal donors. It is therefore difficult to estimate the relevance of these tests in terms of the clinical history. Three other similar cases were reported by Strauss *et al.* (1974), Komiyana *et al.* (1979) and Spitznagel *et al.* (1972); the patients concerned suffered from repeated infections. There was an absence or near absence of specific granules

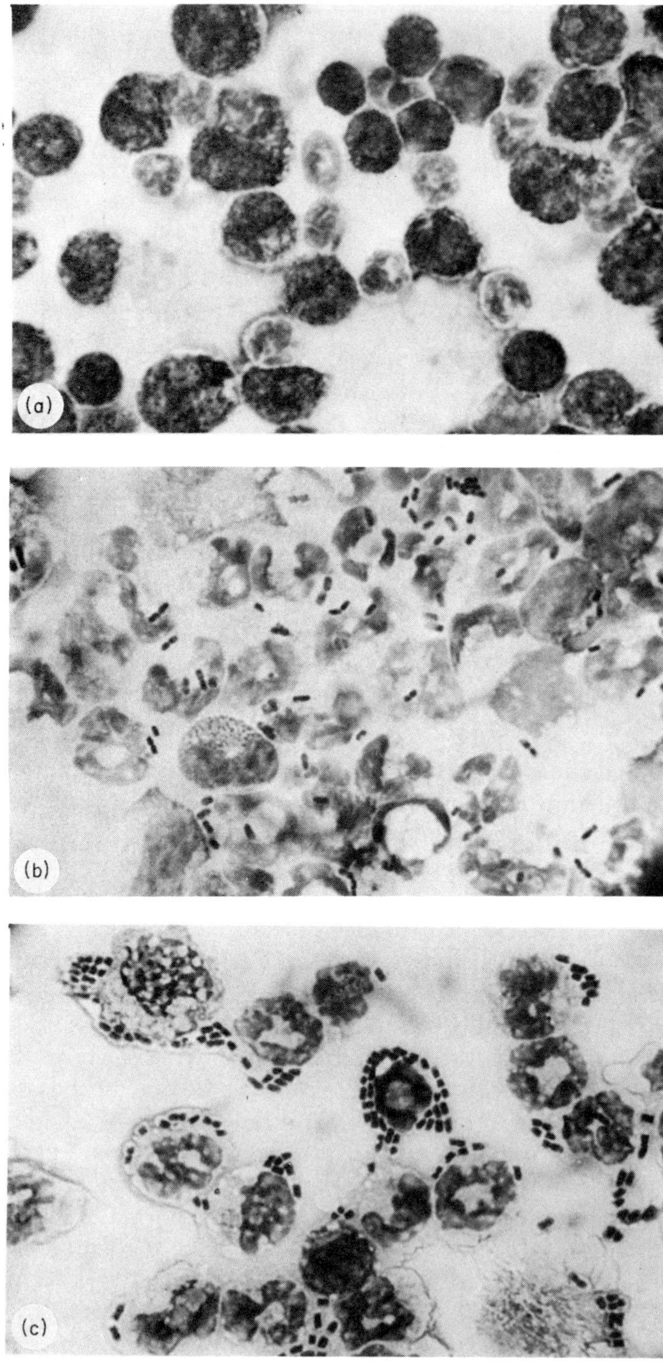
(a)
(b)
(c)

associated with poor *in vitro* killing of some bacteria. In a case described by Parmley *et al.* (1975) there were repeated infections with *E.coli*, *Pseudomonas* and *Klebsiella* species; the specific granules were absent but there was no data on the bactericidal power of the polymorphs.

Miyauchi *et al.* (1983) reported an absence of specific granules in lactoferrin-deficient polymorphs, or polymorphs with low levels of lactoferrin, in patients with leukaemia. This is interesting in view of the known increased susceptibility of these patients to infection and the relatively high levels of saturation of their serum transferrin with iron (see Chapter 7). It is tempting to think that the low levels of lactoferrin derived from the polymorphs could interfere with the development of hypoferraemia mediated by Interleukin 1 and that this is related to the relatively high level of saturation of serum transferrin, which, in turn, could encourage extracellular bacterial growth. This could be exacerbated by poor bactericidal performance of the polymorphs, also associated with a lack of lactoferrin (see above). At present, these suggestions can only be regarded as tentative ideas, but there does seem to be a good case for investigating the whole of this subject in more detail.

3. LACTOFERRIN AND THE CONTROL OF GRANULOPOIESIS

There is good evidence that extracellular lactoferrin released from polymorphs is involved in a negative feedback system controlling the number of circulating polymorphs. Lactoferrin acts as an inhibitor of colony stimulating factor (CSF) produced by monocytes and macrophages which normally stimulate the production of granulocytes. The degree of suppression of CSF activity can be correlated with the degree of saturation of the lactoferrin. Apolactoferrin was active at > 10^{-7} *M*, 8 per cent saturated lactoferrin at 10^{-15} *M* and fully saturated lactoferrin at 10^{-17} *M*. Transferrin had little or no effect (Broxmeyer *et al.*, 1978).

Saturated lactoferrin from a subpopulation of polymorphs (Broxmeyer *et al.*, 1980) binds onto lactoferrin receptors on monocytes and macrophages (Bennett and Davis, 1971; van Snick and Masson, 1976; Broxmeyer, 1978) which controls the production or release of granulocyte–monocyte colony stimulating factor (Broxmeyer *et al.*, 1980). Steinman *et al.* (1982) showed that lactoferrin fully saturated with iron could be taken up by monocytes after 30 minutes of exposure to a 10^{-14} *M* solution of the protein. The lactoferrin appeared as small deposits approximately 110 nm in diameter in the endoplasmic reticulum. The deposits

Figure 14 Peritoneal exudates of mice infected with *Escherichia coli* (after 4.5 hours). (a) Control, bacteria alone. (b) Bacteria plus an apoferritin–antiferritin complex. (c) Bacteria plus a ferritin–antiferritin complex. Note intracellular bacterial growth (× 1000) *From Bullen and Joyce (1982). Reproduced by permission of Blackwell Scientific Publications Limited*

were found only in some monocytes, suggesting that a subpopulation of the cells is involved in the control mechanism.

Some workers (Bagby *et al.*, 1981; Bagby, McCall and Layman, 1983) have suggested that the negative feedback regulation by lactoferrin occurs by control of the release of a specific monokine from mononuclear phagocytes, which in turn stimulates T lymphocytes, endothelial cells and fibroblasts to produce colony-stimulating factor.

Broxmeyer (1978) found that cell-free extracts from human polymorphs could suppress rebound granulopoiesis in mice pretreated with cyclophosphamide. The injection of rabbit lactoferrin into hamsters and rabbits caused a transient neutropenia (Boxer *et al.*, 1982a), while the injection of human lactoferrin into mice suppressed myelopoiesis (Gentile and Broxmeyer, 1983).

Thus links have been established between the release of lactoferrin by polymorphs and the eventual control of granulopoiesis which is essential for regulating the cellular response to infection. The exact details of the mechanisms involved require further clarification.

REFERENCES

Bagby, G.C., McCall, E., and Layman, D.L. (1983). Regulation of colony-stimulating activity production. Interactions of fibroblasts, mononuclear phagocytes and lactoferrin. *Journal of Clinical Investigation*, **71**, 340–344.

Bagby, G.C., Rigas, V.D., Bennett, R.M., Vandenbark, A.A., and Garewall, H.S. (1981). Interaction of lactoferrin, monocytes, and T lymphocyte subsets in the regulation of steady state granulopoiesis in vitro. *Journal of Clinical Investigation*, **68,** 56–63.

Bainton, D.F. (1973). Sequential degranulation of the two types of polymorphonuclear leukocyte granules during phagocytosis of microorganisms. *Journal of Cell Biology*, **58,** 249–264.

Bainton, D.F. (1975). Neutrophil granules. Annotation. *British Journal of Haematology*, **29,** 17–21.

Bennett, R.M., and Davis, J. (1971). Lactoferrin binding to human peripheral blood cells: an interaction with a B-enriched population of lymphocytes and a subpopulation of adherent mononuclear cells. *Journal of Immunology*, **127**, 1211–1215.

Bishop, J.G., Schanbacher, F.L., Ferguson, L.C., and Smith, K.L. (1976). In vitro growth inhibition of mastitis-causing coliform bacteria by bovine apo-lactoferrin and reversal of inhibition by citrate and high concentration of apo-lactoferrin. *Infection and Immunity*, **14,** 911–918.

Boxer, L.A., Bjorksten, B., Bjork, J., Yang, H.H., Allen, J.M., and Baehner, R.L. (1982a). Neutropenia induced by systemic infusion of lactoferrin. *Journal of Laboratory and Clinical Medicine*, **99,** 866–872.

Boxer, L.A., Coates, T.D., Haak, R.A., Wolach, J.B., Hoffstein, S., and Baehner, R.L. (1982b). Lactoferrin deficiency associated with altered granulocyte function. *New England Journal of Medicine*, **303,** 404–410.

Boxer, L.A., Haak, R.A., Yang, H.H., Wolach, J.B., Whitcomb, J.A., Butterick, C.J., and Baehner, R.L. (1982c). Membrane bound lactoferrin alters the surface properties of polymorphonuclear leukocytes. *Journal of Clinical Investigation*, **70,** 1049–1057.

Breton-Gorius, J., Mason, D.Y., Buriot, D., Vilde, J.L., and Griscelli, C. (1980). Lactoferrin deficiency as a consequence of a lack of specific granules in neutrophils from a patient with recurrent infections. *American Journal of Pathology*, **99,** 413–428.

Briggs, R.C., Montiel, M.M, and Wojtkowiak, Z. (1983). Nuclear localization of lactoferrin in the human granulocyte: artifact incurred during slide preparation. *Journal of Histochemistry and Cytochemisty*, **31,** 1152–1162.

Broxmeyer, H.E. (1978). Inhibition in vivo of mouse granulopoiesis by cell free activity derived from human polymorphonuclear neutrophils. *Blood*, **51,** 889–901.

Broxmeyer, H.E., Ralph, P., Bognaxki, J., Kincade, P.W., and de Sousa, M. (1980). A subpopulation of human polymorphonuclear neutrophils contains an active form of lactoferrin capable of binding to human monocytes and inhibiting production of granulocyte-macrophage colony stimulating activities. *Journal of Immunology*, **125,** 903–909.

Broxmeyer, H.E., Smithyman, A., Eger, R.R., Meyers, A., and de Sousa, M. (1978). Identification of lactoferrin as the granulocyte-derived inhibitor of colony-stimulating activity production. *Journal of Experimental Medicine*, **148,** 1052–1067.

Brune, K., Leffell, M.S., and Spitznagel, J.K. (1972). Microbicidal activity of peroxidaseless chicken heterophile leucocytes. *Infection and Immunity*, **5,** 283–287.

Bullen, J.J., and Armstrong, J.A. (1979). The role of lactoferrin in the bactericidal function of polymorphonuclear leucocytes. *Immunology*, **36,** 781–791.

Bullen, J.J., Cushnie, G.H., and Stoner, H.B. (1966). Oxygen uptake by *Clostridium welchii* type A; its possible role in experimental infections in passively immunised animals. *British Journal of Experimental Pathology*, **47**, 488–506.

Bullen, J.J., and Joyce, P.R. (1982). Abolition of the bactericidal function of polymorphs by ferritin–antiferritin complexes. *Immunology*, **46,** 497–505.

Bullen, J.J., Rogers, H.J., and Lewin, J.E. (1971). The bacteriostatic effect of serum on *Pasteurella septica* and its abolition by iron compounds. *Immunology*, **20**, 391–406.

Bullen, J.J., and Wallis, S.N. (1977). Reversal of the bactericidal effect of polymorphs by a ferritin–antibody complex. *FEMS Letters*, **1,** 117–120.

Bullen, J.J., Wallis, S.N., and Griffiths, E. (1976). The effect of antipolymorphonuclear leucocyte serum on *Pseudomonas aeruginosa* infection in rabbits. *Immunology*, **30,** 603–610.

Bullen, J.J., Ward, C.G., and Wallis, S.N. (1974). Virulence and the role of iron in *Pseudomonas aeruginosa* infection. *Infection and Immunity*, **10,** 443–450.

Eaton, J.W., Brandt, P., Mahoney, J.R., and Lee, J.T. (1982). Haptoglobin: a natural bacteriostat. *Science*, **215,** 691–692.

Forsberg, C.M., and Bullen, J.J. (1972). The effect of passage and iron on the virulence of *Pseudomonas aeruginosa*. *Journal of Clinical Pathology*, **25**, 65–68.

Gallin, J.I. (1980). Degranulating stimuli decrease the negative surface charge and increase the adhesiveness of human neutrophils. *Journal of Clinical Investigation*, **65,** 298–306.

Gentile, P., and Broxmeyer, H.E. (1983). Suppression of mouse myelopoiesis by administration of human lactoferrin *in vivo* and the comparative action of human transferrin. Blood **61,** 982–993.

Gladstone, G.P., and Walton, E. (1971). The effect of iron and haematin on the killing of staphyloccoci by rabbit polymorphs. *British Journal of Experimental Pathology*, **52,** 452–464.

Griffiths, E., and Humphreys, J. (1977). Bacteriostatic effect of human milk and bovine colostrum on *Escherichia coli*. *Infection and Immunity*, **15,** 386–401.

Gutteberg, T.J., Haneberg, B., and Jorgensen, T. (1984a). The latency of serum actue phase proteins in meningococcal septicaemia, with special emphasis on lactoferrin. *Clinical Chimica Acta*, **136,** 173–178.

Gutteberg, T.J., Haneberg, B., and Jorgensen, T. (1984b). Lactoferrin in relation to acute phase proteins in sera from newborn infants with severe infections. *European Journal of Pediatrics*, **142,** 37–39.
Harmon, R.J., Schanbacher, F.L., Ferguson, L.C., and Smith, K.L. (1975). Concentration of lactoferrin in milk of normal lactating cows and changes occurring during mastitis. *American Journal of Veterinary Research*, **36,** 1001–1007.
Jensen, M.S., and Bainton, D.F. (1973). Temporal changes in pH within the phagocytic vacuole of the polymorphonuclear leukocyte. *Journal of Cell Biology*, **56**, 379–388.
Klempner, M.S., Dinarello, C.A., and Gallin, J.I. (1978). Human leukocyte pyrogen induces release of specific granule contents from human neutrophils. *Journal of Clinical Investigation*, **61,** 1330–1336.
Komiyama, A., Morosowa, H., Nakahata, T., Miyagawa, Y., and Akabane, T. (1979). Abnormal neutrophil maturation in a neutrophil defect with morphologic abnormality and impaired function. *Journal of Pediatrics*, **94,** 19–25.
Leffell, M.S., and Spitznagel, J.K. (1972). Association of lactoferrin with lysozyme in granules of human polymorphonuclear leukocytes. *Infection and Immunity*, **6,** 761–765.
Leffell, M.S., and Spitznagel, J.K. (1975). Fate of human lactoferrin and myeloperoxidase in phagocytizing human neutrophils: effects of immunoglobulin G subclasses and immune complexes coated on latex beads. *Infection and Immunity*, **12,** 813–820.
Lima, M.F., and Kierszenbaum, F. (1985). Lactoferrin affects phagocytic cell function. 1. Increased uptake and killing of an intracellular parasite by murine macrophages and human monocytes. *Journal of Immunology*, **134,** 4176–4183.
Masson, P.L., Heremans, J.F., and Schonne, E. (1969). Lactoferrin, an iron binding protein in neutrophilic leukocytes. *Journal of Experimental Medicine*, **130,** 643–658.
Miyauchi, J., Watanabe, Y., Enomoto, Y., and Taleuchi, K. (1983). Lactoferrin-deficient neutrophil polymorphonuclear léucocytes in leukaemias: a semiquantitative and ultrastructural cytochemical study. *Journal of Clinical Pathology*, **36**, 1397–1405.
Oseas, R., Yang, H.H., Baehner, R.L., and Boxer, L.A. (1981). Lactoferrin: a promoter of polymorphonuclear adhesiveness. *Blood*, **57**, 939–945.
Padgett, G.A., and Hirsch, J.G. (1967). Lysozyme: its absence in tears and leukocytes of cattle. *Australian Journal of Experimental Biology and Medicine*, **45**, 569–570.
Parmley, R.T., Ogawa, M., Darby, C.P., and Spicer, S.S. (1975). Congenital neutropenia: neutrophil proliferation with abnormal maturation. *Blood*, **46**, 723–734.
Root, R.K., and Cohen, M.S. (1981). The microbicidal mechanisms of human neutrophils and eosinophils. *Reviews of Infectious Diseases*, **3**, 565–598.
Ryter, A., and de Chastellier, C. (1983). Phagocyte–pathogenic microbe interactions. *International Reviews of Cytology*, **85**, 287–327.
Spitznagel, J.K. (1983). Microbial interactions with neutrophils. *Reviews of Infectious Diseases*, **5**, Supplement, 4, 806–822.
Spitznagel, J.K., Cooper, M.R., McCall, A.E., Decatelet, L.R., and Welsh, I.R.H. (1972). Selective deficiency of granules with lysozyme and lactoferrin in human polymorphs (PMN) with reduced microbicidal capacity. *Journal of Clinical Investigation*, **51**, 93a.
Steinman, G., Broxmeyer, H.E., de Harven, E., and Moore, (1982). Immuno-electron microscopic tracing of lactoferrin, a regulator of myelopoesis, into a subpopulation of human peripheral blood monocytes. *British Journal of Haematology*, **50**, 75–84.
Stephenson, M. (1949). *Bacterial Metabolism*, 3rd ed. p.180. Longmans, Green, London.
Stoner, H.B., and Green, H.N. (1948). Bodily reactions to trauma. The effect of ischaemia on muscle protein. *British Journal of Experimental Pathology*, **29**, 121–132.

Strauss, R.G., Boue, K.E., Jones, J.F., Mauer, A.M., and Fulginiti, V.A. (1974). An anomaly of neutrophil morphology with impaired function. *New England Journal of Medicine*, **290**, 478–484.

van Snick, J.L., and Masson, P.L. (1976). The binding of human lactoferrin to mouse peritoneal cells. *Journal of Experimental Medicine*, **144**, 1568–1580.

van Snick, J.L., Masson, P.L., and Heremans, J.F. (1974). The involvement of lactoferrin in the hyposideremia of acute inflammation. *Journal of Experimental Medicine*, **140**, 1068–1084.

Venge, P., Stremberg, A., Braconier, J.H., Roxin, L.E., and Olsson, I. (1978). Neutrophil and eosinophil granulocyte in bacterial infection: sequential studies of cellular and serum levels of granule proteins. *British Journal of Haematology*, **38**, 475–483.

Ward, C.G., Hammond, J.S., and Bullen, J.J. (1986). Effect of iron compounds on the antibacterial function of human polymorphs and plasma. *Infection and Immunity*, **51**, 723–730.

Wolach, B., Coates, T.D., Hugli, T.E., Baehner, R.L., and Boxer, L.A. (1984). Plasma lactoferrin reflects granulocyte activation via complement in burn patients. *Journal of Laboratory and Clinical Medicine*, **103**, 284–293.

Wright, D.G., and Malawista, S.E. (1972). The mobilisation and extracellular release of granular enzymes from human leukocytes during phagocytosis. *Journal of Cell Biology*, **53**, 788–797.

Iron and Infection
Edited by J.J. Bullen and E. Griffiths

Chapter 7

Clinical and physiological aspects

M.J. KLUGER
Department of Physiology,
The University of Michigan Medical School,
Ann Arbor,
Michigan 48109, USA

J.J. BULLEN
Department of Surgery,
University of Miami School of Medicine,
Jackson Memorial Medical Center,
PO Box 016310, Miami,
Florida 33101, USA

Elsewhere in this book the availability of iron has been described as crucial for the growth of bacteria *in vivo*. In this chapter we examine the circumstances in clinical disease where abnormal availability of iron may play a part in stimulating bacterial infection. We also consider some of the physiological responses to infection, particularly those which tend to sequester iron from the micro-environment surrounding the bacteria and thus make it unavailable for bacterial growth.

1. THE CLINICAL CONSEQUENCES OF EXCESS IRON

1.1 The importance of haem compounds

Pathogenic bacteria can utilize the iron in haem compounds, but only after it is made available by some form of tissue damage which releases intracellular material. The lysis of red cells is a good example. Haemoglobin released by red cells dissociates into its subunits (two α-β-chain dimers) and is bound by circulating haptoglobin. One molecule of haptoglobin binds one molecule of haemoglobin to form a saturated complex. This complex is quickly eliminated by reticuloendothelial cells of the liver, bone marrow or spleen. Free haemoglobin appears when the haptoglobin is saturated. The free haemoglobin is easily oxidized and dissociates into ferrihaem and globin. Haemopexin has a higher affinity for ferrihaem than albumin and a haem–haemopexin complex is formed. One molecule of haemopexin binds one molecule of haem. As in the case of the haptoglobin–haemoglobin complex this is rapidly cleared from the circulation by the hepatic parenchymal cells. Excess haem not bound to haemopexin is bound to albumin, each molecule binding two molecules of haem to form methaemalbumin. Methaemalbumin is not cleared form the plasma and is likely to circulate until it is eventually complexed with apohaemopexin. Some of the unbound circulating haemoglobin passes through the glomerular membranes and is absorbed by the renal tubules. When the absorptive capacity of the tubules is exhausted haemoglobin subunits appear in the urine resulting in haemosiderinuria (Muller-Eberhard, 1970; Cederblad, 1979).

Much has been written about the binding of Fe^{3+} by transferrin and its influence on bacterial growth (see Chapters 2, 3 and 5). However, it is only comparatively recently that it has been realized that the formation of a haptoglobin—haemoglobin complex may affect the availability of the iron in the haemoglobin molecule for pathogenic bacteria. Eaton *et al.* (1982) were the first to show the protective effect of haptoglobin. Rats given a normally sublethal dose of 2.5×10^7 *Escherichia coli* died when the bacteria were injected with 20 mg of haemoglobin. If 30 mg of haptoglobin was also included, which was sufficient to bind all the haemoglobin, the majority of the animals survived. Thus when haemoglobin is bound to haptoglobin the bacteria were unable to utilize the haem iron. These results suggested that haptoglobin could have an important bacteriostatic and protective effect *in vivo* (Fig. 1). However, some bacteria can utilize the iron in the haptoglobin–haemoglobin complex. *Vibrio vulnificus* is usually inhibited by human serum but grows rapidly in the presence of 1 mg/ml of

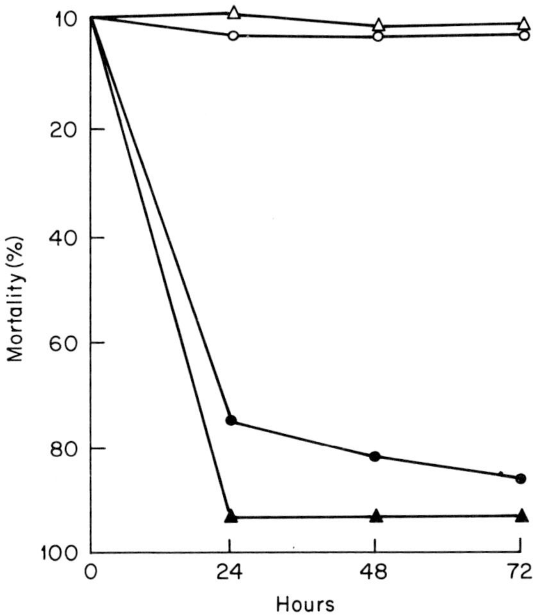

Figure 1 The protective effect of haptoglobin. Mortality in rats inoculated intraperitoneally with: ○ 2.5×10^7 *Escherichia coli*. ● *E.coli* plus 20 mg of haemoglobin. △ *E.coli* plus 20 mg of haemoglobin plus 30 mg of haptoglobin. ▲ *E.coli* plus Fe^{3+}. *From Eaton* et al. *(1982) Reproduced by permission of the American Association for the Advancement of Science*

haemoglobin whether or not it is complexed with haptoglobin (Helms, Oliver and Travis 1984).

The same consideration may apply to the availability of iron in haem. Haematin is highly effective in stimulating bacterial growth in experimental infections with *E.coli* (Bullen, Leigh and Rogers, 1968), *Pasteurella multocida* (Bullen *et al.*, 1968) and *Vibrio vulnificus* (Helms, Oliver and Travis, 1984) but in none of these instances was the degree of saturation of the haem-binding proteins known. However, it has been shown that *Klebsiella pneumoniae* can utilize methaemalbumin even if the saturation of the plasma albumin is as low as 10 per cent (Ward, Hammond and Bullen, 1986). Thus methaemalbumin appears to be a ready source of iron for this particular organism and if this applies to other bacteria it might be important in conditions such as sickle cell anaemia.

The presence of haem, even in very small quantities, could be important in infections involving highly virulent organisms. *Yersinia pestis*, for example, will grow on otherwise inhibitory medium containing the iron-binding protein conalbumen if a minute amount (0.5 pmol) of haemin is present (Perry and Brubaker, 1979). Plague is transmitted from infected rats to man by the flea *Xenopsylla cheopsis*, and after a meal of infected rat blood the bacteria multiply extensively in the flea's proventriculus (the portion of the stomodeum that lies in front of the stomach). When the flea feeds on a fresh host, such as man, some of the contents of the stomach can be injected into the wound (Bacot and Martin, 1914) and it would require only about 1.5×10^{-7} ml of lysed blood to provide 0.5 pmol of haem. Since the stomach of *X.cheopsis* can contain about 0.5 mm^3 of blood (English Plague Commission, 1907) it raises the interesting possibility that a bite could inject relatively large numbers of bacteria together with partially digested blood that might provide enough haem to stimulate rapid bacterial growth. Perry and Brubaker (1979) also suggested that *Y.pestis* might be able to take advantage of circulating haem bound to haemopexin or serum albumin. However, we do net yet know if this organism can utilize haem bound to these proteins. If the amount of haem in a wound exceeded the binding capacity of these proteins locally it obviously could be highly dangerous.

Another and quite distinct means whereby bacteria could acquire iron is by the actual destruction of the proteins that bind Fe^{3+} or haem compounds. Carlsson, Hofling and Sundqvist (1984) reported that some strains of black pigmented *Bacteroides* species can degrade transferrin, haptoglobin, haemopexin and albumin. These bacteria are often associated with mixed infections with other anaerobes and aerobes, and if these proteins are degraded *in vivo* iron could be made available much more readily than usual.

To sum up the present situation, haemoglobin or haem may provide iron for bacteria if present in concentrations that exceed the binding capacity of haptoglobin, haemopexin or albumin. After extensive haemolysis, such as occurs in sickle cell anaemia, the haptoglobin and haemopexin may disappear from the circulation. Some bacteria can utilize the iron in the haptoglobin–haemoglobin complex or in methaemalbumin, and some bacteria can destroy transferrin, haptoglobin, haemopexin and albumin which might affect the availability of iron.

1.2 Bacterial infections in sickle cell anaemia, bartonellosis and malaria

In sickle cell anaemia relatively large amounts of haemoglobin may be present in the plasma. Nauman *et al.* (1971) found that during the crisis of the disease the total plasma haemoglobin in 14 patients was 1.6–40.8 mg per 100 ml (mean 8.5 mg per 100 ml) compared with a mean value of 0.3 mg per 100 ml in 33 control subjects. In the quiescent period of the disease the total plasma haemoglobin had a mean value of 5.9 mg per 100 ml. Methaemalbumin during the crisis varied between <0.1–21.4 mg per 100 ml with a mean value of 1.8 mg per 100 ml while in the quiescent period it was <0.1–6.8 mg per 100 ml with a mean value of 0.5 mg per 100 ml. Methaemalbumin is normally absent in human plasma (Muller-

Eberhard, 1970). Nauman *et al.* (1971) point out that their patients had considerable amounts of circulating haptoglobin–haemoglobin complex with mean values of 4.6 mg per 100 ml during the crisis and 1.9 mg per 100 ml during the quiescent periods. However, free haptoglobin appeared to be absent. Whitten (1962) found that 43 asymptomatic children with sickle cell anaemia had no detectable haptoglobin but the plasma contained haemoglobin with a mean value of 13.5 mg per 100 ml.

Barrett-Connor (1971) provided convincing evidence that patients suffering from sickle cell anaemia were unusually susceptible to infections. This was especially true for those under three years of age. Of 166 patients, 75 had pneumonia involving 169 separate episodes requiring hospitalization. Osteomyelitis occurred in 21, meningitis in 13, and symptomatic urinary tract infection in 10. In addition there was an unusual association between sickle cell anaemia and osteomyelitis caused by *Salmonella*. Over half the cases were caused by *Salmonella*, whereas in osteomyelitis not associated with haemoglobinopathy 80 per cent infections were caused by staphylococci. The increased susceptibility to *Salmonella* osteomyelitis has been recorded many times previously (Hook *et al.*, 1957). Barrett-Connor's (1971) assessment of the increased risk of infection was as follows: approximately 25 times for *Salomonella* infection, over 500 times for pneumococcal meningitis, and over 100 times for *H.influenzae* meningitis. More recent data has confirmed that infection plays a major role in sickle cell disease. Overturf, Powers and Baraff (1977) showed that *Streptococcus pneumoniae* was responsible for 50 cases of meningitis or septicaemia in 422 patients. Thomas, Pattinson and Serjeant (1983) found that in 241 fatal cases of sickle cell anaemia there were 60 cases of acute chest syndrome (pneumonia, embolism or both) with 47 cases of bronchopneumonia. There were 18 cases of meningitis and 13 cases of septicaemia.

Bartonellosis is another disease involving a severe haemolytic anaemia where infections are unusually common. Cuadra (1956) states that uncomplicated bartonellosis has a low mortality. However, secondary infection with *Salmonella* was extremely common (40 per cent), and before the use of chloramphenicol the mortality was over 90 per cent. There was a close relationship between red cell destruction, indicated by anaemia, and susceptibility to infection. If a *Salmonella* bacteraemia occurred during the acute phase of bartonellosis, or immediately afterwards, the prognosis was poor. If the infection occurred long after the acute phase, when the anaemia was slight, and the patient almost well, the prognosis was relatively good even if blood cultures were positive for *Salmonella*.

Cuadra (1956) believed that most patients contracted acute bartonellosis in areas where the disease was endemic, but that these patients had not been born in these areas and presumably had little or no immunity. He also suggested that in the primitive conditions existing in Peruvian villages the chances of contracting *Salmonella* infection in infancy were high and that only those who developed some resistance survived. This immunity, he suggested, could be broken down by bartonellosis.

In sickle cell anaemia and bartonellosis it is difficult to prove that the unusual susceptibility to bacterial infection and to salmonellosis in particular, is due to the liberation of haemoglobin. However, the suspicion that this is so is strongly supported by experimental evidence that haemoglobin and haem stimulate the growth of a wide variety of bacteria in many different hosts (Chapter 1).

The work of Kaye, Gill and Hook (1967) is particularly relevant to *Salmonella* infection. Treatment of mice with phenylhydrazine, which causes the lysis of red cells, or antimouse red cell serum, which has the same effect, enormously enhanced their susceptibility to *Salmonella typhimurium*. The LD 50 fell from 10^4 bacteria to less than 10 organisms. This striking enhancement of virulence was not due to the anaemia itself since anaemia produced by bleeding had no effect. In addition, mice that survived after injection of 10^2–10^3 organisms had counts in their livers and spleens of less than 100 bacteria/g whereas those that had received anti-red cell sera had counts of over 10^8/g in the spleen and liver and over 10^5/ml in the blood.

Plasmodium berghei infections in mice also cause haemolysis and Kaye, Gill and Hook (1967) found that *S.typhimurium* grew faster in mice and was more rapidly lethal if injected intravenously one day before or up to five days after *P.berghei* infection. Death was due to *Salmonella* septicaemia.

In humans, infection with *Plasmodium falciparum* can cause extensive haemolysis. Sears (1967) records a total plasma haem pigment level of over 300 mg per 100 ml, measured by the benzidine method, following a relapse with falciparum malaria. This was accompanied by the disappearance of haptoglobin and haemopexin which began to reappear after five to six days. It is hardly surprising that circumstances of this kind should lead to an increased susceptibility to bacterial infection, and there is a good correlation between malaria and the incidence and severity of salmonellosis, even to the extent that the control of malaria by quinine appears to lead to a spontaneous amelioration of the bacterial infection (Bennett and Hook, 1959).

1.3 The role of trauma

Trauma and haemolysis

By its very nature trauma results in tissue damage and, unless very slight, is frequently accompanied by haemolysis. This may be confined to localized areas such as wounds, but it may also occur systemically such as in severe burns, where up to 25 per cent of the circulating red cells may undergo lysis (Davies, 1982).

In clinical research much attention has been paid to the consequences of the liberation of haemoglobin in the peritoneal cavity following strangulated intestinal obstruction. The mortality from this condition may be as high as 30 per cent, whereas simple mechanical obstruction has a mortality of 10 per cent or less (Yull, Abrahams and Davis, 1962). Strangulated obstruction is characterized by the seepage of blood and bacteria into the peritoneal cavity from the necrotic lesion. This malodorous reddish-black fluid laden with bacteria is lethal when injected into healthy animals (Cohn, 1961) and it has been calculated that as little as 70 ml of blood would be sufficient to have a lethal effect in humans when combined with the bacteria found in the lower intestinal tract (Yull, Abrahams and Davis, 1962).

It has been recognized for a long time that haemoglobin is the virulence-enhancing factor in these peritoneal infections. Davis and Yull (1964) showed that rats tolerated the intraperitoneal injection of 10^8 of a non-haemolytic *E. coli* strain isolated from the human intestinal tract. If the organisms were given with a variety of haem compounds there was a high mortality. The compounds included haemoglobin, haematin, human strangulation fluid containing 10 per cent haemoglobin and blood broth with 3–5 per cent haemoglobin. Bornside and colleagues, (Bornside, Bouis and Cohn, 1968; Bornside and Cohn, 1968) confirmed the importance of free haemoglobin by making the simple observation that intraperitoneal injection of intact red cells and *E.coli* were harmless to mice, but lethal when the red cells were lysed. Bullen, Leigh and Rogers (1968) showed that Fe^{3+} as ferric ammonium citrate in concentrations sufficient to saturate the iron-binding capacity of the serum transferrin for at least six hours was just as effective as lysed red cells or haemoglobin (Fig. 2). Subsequently it was shown that unsaturated transferrin was essential for the bacteriostatic and bactericidal effect against *E.coli* and that this could be reversed by ferric ammonium citrate or haemoglobin (Bullen and Rogers, 1969; Fletcher, 1971).

Exactly the same process appears to operate in the peritoneal cavity. Small numbers of *E.coli* in the peritoneal cavity of guinea-pigs persit for many hours and eventually disappear. In the presence of haemoglobin, haematin or ferric ammonium citrate rapid growth occurs and the animals die from septicaemia (Fig. 2).

Bornside, Bouis and Cohn (1970) confirmed the virulence-enhancing properties of ferric ammonium citrate and found it equally as effective as haemoglobin. Lee *et al.* (1979) showed that an *E.coli* strain isolated from a septic patient was harmless to rats in doses of 10^7 bacteria intraperitoneally, but gave a high mortality if given with haematin, haemoglobin or ferric ammonium citrate. Significantly, haematophorphyrin, which contains no iron, had no effect. Experiments with *Pseduomonas aeruginosa* gave similar results (Bullen, Ward and Wallis, 1974). Non-lethal infections persisted for many hours and then disappeared, but the bacteria grew rapidly if ferric ammonium citrate or haemoglobin were injected at the same time. *In vitro*, peritoneal fluid and unsaturated transferrin approximately halved the normal rate of growth of *Ps aeruginosa* and this effect was reversed by iron. It was also found that although

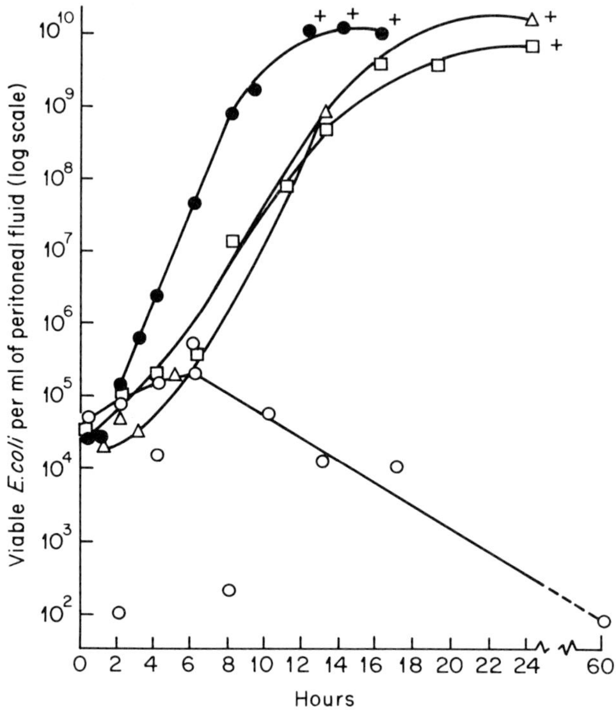

Figure 2 Effect of iron compounds on intraperitoneal infection with *Escherichia coli* in guinea-pigs. Each symbol represents the bacterial count for one guinea-pig. Animals were killed at intervals after infection. *E.coli* plus saline gave 100 per cent survival. *E.coli* plus iron compounds gave 100 per cent mortality. ○ *E.coli* plus saline. ● *E. coli* plus lysed red cells (170 mg of haemoglobin). □ *E.coli* plus haematin hydrochloride (100mg). △ *E.coli* plus Fe^{3+} (5mg of Fe per kg live weight). + Dying animal. *From Bullen, Leigh and Rogers (1968). Reproduced by permission of Blackwell Scientific Publications Limited*

the polymorphs in the peritoneal cavity reached a peak after three hours, between 80 and 90 per cent of all the viable bacteria were extracellular. This was true for both lethal and non-lethal infections and was the same if iron compounds were present or not. Thus the role of the transferrin in the extracellular fluid could be of critical importance in deciding the outcome of these infections.

Some authors have expressed doubts about the growth-promoting power of haemoglobin. Pruett *et al.* (1984) placed *E.coli* and haemoglobin in dialysis bags in the peritoneal cavity of rats and found that the organisms grew no faster than when mixed with albumin. They concluded that haemoglobin does not stimulate the growth of *E.coli in vivo*. However, this technique excluded the plasma transferrin required for the normal inhibition of *E.coli* in plasma or exudates, and it is this bacteriostatic effect that is reversed by the iron in haemoglobin (Bullen, 1981; Eaton *et al.*, 1982; Griffiths, 1983). The experiment with the dialysis bags therefore has little relevance to conditions inside the peritoneal cavity. Pruett *et al.* (1984) attributed the virulence-enhancing effect to the production of leukotoxins from the growth of *E.coli* in the presence of haemoglobin. Leukotoxins may indeed be produced in fluid containing haemoglobin after massive growth of *E.coli*; in this case more than 10^9 bacteria/ml. However, these authors found no evidence that haemoglobin itself had any effect on phagocytic function. This agrees with the observations of others (Eaton *et al.*, 1982). In the peritoneal cavity the presence of haemoglobin stimulates rapid growth from relatively small inocula that can increase by ten-fold in two to three hours (Fig. 2) and there is no evidence that this is due to any antiphagocytic effect (Bullen, 1981). For leukotoxins to be taken seriously in this situation one would need to show that they were produced by incubating small numbers of *E.coli* with haemoglobin for very short periods of an hour or less.

Maskell and Miles (1984) expressed the view that the dangers of enhancement of moderately pathogenic organisms by free iron in tissues are not so great as the literature on experimental infection suggests. In our view their results with guinea-pigs are unsatisfactory for this assessment. The amount of iron injected as Fe^{3+} or as haemoglobin was minute ($\equiv$3 to 10 μg Fe per injection site) and any free Fe^{3+} could be bound by circulating transferrin and any free haemoglobin by circulating haptoglobin. The likelihood that such conditions occur in natural infections in humans is remote since any trauma or underlying disease would be likely to involve a far more generalized lesion that that provided by the intradermal injection of a small amount of iron into a healthy animal.

Finally, it is tempting fate to use haemoglobin as a blood substitute, as has been proposed by de Venuto *et al.* (1979). The advantages claimed for haemoglobin, that it is a component of normal blood, does not require cross-matching, can transport oxygen, has a lower viscosity than blood and can be stored easily, are probably outweighed by the fundamental disadvantage that it can stimulate bacterial growth *in vivo*. There are other disadvantages, described by de Venuto *et al.* (1979) but its effect on bacterial growth should exclude it from therapeutic use.

Trauma and the availability of Fe^{3+}

Wounds in subcutaneous tissue or muscle frequently provide unique conditions for infection. Severe trauma almost invariably results in some local necrosis and the conditions in dead tissue for bacterial growth are quite different from those in healthy tissue. Indeed, conditions in dead tissue resemble to some extent those found in artificial media *in vitro*. If infection is to spread from the local lesion into living tissue the bacteria have to adapt to a different environment, and local conditions in the transition zone between diseased and healthy tissue could be crucial in deciding whether or not invasion of the rest of the body takes place.

Some of these conditions have been explored in experimental gas gangrene in guinea-pigs infected with a virulent and invasive strain of *Clostridium perfringens* type A. In these experiments the effect of toxins was excluded by passive immunization with *Cl.perfringens* type A antiserum which provided high levels of antitoxin in the blood and infected tissues. This applied equally to animals that survived and those that died from overwhelming infection (Bullen and Cushnie, 1962). It was also shown that exudates from passively immunized animals dying from infection were completely nontoxic to normal animals. (Bullen and Cushnie, 1963).

Infection was initiated in the muscles of a hind limb. Passive immunization sometimes protected and sometimes did not. Protection or otherwise was entirely dependent upon the degree of tissue damage at the time of infection. If the damage was severe, such as that produced by injection of the necrotizing agent calcium chloride with the bacteria, then massive bacterial growth occurred with extensive invasion and death from hypovolaemic shock. If the infection was initiated with adrenaline, which causes only a temporary and local fall in the oxidation–reduction potential (*Eh*) of the tissue, and no permanent damage, then bacterial growth ceased after the first four hours and the animal recovered (Rogers, Bullen and Cushnie, 1970). Antiserum was essential for this effect since in its absence bacterial growth continued unchecked until death occurred (Bullen and Cushnie, 1962).

In seeking an explanation for these results it is important to note that both normal and immune sera have a powerful bacteriostatic effect on *Cl.perfringens in vitro*, provided the *Eh* is maintained between 0 and +60 mV, pH 7.5 (Bullen, Dobson and Wilson, 1964). The bacteriostatic effect is dependent upon the presence of unsaturated transferrin (Rogers, 1967). The results obtained *in vitro* were very similar to those seen in guniea-pigs injected with bacteria and adrenaline. There was another similarity. If enough ferric iron was added to saturate the serum transferrin then rapid bacterial growth occurred both *in vitro* (Rogers, 1967) and in animals given adrenaline (Bullen, Cushnie and Rogers, 1967) (Fig. 3). This was effective even if the injection of iron was delayed for six hours when bacterial growth had ceased in the majority of the animals (Bullen, Cushnie and Rogers, 1967). Since saturation of serum transferrin has no effect on complement (Bullen, Rogers and Lewin, 1971; Fletcher, 1971) and does not interfere with phagocytosis or the neutralization of toxins by antibody (Bullen, Cushnie and Rogers, 1967), one must conclude that it is the abolition of the bacteriostatic effect of transferrin and antibody by iron that is responsible for the rapidly fatal infection.

If the bacteriostatic mechanism is as important as the experiments with iron suggest it could explain why the degree of tissue damage is so crucial for survival.

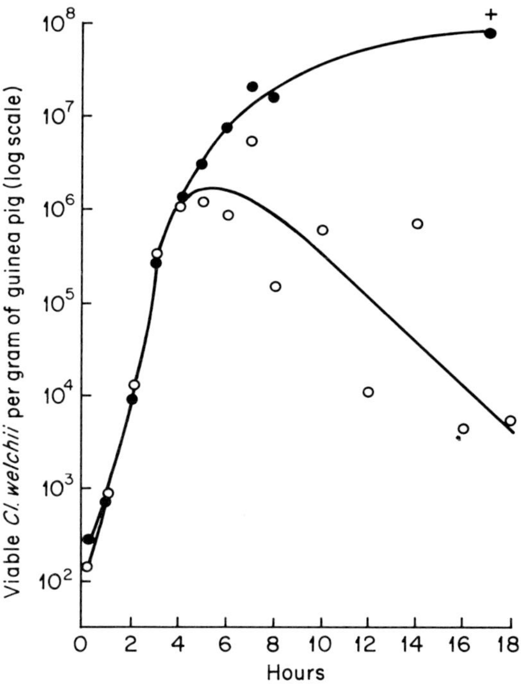

Figure 3 Effect of iron on infection with *Clostridium perfringens* (originally known as *Cl. welchii*) in guinea-pigs passively immunized with antiserum. Infection initiated with adrenaline. Each symbol represents the bacterial count for one guinea-pig. Animals were killed at intervals. *Cl. perfringens* without iron gave 100 per cent survival. *Cl. perfringens* plus iron gave 100 per cent mortality. ○ *Cl.perfringens* plus adrenaline. ● *Cl. perfringens* plus adrenaline plus iron (5 mg of Fe per kg live weight). + Dying animal. *From Bullen, Cushnie and Rogers (1967). Reproduced by permission of Blackwell Scientific Publications Limited*

Measurements of tissue *Eh* made during the course of infection (Rogers, Bullen and Cushnie, 1970) suggest why this should be so. In passively immunized animals given adrenaline and *Cl.perfringens* the *Eh* fell to nearly −400mV by six hours, but adrenaline produces no permanent damage and the *Eh* rose steadily after eight hours (Fig. 4). Since bacterial growth ceased at four hours, one must assume that conditions at the periphery of the lesion were suitable for bacteriostasis. Exactly where this occurs is not known but there must be a gradient in *Eh* from the centre of the lesion (−400 mV) to healthy tissue (approximately +300 mV) outside the infected area (Rogers, Bullen and Cushnie, 1970). Bacteriostasis could occur anywhere where the *Eh* was at +60 mV (pH.7.5) or above

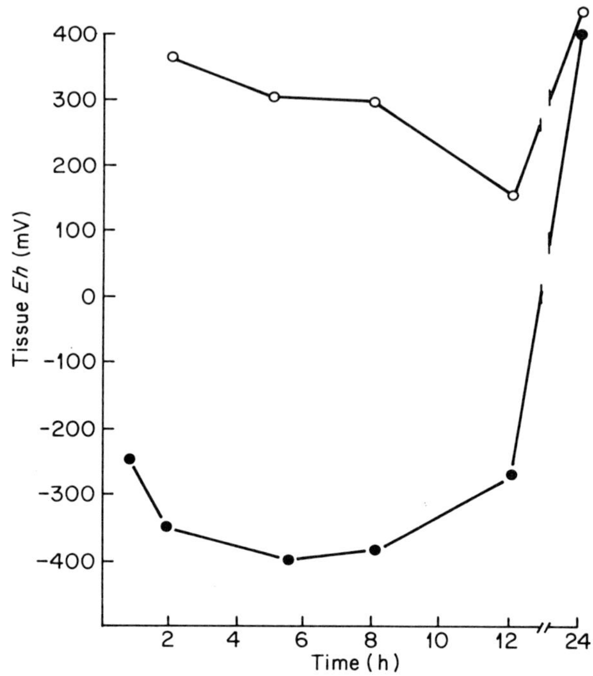

Figure 4 *E*h of tissue in non-fatal infection with *Clostridium perfringens* in passively immunized guinea-pig. Infection initiated with adrenaline. *Eh* measurement at: ● injection site (limb), ○ inguinal region. *From Rogers, Bullen and Cushnie (1970). Reproduced by permission of Blackwell Scientific Publications Limited*

(Bullen, Dobson and Wilson, 1964; Rogers, 1967). Once bacterial growth had stopped the *Eh* at the site of the infection rose to the level found in normal tissue. Clinical improvement occurred after seven hours and the *Eh* in the inguinal region remained high throughout (Fig. 4) (Rogers, Bullen and Cushnie, 1970).

The importance of suitable conditions for bacterial multiplication is brought out by experiments with iron (Figs. 3 and 5). Saturation of the serum transferrin abolishes bacteriostasis and would allow rapid multiplication to occur at the periphery of the lesion, even at a relatively high *Eh* (+60 mV or below, pH 7.5) (Rogers, 1967; Bullen, Cushnie and Rogers, 1967). This would allow the infection to spread and as the bacterial numbers increased so would the tissue *Eh* tend to fall. This is what appears to happen (Fig. 5). Not only did the *Eh* at the site of the infection remain low (−400 mV) but eventually the infection spread to the inguinal region and iliac crest with a characteristically sudden fall in *Eh*.

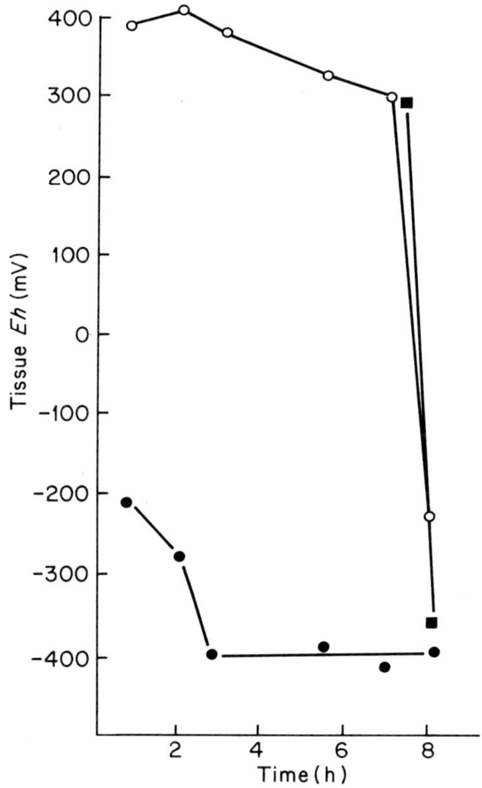

Figure 5 *E*h of tissue in fatal infection with *Clostridium perfringens* in passively immunized guinea-pig receiving 5 mg of Fe^{3+} per kg. Infection initiated with adrenaline. *E*h measurement at: ● injection site (limb), ○ inguinal region, ■ iliac crest. *From Rogers, Bullen and Cushnie (1970). Reproduced by permission of Blackwell Scientific Publications Limited*

In severely damaged tissue such as the necrotic lesion produced by the injection of calcium chloride, or in clinical gas gangrene following wounds there is a rapid and persistent fall in *Eh* (Fildes, 1929; Oakley, 1954) and pH (Stoner and Green, 1948). This lesion would provide the focus for the further spread of infection since it acts as a permanent area of low pH and *Eh* where the bacteria could multiply. Large numbers of *Cl.perfringens* in an environment of low *Eh* can consume large amounts of oxygen and cause a rapid fall of oxygen tension in living tissue (Bullen, Cushnie and Stoner, 1966). At the periphery of the lesion this could provide conditions for the extension of bacterial growth since once the *Eh* falls below −140 mV (pH 7.5) the Fe^{3+} on transferrin is reduced to Fe^{2+} and is no longer bound by the protein (Rogers, Bullen and Cushnie, 1970). The iron would then be available for bacterial growth. Further bacterial growth would extend the area of low oxygen tension and low *Eh*. This process would provide the means for a continuous extension of infection into healthy tissue. It would also explain why the disease advances in spite of the presence of large amounts of specific antitoxin (MacLennan and MacFarlane, 1945; Bullen and Cushnie, 1962). Although no toxin is present, the tissue probably dies from anoxia following a gradual encroachment by large numbers of bacteria. This severe local anoxia leads to a rapid breakdown of vascular permeability, which, if prolonged, results in death from hypovolaemic shock (Stoner *et al.*, 1967).

In clinical terms the importance of removing necrotic tissue was well expressed by van Heyningen (1955). Referring to the fact that the patient with gas gangrene can be saved by radical surgery, he said, 'The recovery that takes place is dramatic, heartening, and instructive. A source of poison appears to have been removed, and this poison does not seem to be the alpha toxin.' Oakley (1954) states that almost all accounts of gas gangrene in man insist on the importance of radical surgery (Jeffrey and Thomson, 1944; North, 1947). He also says that it is scarcely surprising that radical surgery is effective in treatment since this would remove the great bulk of infecting organisms and the *Eh* in the adequately vascularized muscle would be far too high to allow remaining organisms to grow. The data presented above suggest that the reasons go further than this. Removal of all the infected tissue would prevent local anoxia and thus remove the means of extending the infection at the edge of the lesion. It would also provide good conditions for the bacteriostatic reaction. In addition, removal of a source of anoxia would tend to alleviate shock brought about by changes in vascular permeability. In this context it is interesting that hyperbaric oxygen can prevent the shock induced by intraperitoneal injection of very large numbers of *Cl.perfringens* in passively immunized animals, provided that treatment was started within one hour of infection. This halted bacterial growth (Bullen, Cushnie and Stoner, 1966).

1.4 Effects of increased saturation of transferrin

Apart from haem compounds, the other main source of iron for bacterial growth is Fe^{3+} normally bound to transferrin or lactoferrin. As explained in Chapters 2 and 3, the iron-binding proteins have a normal level of saturation of about 30 per cent and the amount of free Fe^{3+} in equilibrium with the bound iron is about $10^{-18}M$, which is far too low for normal bacterial growth. The role of lactoferrin released from polymorphs in inducing hypoferraemia is discussed later in this chapter, but comparatively little is known about the influence of locally released lactoferrin on infection. Any condition that fully saturates the iron-binding proteins makes Fe^{3+} freely available to bacteria, while even an increase in saturation may make it more easily available to some organisms. Thus a 90 per cent saturation of rabbit transferrin is just as effective as 200 per cent saturation in abolishing the bacteriostatic effect of antibody and transferrin against *Pasteurella multocida* (Bullen, Rogers and Lewin, 1971). Similarly, human serum with a 50 per cent saturation with iron had a bacteriostatic effect for 18 hours against *Candida albicans* which was abolished by raising the saturation to 90 per cent. A further increase to 120 per cent resulted in an increase in fungal growth by about thirty-fold (Caroline *et al.*, 1964).

Several instances are recorded where excess iron has been made available accidentally, or as a consequence of treatment. In young children, infection with *Yersinia enterocolitica* usually results in a self-limiting gastroenteritis, and septicaemia is rare. Two children (20–21 months) who had ingested large amounts of iron as ferrous carbonate or fumarate and had received desferrioxamine both orally and intramuscularly developed a severe gastrointestinal illness with septicaemia (Melby *et al.*, 1982). Since *Y.enterocolitica* can grow in the presence of iron-binding proteins (conalbumen or human serum) if desferrioxamine is present (Perry and Brubaker, 1979; Brock and Ng, 1983), there is a possibility that treatment with this drug following ingestion of iron stimulated bacterial growth. Desferrioxamine enhances the virulence of *Y.enterocolitica* for mice (Robins-Browne and Prpic, 1985). However, it is as well to remember that haemin was the most effective source of Fe for *Y.enterocolitica* (Perry and Brubaker, 1979) and it is possible that local bleeding caused by a high concentration of iron salts could have provided enough haem for rapid bacterial growth as well as making a portal for entry (Melby *et al.*, 1982). It is also possible, of course, that both mechanisms could have stimulated bacterial growth simultaneously. As for desferrioxamine, this iron chelator can also enhance the susceptibility of mice to virulent *Salmonella typhimurium* in both normal and iron-overloaded animals (Jones *et al.*, 1977). Desferrioxamine enhances the virulence of *Vibrio vulnificius* for mice by a factor of approximately 10,000-fold, and can also reverse the inhibitory effect of serum for this organism (Wright, Simpson and Oliver, 1981). For all these reasons this drug should be used with care.

Direct injection of iron compounds can also cause problems. Briggs, Kennedy and Goldberg (1963) reported that injection of iron sorbitol citrate (Jectofer) caused a doubling in the number of leukocytes in the urine of patients with urinary tract infections. This was almost certainly due to an exacerbation of the infection since no such increase occurred in patients with noninfectious renal disease or in normal controls. Interestingly enough, the ability of iron sorbitol citrate to stimulate the growth of *E.coli* in the kidney was elegantly demonstrated by Fletcher and Goldstein (1970). Not only did iron sorbitol citrate (MW $< 5{,}000$) stimulate bacterial growth and abscess formation in the kidney but large deposits of iron could be seen in the cells of the proximal tubules and some in the collecting ducts and distal tubules. Neither iron dextran (MW 180,000) nor iron dextrin (MW 230,000) stimulated renal infection, and neither passed through the glomerulus. Since the iron sorbitol citrate was injected 24 hours after the bacteria had been given intravenously, one must assume that the iron stimulated bacteria already lodged in the kidney. As the authors point out, these results could not be attributed to blockade of the reticuloendothelial system since both iron dextran and iron dextrin are taken up by this system and had no effect on bacterial growth. The use of Jectofer in patients with suspected pyelonephritis would therefore appear to be contraindicated. The injection of iron dextran may be harmful where more generalized infections are involved. Barry and Reeve (1977) found that the incidence of neonatal sepsis among Polynesian infants injected with iron dextran for five days from the second day of birth was approximately twenty times that of European infants born at the same time who did not receive iron. The high incidence of infection ceased when the treatment with iron was stopped. These data do not prove that the injection of iron was responsible but this conclusion fits in well with experimental evidence. Becroft, Dix and Farmer (1977) examined blood from seven infants treated with 1 ml of iron dextran (Imferon) on two consecutive days. Blood samples were obtained an hour before treatment and 24 hours after the last injection. The post-treatment sera contained approximately thirty times as much iron as that before treatment although the saturation of the transferrin was not measured. None of the post-treatment samples showed any apparent reduction in the bactericidal power of the blood phagocytes, but the majority of sera had a greatly reduced bacteriostatic effect against *E.coli*.

Hypoferraemia is one of the most common findings of chronic disease (Roeser, 1980). However, leukaemia appears to be an exception. Caroline, Rosner and Kozinn (1969) showed that of thirty-four patients with acute myeloid leukaemia, twenty-one had high levels of serum iron ($>120\,\mu g$ per 100 ml) and in seventeen the transferrin was fully saturated. Two patients had systemic candidiasis. Of six patients with acute lymphoblastic leukaemia two had high levels of serum iron and fully saturated transferrin. One of these patients had systemic candidiasis, as did one with normal serum iron and unsaturated transferrin. Of ten patients with chronic myeloid leukaemia two had high levels of serum iron and fully saturated or nearly saturated transferrin. Of thirty-six cases of chronic lymphocytic leukaemia, polycythemia vera and multiple myeloma none had raised serum iron or abnormal iron-binding capacity. Two out of fourteen patients with lymphoma had high levels of serum iron and fully saturated transferrin.

Patients with leukaemia are unusually susceptible to infection (Caroline, Rosner and Kozinn, 1969; Estey *et al.*, 1982; Hunter *et al.*, 1983). Estey *et al.* (1982) record that of 161 failures in the treatment of 378 patients with acute leukaemia 36 were considered therapeutic failures and in the rest (125) death was largely attributable to infection. The bacteria involved included *Klebsiella* species, *Pseudomonas* species, and enterococci. Thirty-seven per cent of fatal infections were due to fungi, of which the majority were caused by *C.albicans*. In addition, the relatively poor results obtained with patients over 50 years of age (45 per cent complete remission compared with 70 per cent in those younger) were largely due to early deaths from infection and this experience was similar to that of the Medical Research Council's Working Party on Leukaemia in Adults (1974).

Hunter *et al.* (1983) found that twenty-eight out of forty-seven adults (60 per cent) with acute myeloid leukaemia had levels of transferrin saturation above 50 per cent. Some patients had low levels of transferrin. It was shown that the highly saturated sera had far less ability to inhibit a strain of *Ps.aeruginosa* than did normal sera and that the higher the saturation the less the inhibition. Caroline, Rosner and Kozinn (1969) found that leukaemic sera (96–100 per cent saturation) was far less able to inhibit *C.albicans* than normal sera and gave counts approximately 1,000 times greater after 48 hours of incubation. The addition of human transferrin to the leukaemic sera restored its inhibitory power to normal levels. This was reversed by adding iron.

These results strongly suggest that sera with highly saturated transferrin may predispose leukaemic patients to infection, especially with *C.albicans*. It could be argued that neutropenia could also play a role in reducing resistance, and this may well be a contributary factor. However, it has been shown that even with normal polymorphs saturation of the serum transferrin can lead to rapid extra cellular growth which eventually overwhelms the phagocytic cells (Bullen, Ward and Wallis, 1974; Ward, Hammond and Bullen, 1986).

In thalassaemia there is a marked tendency for an increased saturation of the serum transferrin. This is increased by splenectomy. Pootrakul, Rugkiatsakul and Wasi (1980) showed that in sixty-one normal controls the mean saturation of serum transferrin with iron was 35.8 ± 8.9 per cent. For forty-six patients with Hb H disease it was 61.4 ± 24.7 per cent, and for eighty-four patients with B-thalassaemia/Hb E disease it was 67.3 ± 25.0 per cent. After splenectomy of thirty-five B-thalassaemia/Hb E patients saturation rose to 90.5 ± 15.6 per cent. In addition, among the last three groups, there were thirty-one patients with 100 per cent saturation of the serum transferrin with iron.

According to Eraklis (1967) the influence of splenectomy on the likelihood of severe infection depends upon the underlying disease. Splenectomy does not encourage infection if performed for trauma, idopathic thrombocytopaenic purpura, extrahepatic portal vein thrombosis, portal hypertension or localized tumours. The risk is also minimal for children with hereditary spherocytosis or with hypoplastic or aplastic anaemia.

Where splenectomy accompanies hepatitis, cirrhosis, thallassaemia major, Wiscott Aldrich's syndrome, histiocytosis or inborn errors of metabolism, the risk of infection is high, with a 21 per cent death rate among ninety-seven patients. Clinically, the course of infection was characteristic. In 60 per cent of cases there was a sudden and overwhelming meningitis and septicaemia with death in 12 to 24 hours after the onset of symptoms. In the remainder there was an acute and fulminating pneumonia with septicaemia. Over half of these deaths were due to pneumococcal infection; the rest to meningococci and *H. influenzae*.

Caroline *et al.* (1969) attempted to explore the reasons for the predisposition to infection in splenectomized patients. There was no significant alteration in the level of serum globulins and no depression of leukocyte function. However, using *C. albicans* as a test organism it was found that thalassaemic sera with 100 per cent saturation of serum transferrin gave viable counts for the fungus many thousands of times greater than did normal sera after 48 hours of incubation. This was almost certainly related to the saturation of the iron-binding protein since growth could be prevented by adding unsaturated sera or purified iron-free transferrin. This circumstantial evidence does not prove that the increase in saturation is the reason for the patient's increased susceptibility. However, as Eraklis (1967) points out, in several diseases splenectomy itself does not predispose to infection. This suggests that the removal of this organ has little effect *per se*. In thalassaemic patients splenectomy is accompanied by a significant rise in saturation of transferrin superimposed on an already existing tendency for higher saturation than normal (Pootrakul, Rugkiatsakul and Wasi, 1980). This may be sufficient to tip the balance towards the fulminating infections described by Eraklis (1967).

Infections with *Yersinia enterocolitica* are frequently associated with conditions that have a tendency for raised serum iron or low levels of transferrin. These include cirrhosis, with or without haemochromatosis, and thalassaemia (Bouza *et al.*, 1980; Rabson, Hallett and Koornhof, 1975.) Robins-Browne, Rabson and Koornhof (1979) reported fourteen cases of *Yersinia enterocolitica* infections in Johannesburg in which all but one had some underlying disease. Ten had cirrhosis, one thalassaemia, one congenital hypoplastic kidneys and one kwashiorkor. In three autopsies there were widespread deposits of haemosiderin characteristic of Bantu siderosis. Bantu siderosis results from a high intake of iron from home-brewed beer or other beverages brewed in iron utensils (Bothwell *et al.*, 1964). Buchanan (1971) considered that the severe shock sometimes associated with Bantu siderosis might be due to infection, particularly with *Klebsiella* species and *E. coli*. Four out of five patients with these symptoms had very high levels of serum iron and acute liver necrosis.

In haemochromatosis the elevation of serum iron to above 200 μg per 100 ml is accompanied by a reduction in total iron-binding capacity and almost complete saturation of the serum transferrin (Walker and Williams, 1974). The sera of these patients also contains a pool of freely available iron present as a complex with a molecular weight of less than 10,000. These complexes are not present in normal sera (Gutteridge *et al.*, 1985). Patients with haemchromatosis, or other diseases with high levels of serum iron are unusually sensitive to infection with *Vibrio vulnificus* (Blake *et al.*, 1979). Chart and Griffiths (1985) showed that *V. vulnificus* can grow rapidly in sera from patients with haemochromatosis and that this is due to the presence of freely available iron. Growth in normal sera was inhibited. The growth in haemochromatosis sera can be inhibited by the addition of human apotransferrin (Chart and Griffiths, personal communication). However, not all infections with *V. vulnificus* are in haemochromatosis patients. Wound infections occur in patients with normal sera (Blake *et al.*, 1979; Tacket, Brenner and Blake, 1984). The most likely source of iron in these cases is haemoglobin. Experimental infections with *V. vulnificus* can be greatly enhanced by haemoglobin or haematin (Helms, Oliver and Travis, 1984). Infection with *Yersinia pseudotuberculosis* is also closely associated with haemochromatosis. Yamashiro *et al.* (1971) reviewed the literature and described eighteen cases of septicaemia caused by *Y. pseudotuberculosis* (not normally a human pathogen). Six patients had liver disease, two alcoholic cirrhosis and the rest haemochromatosis.

Jones (1962) described several cases of irreversible shock in haemochromatosis which might be due to infection. In animals Rehg *et al.* (1980) point out that the rock hyrax (*Procavia capensis*) can suffer from lesions resembling haemochromatosis and the majority that died had evidence of infection.

Protozoan infections, such as malaria, can be exacerbated by the increased availability of Fe^{3+} which follows an increase in saturation of serum transferrin. Murray *et al.* (1975) described 74 attacks of malaria among 181 individuals who had been starved previously by famine and then refed. Parasitized red cells (2 per cent) and reticulocytes (2.3 per cent) were low in patients admitted to hospital, but reached a peak (15 and 17 per cent respectively) after five days of refeeding. The serum transferrin, although relatively highly saturated on admission (54 per cent), was almost completely saturated (96 per cent) within 48 hours of refeeding. Attacks of malaria reached a peak by the fifth day. These were treated promptly with chloroquine and both the transferrin saturation and the number of parasitized cells declined thereafter. The suggestion that high levels of iron were to blame for the recrudescence of malaria is supported by animal experiments. Rats given 10 mg of iron dextran 14 days before infection with *P. berghei* had a 98 per cent saturation of transferrin compared with 43 per cent in controls and higher levels of parasitized red blood cells. The animals treated with iron also died earlier than the controls.

In another study by Murray *et al.* (1978) the subjects were nomads who normally suffer from chronic iron deficiency due to a diet of milk. Only those who were in a stable nutritional state were studied; i.e. those who were neither suffering from malnutrition nor being actively refed. Seventy-one received oral ferrous sulphate, sixty-six a placebo. The controls had a mean serum iron concentration of 3.4 μmol/litre and a transferrin saturation of 7 per cent. This was unchanged after 30 days. The test group initially had a mean serum Fe of 3.9 μmol/litre which rose to 13.1 μmol/litre, and a transferrin saturation of 8 per cent which rose to 31 per cent. In the controls two showed positive smears for malaria and there was one clincial attack. In the treated group there were twenty-one positive smears for malaria, thirteen of which were associated with clinical attacks. These figures are quite striking and support the previous evidence that a rise in the saturation of serum transferrin is accompanied by an increase in susceptibility to malaria. It also appears that it is the rise in serum saturation that is important and not the absolute values for Fe, since the figures for the nomads (Murray *et al.*, 1978) were very much lower than those for natives from Eastern Niger (Murray *et al.*, 1975) and in the nomads the percentage saturation after receiving iron corresponded closely to the generally accepted normal level (about 30 per cent).

Byles and D'sa (1970) pointed out that in areas where malaria is endemic the injection of iron dextran significantly increases the number of circulating parasites in pregnant women. Thirty-nine patients from a group of 455 had generalized reactions following the infusion of iron dextran. Eleven of these (28 percent) had malarial parasites in the blood. Only seven patients out of 462 had generalized reactions from the same dose of iron given with the antimalarial drug chloroquine. None of these had circulating malarial parasites.

In a different context, Murray, Murray and Murray (1980) suggested that the unusual freedom of Masai tribesmen from *Entamoeba histolytica* infections could be due to their predominant milk diet which gives a low serum iron and, probably, low levels of free iron in the gut. This idea was supported by the observation that oral treatment with Fe gave rise to a significant rise in the number of ameobic cysts, amoebae, and the number of positive sera in thirty-five Masai compared with the same number of controls.

Finally, there is evidence that in deficiency diseases such as kwashiorkor the level of transferrin can be crucial. McFarlane *et al.* (1970) found that in forty children suffering from kwashiorkor the initial mean level of serum albumin in those that eventually died was similar to those that survived, whereas the mean transferrin value was only one-third of those that survived. Similarly, after treatment with a high protein diet and iron, those that survived had mean values for transferrin (1.3 mg/ml) approximately four times those that died (0.33 mg/ml). In this instance the giving of iron to those with low levels of transferrin could have predisposed them to infection, and it is well known that a high proportion of those that die from kwashiorkor suffer from acute infections (Soltys and Brody, 1970).

1.5 Summary

In attempting to summarize the clinical consequences of increased availability of iron there are a number of points that need emphasizing. The first is that the liberation of haem compounds, either from concomitant disease or as a result of trauma, is potentially dangerous. The degree of danger depends upon the concentration of haem available. This may depend in part on the presence of haemoglobin-binding and haem-binding proteins which may provide some protective effects by denying bacteria access to the iron in the haem. The exact role of these proteins requires further investigation.

Second, raised levels of freely available Fe in humans increase the likelihood of infection. This suggestion is strongly supported by experimental evidence. Much of the clinical evidence is circumstantial but it is quite consistent and increasingly convincing.

Third, the administration of iron-chelating agents like desferrioxamine, which can transport iron to some bacteria, can be dangerous, especially in patients already overloaded with iron.

Fourth, more work is required on the role of iron in wounds, either as haem compounds or as free Fe^{2+} or Fe^{3+}, which may become available as a result of trauma. We also need to know more about the local role of lactoferrin. However, as the work on gas gangrene suggests, iron in wounds may play a far greater role than is generally recognized. There is an urgent need for more data and more experimental work in this field.

2. HOST RESPONSE TO INFECTION

The first part of this chapter describes the enhancement of infection by an increase in the availability of iron. We now consider some physiological responses that have the opposite effect and tend to withhold iron from invading bacteria.

2.1 Interleukin-1 and the initiation of a coordinated response to infection

Physiological responses to infection are initiated, in part, by hormones synthesized and released by phagocytic cells. As a result of a number of local and systemic changes induced by these hormones, resistance is increased. This coordinated response is of the greatest importance for survival, and if suppressed or subverted, invariably leads to an increase in susceptibility to infection, often with fatal results.

Over the past few years, it has become apparent that one of the most important non-specific responses to bacterial infection is the release of the hormone interleukin-1. This hormone had been called 'endogenous pyrogen' by biologists studying fever and 'leukocyte endogenous mediator' by those studying the metabolic changes that occur with infection. Through the 1970s, investigators characterized factors (monokines) released from macrophages which stimulated various immunologically non-specific responses in thymocytes and splenocytes. Each monokine was named for its effect in the particular bioassay under investigation—e.g. lymphocyte activating factor (Gery, Gershon and Waksman, 1972), B-cell differentiation factor (Hoffman *et al.*, 1979), etc. These monokines appear to be very similar biochemically and a number of studies indicate that the diverse activities may all be triggered by a common mediator (Koopman, Farrar and Fuller-Bonar, 1978; Rosenwasser, Dinarello and Rosenthal, 1979; Murphy, Simon and Willoughby, 1980; Sztein *et al.*, 1981). The Second International Lymphokine Workshop (Ermatingen, Switzerland, 1979) established the term 'interleukin-1' to refer to the products of macrophages which act as messengers between different leukocyte populations (Mizel and Farrar, 1979). For an overview on the general subject of interleukin-1 see Dinarello (1984) and the Proceedings of the Symposium in Ann Arbor, Michigan, *The Physiologic, Metabolic, and Immunologic Actions of Interleukin-1* (Kluger, Oppenheim and Powanda, 1985).

The many non-immunological actions of interleukin-1 include the development of fever, reductions in plasma concentrations of iron and zinc, elevations in plasma concentration of many proteins such as C-reactive protein, haptoglobin and fibrinogen, leukocytosis, and other 'acute phase' changes (Kampschmidt, 1980; Powanda and Canonico, 1981; Bornstein, 1982).

A variety of stimuli result in the production and release of interleukin-1. For example, interaction of the macrophage with the lipopolysaccharide component of Gram-negative bacteria (primarily the lipid A component) initiates the synthesis and release of interleukin-1 (Kenedi *et al.*, 1982). Hypersensitivity reactions appear to induce the production of interleukin-1 via the production of a lymphokine acting as a messenger between the lymphocyte and the macrophage (e.g. see the review by Dinarello, 1982). Interleukin-1 is also released during and following exercise; however, the precise stimulus for release is unknown at present (Cannon and Kluger, 1983; Cannon and Dinarello, 1984).

There is considerable evidence that the release of an interleukin-1-like hormone has a long phylogenetic history; i.e. many of the changes brought about by interleukin-1 in mammals are also found in 'lower' vertebrates. For example, fever in response to infectious agents in common throughout the vertebrates (Kluger, 1979). Whether an organism is 'warm-blooded' and regulates its body temperature largely by physiological means, or 'cold-blooded' and as a result has to rely on behaviour to regulate its body temperature, contact with bacteria or bacterial products will result in an elevation in the thermoregulatory 'set-point' and, when possible, a rise in body temperature by behavioural or physiological mechanisms. For example, injection of lipopolysaccharide into the laboratory rabbit results in the production of interleukin-1. This hormone presumably travels to the hypothalamus where it acts, probably indirectly, to raise the thermoregulatory 'set-point'. As a result, the rabbit decreases its skin blood flow and huddles, both responses that help the rabbit to conserve heat, and increases its metabolic heat production by shivering. As a result, body temperature will rise the 1, 2 or 3°C necessary to reach the elevated thermoregulatory 'set-point'. Injection of lipopolysaccharide into the 'cold-blooded' lizard, the desert iguana, will also result in an elevation in body temperature. However, in the lizard this elevation in temperature is almost entirely by behavioural means. The lizard will spend greater lengths of time under a heat lamp or other source of heat and as a result its body temperature will rise to reach its elevated 'set-point' temperature. Injection of desert iguanas with a crude preparation of interleukin-1 isolated from peritoneal macrophages of rabbits also results in the development of a fever (Bernheim and Kluger, 1977).

Another non-specific host response to infection triggered by interleukin-1, which also appears to have a long phylogenetic history, is the reduction in plasma iron and zinc concentration. Not only do infected mammals show the classic hypoferraemic and hypozincaemic responses, but so do reptiles (Grieger and Kluger, 1978; Hacker, Rothenburg and Kluger, 1981), presumably the result of a release of interleukin-1. Interleukin-1 is also thought to stimulate the synthesis of C-reactive protein in teleost fishes and birds as well as in mammals (Pepys, 1981).

The elevation of circulating levels of interleukin-1 during infection or injury is thought to enhance non-specific host defence responses, and non-specific and specific immunity (e.g. see Powanda and Beisel, 1982). For example, Kampschmidt and Pulliam (1974) showed that injection of rats with partially purified interleukin-1 24 hours prior to infection with *S.typhimurium* led to significant enhancement in survival rate. Heating the interleukin-1, presumably as the result of denaturing the protein, led to the loss of its protective action. In experimental animals and in people, protein deprivation has been shown to reduce the production of interleukin-1 and to increase mortality rate in response to infection with *Pasteurella multocida* (Hoffman-Goetz and Kluger, 1979; Hoffman-Goetz *et al.*, 1980). Survival in critically ill malnurished patients has been correlated with the ability of these patients to synthesize interleukin-1 (Keenan *et al.*, 1982).

The mechanisms responsible for the protective effect of interleukin-1 appear to be numerous (see Powanda and Canonico, 1981, for a review) (Fig. 6). Granulocytosis, hepatic synthesis of acute phase proteins, such as fibrinogen and haptoglobin, and activation of T lymphocytes are just some of the biological effects initiated by interleukin-1. Two additional effects that are thought to be important components of the non-specific host response to infection are the development of fever and the reduction in the plasma concentration of iron.

2.2 Fever

As mentioned above, interleukin-1 is thought to induce a fever by elevating the thermoregulatory 'set-point' in the anterior hypothalamus. The action of this hormone on the hypothalamus is thought to be indirect since there is no evidence that interleukin-1 can actually cross the blood brain barrier, although this is currently an area of investigation (Blatteis *et al.*, 1983). Most investigators believe that the specific signal for raising the 'set-point' comes from a prostaglandin or other metabolite of arachidonic acid (e.g. see Feldberg and Milton, 1978).

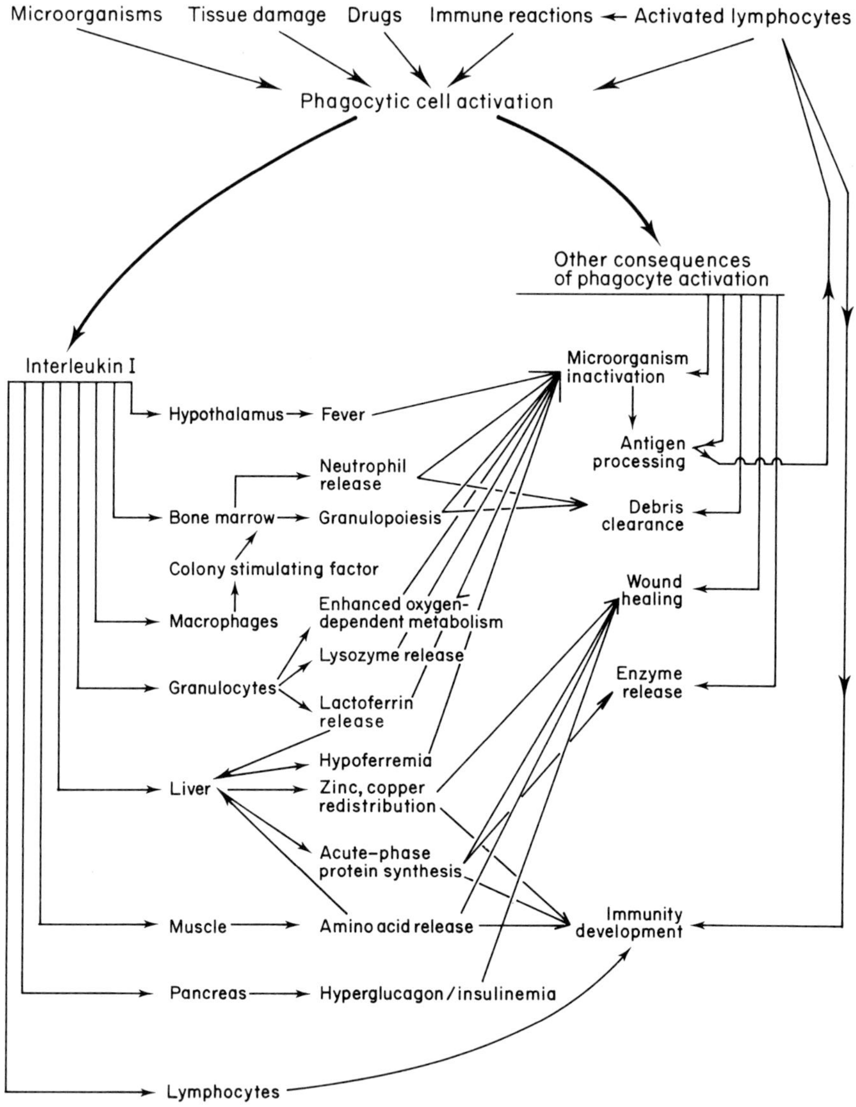

Figure 6 Postulated interactions among various aspects of non-specific and specific immunity modulated by interleukin-1. *From Powanda* and *Beisel (1982). Reproduced by permission of the American Society for Clinical Nutrition*

The idea that prostaglandins play a role in the intitiation of a fever is based on several studies. Prostaglandins occur naturally in the hypothalamus and the concentration of these chemicals rise during infection. Injection of minute amounts of prostaglandins of the E series into the anterior hypothalamus results in a fever; in addition, antipyretic drugs such as aspirin and acetaminophen are potent inhibitors of prostaglandin synthesis. Many studies have shown than an injection of a small amount of an antipyretic drug into the hypothalamus is more effective in reducing fever than ingestion or intravenous injection of a much larger dose. These data are interpreted as indicating that the antipyresis (and therefore the prostaglandin inhibitory effect) occur at the level of the hypothalamus. Despite the seemingly overwhelming evidence in favour of prostaglandins playing a crucial role in the development of fever, there are some data indicating that prostaglandins may not be involved in all fevers (see reviews in Feldberg and Milton, 1978, and Kluger, 1979).

There is considerable evidence that moderate fevers are adaptive to the infected host. As mentioned above, fever in response to infectious agents occurs throughout the vertebrates. The long phylogenetic history of fever, by itself, suggests that fever is adaptive. This is because, regardless of whether an organism is an endotherm or an ectotherm, a rise in body temperature results in a substantial increase in metabolic heat production, and therefore energy expenditure. Most biochemical reactions have a Q_{10} of approximately 2–3. This means that for every 1°C rise in body temperature, metabolic rate increases about 10 per cent or more. It is unlikely that a large increase in energy expenditure associated with fever would have evolved and been retained had it no survival value. Maladaptations, which occasionally occur, are clearly selected against.

Occasionally the argument is made that some host responses to infection are harmful. There are few, if any, physiological or immunological responses that are predominantly maladaptive. Although certain inflammatory responses are thought to be injurious (such as inflammation in knee joints or allergic reactions to pollen), it is generally agreed that the inflammatory response is essential to survival in a hostile world. Without the movement of phagocytes into a damaged area to destroy or inactivate the pathogens and the subsequent activation of repair mechanisms, minor breaks in the epithelial linings could result in massive infection and death.

In addition to the above argument based on evolutionary biology, reptiles and fishes have provided excellent animal models to investigate directly the biological role of fever. Moderate fevers following injection of lizards (Kluger, Ringler and Anver, 1975) or goldfish (Covert and Reynolds, 1977) with live bacteria have shown that the elevation in body temperature increases the survival rate (Fig. 7).

Studies using newborn mammals (Teisner and Haahr, 1974; Carmichael, Barnes and Percy, 1979) have also shown that moderate fevers decrease morbidity, mortality, or both, during viral infections. When an aspirin-like drug was used to lower fevers in bacterially infected rabbits, mortality rate increased (Vaughn, Veale and Cooper, 1980). Furthermore, ferrets infected with influenza virus and given sodium salicylate to reduce their fevers had higher titres of

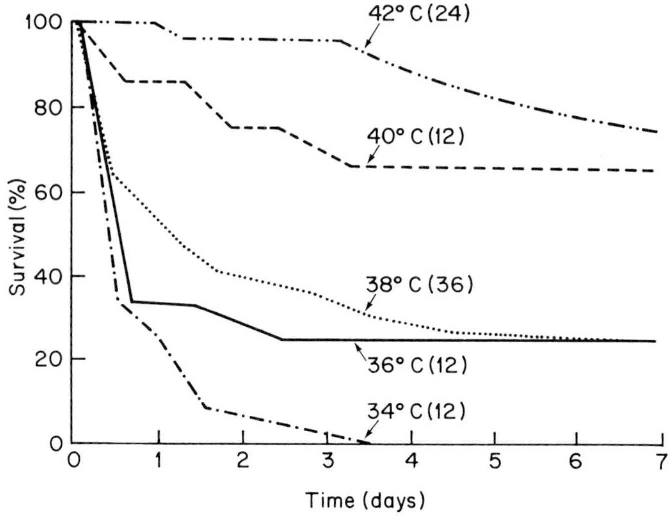

Figure 7 Relationship between temperture and percentage survival of desert iguanas infected with *Aeromonas hydrophila*. The numbers in parenthesis represent the sample size. The normal non-infected body temperature of these lizards is about 38°C. During infection these lizards regulate their body temperature between 40° and 42°C by changing their position within the environment. *From Kluger, Ringler and Anver (1975). Reproduced by permission of the American Society for the Advancement of Science*

virus in their upper respiratory system compared to ferrets not given the antipyretic drug (Husseini *et al.*, 1982).

Many components of the host defence system appear to be enhanced by small elevations in body temperature. For example, there is considerable evidence that the mobility of some types of leukocytes increases with increasing temperature in the ranges of temperature normally encountered during infection (Bryant *et al.*, 1966; Phelps and Stanislaw, 1969; Nahas, Tannieres and Lennon, 1971; Berheim *et al.*, 1978; van Oss *et al.*, 1980). Not only must leukocytes engulf pathogenic microorganisms but, to be effective, they must kill these pathogens. Some evidence points towards increased killing of some species of bacteria at temperatures simulating fever (Roberts and Steigbigel, 1977; Sebag, Reed and Williams, 1977).

In response to various stimulants or activators, lymphocytes undergo proliferation and transformation and as a result are then capable of participating in various aspects of the immune response. It has recently been shown that temperatures corresponding to moderate fevers result in an enhancement and, in some cases, an acceleration of lymphocyte transformation (Ashman and Nahmias, 1977; Roberts and Steigbigel, 1977; Gupta and Agarwal, 1980). In addition to the enhancement in non-specific host defence responses described above, there have recently been reports that the effects of interleukin-1 on activation of thymocytes are enhanced at 38°C compared to 32°C (Hanson *et al.*, 1983). Using more physiologically relevant temperatures, Duff and Durum (1982) have also found that T cell proliferation is enhanced by elevated temperature. In addition, Jampel *et al.* (1983) have shown that elevated temperatures augments helper T cell activation.

The antiviral (Heron and Berg, 1978) and antitumour (Heron and Berg, 1978; Yerushalmi, Tovey and Gresser, 1982) effects of interferon are also enhanced at elevated temperatures. In addition, the *in vivo* production of interferon in the rhesus monkey is increased at febrile temperatures (Downing *et al.*, 1984). Not only does the production and activity of interferon increase at febrile temperatures, but interferon, itself, appears to be pyrogenic, perhaps via the production of interleukin-1 (Dinarello *et al.*, 1984; Feldberg and Scott, 1984). These, along with the above studies, indicate that small elevations in temperature can enhance both non-specific and immunological defences against pathogens.

2.3 Hypoferraemia during infection and inflammation

Infection and inflammation generally results in a reduction in the plasma concentration of iron. This decrease is thought to be attributable primarily to increased storage of iron in the liver (see the review by Bezkorovainy, 1980) and to a lesser extent to decreased absorption of iron across the gut epithelium. Increased excretion of iron via the urinary tract apparently has only a minor role in reducing the plasma concentration of iron (Klaiman *et al.*, 1981).

Two pools of iron are likely candidates for the increased liver concentration of iron—a large pool of iron in red blood cells and a smaller pool of iron bound to transferrin. Red blood cells have an average lifespan of about 120 days, and senescent or damaged erythrocytes are phagocytized by the reticuloendothelial cells. During the next several days the iron from haemoglobin is released into the general circulation where it can be used to produce new red blood cells or is stored as ferritin. While the amount of iron bound to transferrin is relatively small compared to that in haemoglobin, the turnover rate of the plasma transferrin–iron pool is relatively rapid. For example, the half-life of iron bound to circulating transferrin is approximately one hour in humans (Cavill and Ricketts, 1980) and 0.7 hours in mice (Letendere and Holbein, 1983).

Most evidence indicates that the hypoferraemia of infection or inflammation is the result of decreased release of iron from the reticuloendothelial system, rather than the increased uptake from the plasma transferrin–iron pool (Freireich *et al.*, 1957; Quastel and Ross, 1966). Lee (1983) has published an excellent review on iron metabolism during infection and inflammation and has described two likely mechanisms for this increased storage of iron in the liver: (1)

release of lactoferrin from neutrophils and (2) increased synthesis of ferritin. Both appear to participate in the hypoferraemic response.

Lactoferrin is a glycoprotein that at low pH has a greater affinity for iron than does transferrin. Van Snick, Masson and Heremans (1974) proposed that the hypoferraemia of infection and inflammation was the result of the release of lactoferrin from neutrophils, the subsequent transfer of iron from transferrin to lactoferrin and the selective uptake of the lactoferrin–iron complex by the reticuloendothelial system. This theory is supported by data by Klempner, Dinarello and Gallin (1978), indicating that interleukin-1 does result in neutrophil release of lactoferrin. The problem with lactoferrin being responsible for the general hypoferraemia observed during local inflammation is that the amount of lactoferrin–iron taken up by the reticuloendothelial system from the general circulation, where the pH is generally about 7.4, is probably too small to account for the large fall in plasma iron concentration. Rather than the circulating lactoferrin–iron complex being picked up by the liver macrophages, it is possible that in response to the synthesis and release of interleukin-1, lactoferrin is released from neutrophils, complexes to iron and remains at or near its site of release. This lactoferrin–iron is then picked up by circulating or fixed macrophages, resulting in localized hypoferraemia. Systemic hypoferraemia resulting in increased storage of iron in the liver may be brought about during general infections where interleukin-1 is released by Kupffer cells in the liver.

The other theory to explain the hypoferraemia of infection and inflammation is that synthesis of ferritin, an iron-storage protein, is increased in the liver (Konijn and Hershko, 1977). Konijn and Hershko showed that in rats injected with turpentine, hepatic ferritin synthesis increased and that this increase clearly preceded the decline in plasma iron concentration, suggesting that the ferritin had bound free iron and led to the hypoferraemia of infection and inflammation. They proposed that along with the other acute phase proteins synthesized by the liver (e.g. fibrinogen, C-reactive protein, alpha-2-glycoprotein, etc.) ferritin synthesis is also a non-specific response to inflammation. In a fascinating study, Letendre and Holbein (1984) have shown that in mice infected with *Neisseria meningitidis* the hypoferraemic response was associated with a preferential incorporation of haem-derived iron into the intracellular hepatic ferritin pool.

As described earlier, the artificial elevation of plasma iron generally results in increased severity of infection. It is also generally assumed that the hypoferraemia of infection is an adaptive host defence response. Despite these overwhelming data supporting a beneficial role for the hypoferraemia of infection, no experiments have been done to show that prevention of the reduction in iron at the actual time of infection has any effect on mortality or morbidity due to that infection. However, based on the above data one would certainly suppose that this would adversely affect the host.

Besides the role of hypoferraemia in reducing bacterial growth, iron is thought to have a role in modulating the inflammatory response. Neutrophils produce superoxide anion (O_2^-) and hydrogen peroxide (H_2H_2). In the presence of Fe^{3+} the O_2^- is converted to O_2 and Fe^{2+} (Haber and Weiss, 1934). The Fe^{2+} and the H_2O_2 result in the formation of Fe^{3+} and OH· (hydroxyl radical), and OH^- (see Chapter 1). The hydroxyl radical is a potent oxidant and can contribute to bacterial killing during infection (Ambruso and Johnston, 1981) as well as to acute damage during inflammation (Sacks *et al.*, 1981). In an *in vitro* study, Ambruso and Johnston (1981) have shown that lactoferrin enhances hydroxyl radical formation. It may be worth noting that exercise results in the release of interleukin-1 (Cannon and Kluger, 1983). Inflammation and tissue damage in joints due to exercise may in part be attributable to the localized release of interleukin-1 (Wood *et al.*, 1983) and its subsequent induction of the release of lactoferrin (Klempner, Dinarello and Gallin, 1978; Smith, Bowman and Speziale, 1985) and enhanced hydroxyl radical formation.

In an *in vivo* study, Ward *et al.* (1983) have shown that infusion of lactoferrin or Desferal into rats given the inflammatory agent cobra venom factor led to reduced lung damage, presumably due to a decrease in the extracellular concentration of iron. Infusion of iron, particularly Fe^{3+}, resulted in greater lung damage.

2.4 Synergism between fever and hypoferraemia

There is evidence that fever and hypoferraemia combine to form a synergistic protective mechanism. In this section, we will review the evidence that these two acute responses to infection, both triggered by the release of interleukin-1, enhance resistance to infection. At the outset, it is important to emphasize that the reduction in plasma iron is not the result of the elevation of the body temperature. For example, in the lizard, *Dipsosaurus dorsalis*, injection with bacteria results in both fever and hypoferraemia (Grieger and Kluger, 1978). Prevention of the rise in body temperature does not affect the development of hypoferraemia. Conversely, making lizards hyperthermic, without injection with bacteria or other inducers of interleukin-1, does not result in lowering of plasma iron concentration. In rats, fever in response to endotoxin can be effectively blocked using sodium silicylate, yet hypoferraemia still occurs (Tocco *et al.*, 1983). In a study by Cremades *et al.* (1982) using rabbits, antipyretic drugs by themselves led to a slight rise in serum iron, but the effect of these drugs on serum iron concentration was not dependent on their capacity to block fever in response to an injection of endotoxin. Cremades *et al.* (1982) suggested that a potentially harmful effect of antipyretic drugs may be their effect on extracellular iron concentration. Tocco *et al.* (1983) found a similar small rise in plasma iron concentration in rats in reponse to injection with sodium salicylate.

Garibaldi (1972) showed that there is a synergistic response between fever and hypoferraemia. The biosynthesis of iron-transport compounds (enterochelin) by *S. typhimurium* is inhibited by temperatures simulating fever. For example, at

40.3°C the growth of *S.typhimurium* was reduced (compared to 36.9°C) unless the growth medium was supplemented with bacterial siderophores (i.e. phenolate iron-transport compounds). Kochan (1977) has shown similar results for *E.coli*. In a more recent study using radiolabelled iron bound to enterochelin, Worsham and Konisky (1984) found that the production of enterochelin by *S.typhimurium* was reduced at elevated temperatures; however, they found no reduction in enterochelin production by a variety of strains of *E.coli* at temperatures simulating fever. Muller, Edwards and Smith (1983) found that the *in vitro* growth of *Legionella pneumophila* was reduced at low levels of free iron and at incubation temperatures greater than 39°C. Production of iron-transport compounds was not measured.

Grieger and Kluger (1978) have shown that when the iron concentration of a growth medium (Trypticase soy broth) was high, the *in vitro* growth of *Aeromonas hydrophila* was similar at temperatures simulating afebrile (38°C) and febrile (41°C) conditions for infected desert iguanas. However, when the iron concentration in the medium was reduced to levels found during infection, growth of *A.hydrophila* was markedly inhibited providing the incubation temperature was at the febrile temperature of 41°C. Grieger and Kluger also showed that injection of these lizards with iron increased their mortality rate, even when the lizards were maintained at their febrile temperature of 41°C. In an earlier study, Kluger, Ringler and Anver (1975) had shown that maintenance of these lizards at febrile tempertures reduced the mortality rate during infection with *A.hydrophila*. Kluger and Rothenburg (1979) found similar results for the *in vitro* growth of *Pasteurella multocida* when grown in a medium containing an iron concentration similar to that found in infected rabbits. Vaughn, Veale and Cooper (1980) have shown that moderate fevers in rabbits were associated with increased survival rate during infection with *P.multocida*. The combination of these *in vitro* and *in vivo* studies suggests that fever coupled with hypoferraemia enhance resistance to bacterial infection.

2.5 Circadian variations in body temperature and plasma iron concentration

Changes in body temperature (Wever, 1979) and plasma iron can also occur on a circadian basis (Hamilton *et al.*, 1950; Lynch *et al.*, 1973). In male Sprague Dawley rats the highest body temperatures during the day occur when the plasma iron concentration is lowest (Ucar, Tocco and Kluger, 1983) (Fig. 8). It was considered that part of the elevation in body temperature and reduction in plasma iron concentration oberved at night (when the rats are active) might be the result of a circadian release of interleukin-1. To test this hypothesis, rats were injected with sodium salicylate to determine whether this antipyretic drug would reduce body temperature at night. A significant reduction in body temperature occurred. In addition, a circulating pyrogen has been found in the plasma of rats at night that was absent from the plasma of rats during

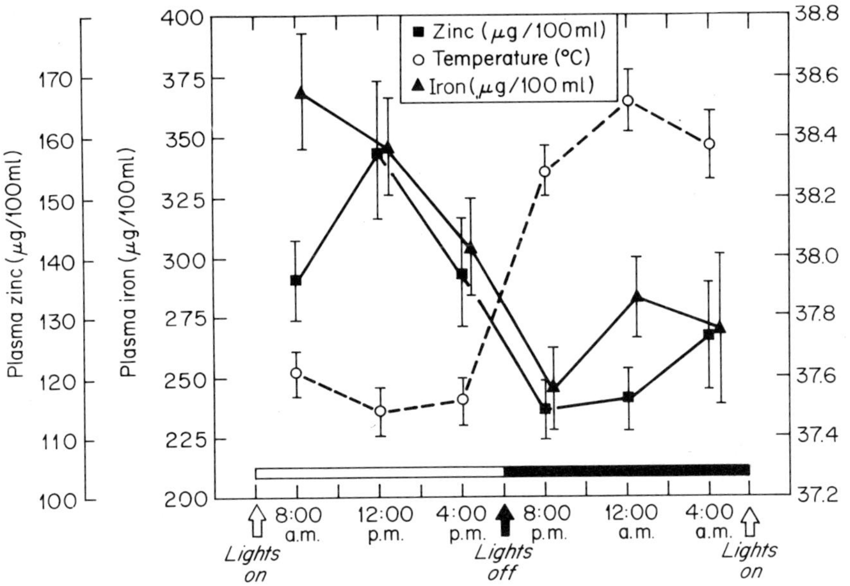

Figure 8 The normal circadian variation in rectal temperature (°C) and plasma concentrations of iron and zinc in male Sprague-Dawley rats ($N = 8$ for each time point). Values represent mean ± 1 Standard error of the mean. *From Ucar, Tocco and Kluger (1983). Reproduced by permission of the Society for Experimental Biology and Medicine*

the day. In the light of evidence presented above regarding the synergism between fever and hypoferraemia reducing the severity of bacterial infection, plus many of the other beneficial effects induced by interleukin-1, it was thought that if the pyrogen were interleukin-1 then rats infected at night should have increased resistance to infection. To test this hypothesis, rats were injected with *S.typhimurium*—one group at midnight during the period of greatest activity and one group at noon during the period of least activity. The mortality rate measured at 72 hours was 25 per cent (5 of 20) in the group infected at midnight and 60 per cent (12 of 20) in the group injected at noon. These data support the hypothesis that the immune defence system of rats to *S.typhimurium* is more effective at night, and this may be related to an increased level of interleukin-1. Whether the enhanced survival is related to the effect of interleukin-1 on body temperature and plasma iron levels or to some other circadian variation is not yet known.

REFERENCES

Ambruso, D.R., and Johnston, Jr., R.B. (1981). Lactoferrin enhances hydroxyl radical production by human neutrophils, neutrophil particulate fractions, and an enzymatic generating system. *Journal of Clinical Investigation*, **67**, 352–360.

Ashman, R.B., and Nahmias, A.J. (1977). Enhancement of human lymphocyte responses to phytomitogens *in vitro* by incubation at elevated temperatures. *Clinical and Experimental Immunology*, **29**, 464–467.

Bacot, A.W., and Martin, C.J. (1914). Observations on the mechanism of the transmission of plague by fleas. *Journal of Hygiene*. Plague, Supplement 3, 423–439.

Barrett-Connor, E. (1971). Bacterial infection and sickle cell anaemia. An analysis of 250 infections in 166 patients and a review of the literature. *Medicine*, **50**, 97–112.

Barry, D.J.M., and Reeve, A.W. (1977) Increased incidence of gram negative neonatal sepsis with intramuscular iron administration. *Pediatrics*, **60**, 902–912.

Becroft, D.M.O., Dix, M.R. and Farmer, K. (1977). Intramuscular iron-dextran and susceptibility of neonates to bacterial infections. *Archives of Diseases of Childhood*, **52**, 778–781.

Bennett, I.L., and Hook, E.W. (1959). Infectious diseases (some aspects of salmonellosis). *Annual Review of Medicine*, **10**, 1–20.

Bernheim, H.A., Bodel, P.T., Askenase, P., and Atkins, E., (1978). Effects of fever on host defence mechanisms after infection in the lizard *Dipsosaurus dorsalis*. *British Journal of Experimental Pathology* **59**, 76–84.

Bernheim, H.A., and Kluger, M.J. (1977). Endogenous pyrogen-like substance produced by reptiles. *Journal of Physiology (London)*, **276**, 659–666.

Bezkorovainy, A. (1980). *Biochemistry of Nonheme Iron*. Plenum Press, New York.

Blake, P.A., Merson, M.H., Weaver, R.E., Hollis, D.G., and Heublein, P.C. (1979). Disease caused by a marine *Vibrio*: clinical characteristics and epidemiology. *New England Journal of Medicine*, **300**, 1–5.

Blatteis, C.M., Bealer, S.L. Hunter, W.S. Llanos-Q, J., Ahokas, R.A., and Mashburn, Jr., T.A. (1983). Suppression of fever after lesions of the anteroventral third ventricle in guinea pigs. *Brain Research Bulletin*, 11:519–526.

Bornside, G.H., Bouis, P.J., and Cohn, I. (1968). Haemoglobin and *Escherichia coli*, a lethal intraperitoneal combination. *Journal of Bacteriology*, **95**, 1567–1571.

Bornside, G.H., Bouis, P.J., and Cohn, I. (1970) Enhancement of *Escherichia coli* infection and endotoxic activity by haemoglobin and ferric ammonium citrate. *Surgery*, **68**, 350–355.

Bornside, G.H., and Cohn, I. (1968). Haemoglobin as a bacterial virulence enhancing factor in fluids produced in strangulation intestinal obstruction. *American Surgeon*, **34**, 63–67.

Bornstein, D.L. (1982). Leukocytic pyrogen: a major mediator of the acute phase reaction. *Annals of the New York Academy of Science*, **389**, 323–336.

Bothwell, T.H., Seftel, H., Jacobs, P., Torrance, J.D., and Baumslag, N. (1964). Iron overload in Bantu subjects. Studies on the availability of iron in Bantu beer. *American Journal of Clinical Nutrition*, **14**, 44–51.

Bouza, E., Dominguez, A. Meseguer, M. Buzon, L. Boixeda, D. Revello, M.J., de Rafael, L., and Martinez-Beltran, J. (1980). *Yersinia enterocolitica* septicemia. *American Journal of Clinical Pathology*, **74**, (4), 404–409.

Briggs, J.D., Kennedy, A.C., and Goldberg, A. (1963). Urinary white cell excretion after iron sorbitol citric acid. *British Medical Journal*, **2**, 352–354.

Brock, J.H., and Ng, J. (1983). The effect of desferrioxamine on the growth of *Staphylococcus aureus*, *Yersinia enterocolitica*, and *Streptococcus faecalis* in human serum: uptake of desferrioxamine-bound iron. *FEMS Microbiology*, Letters, **20**, 439–442.

Bryant, R.E., DesPrez, R.M. VanWay, M.H. and Rogers, D.E. (1966). Studies on human leukocyte motility. I. Effects of alterations in pH, electrolyte concentration, and phagocytosis on leukocyte migration, adhesiveness, and aggregation. *Journal of Experimental Medicine*, **124**, 483–499.

Buchanan, W.M. (1971). Shock in Bantu siderosis. *American Journal of Clinical Pathology*, **55**, 401–406.
Bullen, J.J. (1981). The significance of iron in infection. *Reviews of Infectious Diseases*, **3**, 1127–1138.
Bullen, J.J., and Cushnie, G.H. (1962). Experimental gas gangrene: the effect of antiserum on the growth of *Clostridium welchii* type A. *Journal of Pathology and Bacteriology*, **84**, 177–192.
Bullen, J.J., and Cushnie, G.H. (1963). The failure of antitoxin to protect guinea pigs against intraperitoneal infection with *Clostridium welchii* type A. *Journal of Pathology and Bacteriology*, **86**, 345–360.
Bullen, J.J., Cushnie, G.H., and Rogers, H.J. (1967). The abolition of the protective effect of *Clostridium welchii* type A antiserum by ferric iron. *Immunology*, **12**, 303–312.
Bullen, J.J., Cushnie, G.H., and Stoner, H.B. (1966). Oxygen uptake by *Clostridium welchii* type A. Its possible role in experimental infection in passively immunised animals. *British Journal of Experimental Pathology*, **47**, 488–506.
Bullen, J.J., Dobson, A., and Wilson, A.B. (1964). Bacteriostatic effects of horse antiserum on *Clostridium welchii* type A. The role of *Eh* and pH. *Journal of General Microbiology*, **35**, 175–182.
Bullen, J.J., Leigh, L.C., and Rogers, H.J. (1968). The effect of iron compounds on the virulence of *Escherichia coli* for guinea pigs. *Immunology*, **15**, 581–588.
Bullen, J.J., and Rogers, H.J. (1969). Bacterial iron metabolism and immunity to *Pasteurella septica* and *Escherichia coli*. *Nature*, **224**, 380–382.
Bullen, J.J., Rogers, H.J., and Lewin J.E. (1971). The bacteriostatic effect of serum on *Pasteurella septica* and its abolition by iron compounds. *Immunology*, **20** 391–406.
Bullen, J.J., Ward, C.G., and Wallis, S.N. (1974). Virulence and the role of iron in *Pseudomonas aeruginosa* infection. *Infection and Immunity*, **10**, 443–450.
Bullen, J.J., Wilson, A.B, Cushnie, G.H., and Rogers, H.J. (1968). The abolition of the protective effect of *Pasteurella septica* antiserum by iron compounds. *Immunology*, **14**, 889–898.
Byles, A.B., and D'sa, A. (1970). Reduction in reaction due to iron dextran infusion using chloroquine. *British Medical Journal*, **3**, 625–627.
Cannon, J.G., and Dinarello, C.A. (1984) Interleukin-1 activity in human plasma. *Federation Proceedings*, **43**(3), 462.
Cannon, J.G., and Kluger, M.J. (1983). Endogenous pyrogen activity in human plasma after exercise. *Science*, **220**, 617–619.
Carlsson, J., Hofling, J.F. and Sundqvist, C.K. (1984). Degradation of albumin, haemopexin, haptoglobin, and transferrin by black pigmented *Bacteriodes* species. *Journal of Medical Microbiology*, **18**, 39–46.
Carmichael, L.E., Barnes, F.D. and Percy, D.H. (1979). Temperature as a factor in resistance of young puppies. *Journal of Infectious Diseases*, **120**, 669–678.
Caroline, L., Kozinn, P.J., Feldman, F, Stiefel E.H., and Lichtman, H. (1969). Infection and iron overload in thalassaemia. *Annals of the New York Academy of Science*, **165**, 148–155.
Caroline, L., Rosner, F. and Kozinn, P.J. (1969). Elevated serum iron, low blood transferrin, and candidiasis in acute leukemia. *Blood*, **34**, 441–451.
Caroline, L., Taschdjian, C.L., Kozinn, P.J, and Schade, A.L. (1964). Reversal of serum fungistasis by adding iron. *Journal of Investigative Dermatology*, **42**, 415–419.
Cavill, I., and Ricketts, C. (1980). Human iron kinetics. In *Iron in Biochemistry and Medicine* (Eds. A. Jacobs and M. Worwood), Vol. II, pp. 573–604. Academic Press, New York.
Cederblad, G. (1979). Plasma proteins involved in haem metabolism and transport of metal, hormones, and vitamins. In *Plasma Proteins* (Eds. B. Blomack and L.A.

Hanson), pp.94–117. John Wiley and Sons, Chichester.
Chart, H., and Griffiths, E. (1985). The availability of iron and the growth of *Vibrio vulnificus* in sera from patients with haemochromatosis. *FEMS Microbiology Letters*, **26**, 227–231.
Cohn, I. (1961). *Strangulation Obstruction*. C.C. Thomas, Springfield, Illinois.
Covert, J.B., and Reynolds, W.W. (1977). Survival value of fever in fish. *Nature*, **267**, 43–45.
Cremades, A., Garcia, F., Del Rio, J., and Brugger, A.J. (1982). Fever, antipyretics and serum iron levels in rabbits. *European Journal of Pharmacology,* **83**, 199–205.
Caudra, M. (1956). Salmonellosis complication in human bartonellosis. *Texas Reports of Biology and Medicine*, **14**, 97–113.
Davies, J.W.L. (1982). *Physiological Responses to Burning Injury*, pp. 393–423. Academic Press, London.
Davis, J.H., and Yull, A.B. (1964). A toxic factor in abdominal injury. II. The role of the red cell component. *Journal of Trauma*, **4**, 84–87.
De Venuto, F., Friedman, H.I., Neville, J.R., and Peck, C.C. (1979). Appraisal of hemoglobin as a blood substitute. *Surgery, Gynecology and Obstetrics*, **149**, 417–436.
Dinarello, C.A. (1982). Leukocytic pyrogen. In *Lymphokines*, Vol. 7 (Pick, E. and Landy, M., Eds.) pp. 23–74. Academic Press, New York.
Dinarello, C.A. (1984). Interleukin–1. *Reviews of Infectious Diseases*, **6**, 51–95.
Dinarello, C.A., Bernheim, H.A., Duff, G.W., Le, H.V., Nagabhushan, T.L., Hamilton, N.C., and Coceani, F. (1984). Mechanisms of fever induction by recombinant interferon. *Journal of Clinical Investigation*, **74**, 906–913.
Downing, J.F., Martinez-Valdez, H. Long, T. Elizondo, R., and Taylor, M.W. (1984). *In vivo* induction of IFN-gamma at febrile temperatures. In *The Biology of the Interferon System* (Eds. H. Kirchner and H. Schellekens), pp. 429–432. Elsevier Science Publishing B.V.
Duff, G.W., and Durum, S.K. (1982). T cell proliferation induced by interleukin 1 is greatly increased by hyperthermia. *Clinical Research*, **30**, 694A.
Eaton, J.W., Brandt, P., Mahoney, J.R., and Lee, J.T. (1982). Haptoglobin: a natural bacteriostat. *Science*, **215**, 691–692.
English Plague Commission (1907). Further observations on the transmission of plague by fleas, with special reference to the fate of the plague bacillus in the body of the rat flea. *Journal of Hygiene*, **7**, 395–420.
Eraklis, A.J., Kevy, S.V., Diamond, L.K, and Gross, R.E. (1967). Hazard of overwhelming infection after splenectomy in childhood. *New England Journal of Medicine*, **276** (22), 1225–1229.
Estey, E.H., Keating, M.J., McCredie, K.B., Bodey, G.P., and Freireich, E.J. (1982) Causes of initial remission induction failure in acute myelogenous leukemia. *Blood*, **60** (2), 209–315.
Feldberg, W., and Milton, A.S. (1978). Prostaglandins and body temperature. In *Handbook of Experimental Pharmacology*, Vol. 50, *Inflammation* (Eds. J.R. Vane and S.H. Ferreira), pp. 617–656. Springer-Verlag, Berlin.
Feldberg, W., and Scott, G.M. (1984). Interferon fever in cats. *Journal of Physiology (London)*, **355**, 28P.
Fildes, P. (1929). Tetanus 1X: The oxidation-reduction potential of the subcutaneous tissue fluid of the guinea-pig; its effect on infection, *British Journal of Experimental Pathology*, **10**, 197–204.
Fletcher, J. (1971). The effect of iron and transferrin on the killing of *Escherichia coli* in fresh serum. *Immunology*, **20**, 493–500.
Fletcher, J., and Goldstein, E. (1970). The effect of parenteral iron prepartion on experimental pyelonephritis. *British Journal of Experimental Pathology*, **51**, 280–285.

Freireich, E.J., Miller, A., Emerson, C.P., and Ross, J.F. (1957). The effect of inflammation on the utilization of erythrocyte and transferrin bound radioiron for red cell production. *Blood*, **12**, 972–983.

Garibaldi, J.A. (1972) Influence of temperature on the biosynthesis of iron transport compounds by *Salmonella typhimurium*. *Journal of Bacteriology*, **110**, 262–265.

Gery, I., Gershon, R.K., and Waksman, B.H. (1972). Potentiation of the T-lymphocyte response to mitogens. I. The responding cell. *Journal of Experimental Medicine*, **136**, 128–142.

Grieger, T.A., and Kluger, M.J. (1978). Fever and survival: the role of serum iron. *Journal of Physiology (London)*, **279**, 187–196.

Griffiths, E. (1983). Adaptation and multiplication of bacteria in host tissues. *Philosophical Transactions of the Royal Society of London*, Series B, **303**, 85–96.

Gupta, S., and Agarwal, S.S. (1980). Effect of hyperthermia on *in vitro* proliferative response of lymphocyte subpopulations. *Federation Proceedings*, **39**, 916.

Gutteridge, J.M.C., Rowley, D.A., Griffiths, E., and Halliwell, B. (1985). Low molecular weight iron complexes and oxygen radical reactions in idiopathic haemochromatosis. *Clinical Science*, **68**, 463–467.

Haber, F., and Weiss, J. (1934). The catalytic decomposition of hydrogen peroxide by iron salts. *Proceedings of the Royal Society of Edinburgh. Section (Maths. Phys. Sci.)*, **147**, 332–351.

Hacker, M.R., Rothenburg, B.A., and Kluger, M.J. (1981). Plasma iron, copper, and zinc in lizard *Dipsosaurus dorsalis*: effects of bacteria injection. *American Journal of Physiology*, **240**, R272–R275.

Hamilton, L.D., Gubler, C.J., Cartwright, G.E., and Wintrobe, M.M., (1950). Diurnal variation in the plasma iron level of man. *Proceedings of the Society for Experimental Biology and Medicine*, **75**, 65–68.

Hanson, D.F., Murphy, P.A., Silicano, R., and Shin, H.S. (1983). The effect of temperature on the activation of thymocytes by interleukins I and II. *Journal of Immunology*, **130**, 216–221.

Helms, S.D., Oliver, J.D., and Travis, J.C. (1984). Role of heme compounds and haptoglobin in *Vibrio vulnificus* pathogenicity. *Infection and Immunity*, **45**, (2), 345–349.

Heron, I., and Berg, K. (1978). The actions of interferon are potentiated at elevated temperature. *Nature*, **274**, 508–510.

Hoffman, M.K., Koenig, S., Mittler, R.S., Oettgen, H.F., Ralph, P., Galanos, C., and Hammerling, U. (1979). Macrophage factor controlling differentiation of B cells. *Journal of Immunology*, **122**, 497–502.

Hoffman-Goetz, L., and Kluger, M.J. (1979). Protein deprivation: its effects on fever and plasma iron during bacterial infection in rabbits. *Journal of Physiology (London)*, **295**, 263–272.

Hoffman-Goetz, L., McFarlane, D., Bistrian, B.R., and Blackburn, G.L., (1980). Restoration of reduced production of leukocytic endogenous mediator by peripheral blood leukocytes of patients with kwashiorkor by short-term nutritional support. *American College of Surgeons 1980 Surgical Forum*, **31**, 108–110.

Hook, E.W., Campbell, C.G., Weens, H.S., and Cooper, G.R. (1957). *Salmonella* osteomyelitis in patients with sickle cell anaemia. *New England Journal of Medicine*, **257**, 403–407.

Hunter, R.L., Bennett, B., Towns, M., and Vogler, W.R. (1984). Transferrin and Disease. I. Defects in the regulation of transferrin satuaration with iron contribute to susceptibility to infection. *American Journal of Clinical Pathology*, **81**, 748–753.

Husseini, R.H., Sweet, C., Collie, M.H., and Smith, H. (1982). Elevation of nasal viral levels by suppression of fever in ferrets infected with influenza viruses of differing virulence. *Journal of Infectious Diseases*, **145**, 520–524.

Jampel, H.D., Duff, G.W., Gershon, R.K., Atkins, E., and Durum, S.K., (1983). Fever and immunoregulation. III. Hyperthermia augments the primary *in vitro* humoral immune response. *Journal of Experimental Medicine*, **157**, 1229–1238.

Jeffrey, J.S., and Thomson, S. (1944). Gas gangrene in Italy. A study of 33 cases treated with penicillin. *British Journal of Surgey*, **32**, 159–167.

Jones, N.L. (1962). Irreversible shock in haemochromatosis. *Lancet*, I, 569–572.

Jones, R.L., Peterson, C.M., Grady, R.W., Kumbaraci, T., Cerami, A., and Graziano, J.H. (1977). Effect of iron chelates and iron overload on *Salmonella* infection. *Nature*, **267**, 63–64.

Kampschmidt, R.F. (1980). Biological manifestations of leukocytic endogenous mediator. In *Microbiology—1980* (Ed. D. Schlessinger), pp. 1113–1115. American Society for Microbiology, Washington, DC.

Kampschmidt, R.F., and Pulliam, L.A. (1975). Stimulating of antimicrobial activity in the rat with leukocytic endogenous mediator. *Journal of the Reticuloendothelial Society*, **17**, 162–169.

Kaye, D., Gill, F.A., and Hook, E.W. (1967). Factors influencing host resistance to *Salmonella* infections: the effects of haemolysis and erythrophagocytosis. *American Journal of Medical Science*, **254**, 205–215.

Keenan, R.A., Moldawer, L.L., Yang, R.D., Kawamura, I., Blackburn, G.L., and Bistrian, B.R. (1982). An altered response by peripheral leukocytes to synthesize or release leukocyte endogenous mediator in critically ill, protein-malnourished patients. *Journal of Laboratory and Clinical Medicine*, **100**, 844–857.

Kenedi, E., Laburn, H., Mitchell, D., and Ross, F.P. (1982). On the pyrogenic action of intravenous lipid A in rabbits. *Journal of Physiology (London)*, **328**, 361–370.

Klaiman, A.P., Victery, W., Kluger, M.J., and Vander, A.J., (1981). Urinary excretion of zinc and iron following acute injection of dead bacteria in dog. *Proceedings of the Society for Experimental Biology and Medicine*, **167**, 165–171.

Klempner, M.S., Dinarello, C.A., and Gallin, J.I. (1978). Human leukocytic pyrogen induces release of specific granule contents from human neutrophils. *Journal of Clinical Investigation*, **61**, 1330–1336.

Kluger, M.J. (1979). *Fever: Its Biology, Evolution and Function*. Princeton University Press, Princeton, New Jersey.

Kluger, M.J., Oppenheim, J.J., and Powanda, M.C., (Eds.) (1985). *Proceedings of the symposium: the physiologic, metabolic and immunologic actions of interleukin—1*. In the series *Progress in Leukocyte Biology*. Alan Liss, New York.

Kluger, M.J., Ringler, D.H., and Anver, M.R. (1975). Fever and survival. *Science*, **188**, 166–168.

Kluger, M.J., and Rothenburg, B.A. (1979). Fever and reduced iron: their interaction as a host defense response to bacterial infection. *Science*, **203**, 374–376.

Kochan, I. (1977). Role of siderophores in nutritional immunity and bacterial parasitism. In *Microorganisms and Minerals*, pp. 251–288. M. Dekker, New York.

Konijn, A.M., and Hershko, C. (1977). Ferritin synthesis in inflammation. I. Pathogenesis of impaired iron release. *British Journal of Haematology*, **37**, 7–16.

Koopman, W.J., Farrar, J.J., and Fuller-Bonar, J. (1978). Evidence for the identification of lymphocyte activating factor as the adherent cell-derived mediator responsible for enhanced antibody synthesis by nude mouse spleen cells. *Cellular Immunology*, **35**, 92–98.

Lee, G.R. (1983) The anemia of chronic disease. *Seminars in Hematology*, **20**, 61–80.

Lee, J.T., Arenholz, D.A., Nelson, R.D., and Simmonds, R.L. (1979) Mechanism of the adjuvant effect of haemoglobin in experimental peritonitis. V. The significance of the coordinated iron component. *Surgery*, **86**, 41–47.

Letendre, E.D., and Holbein, B.E., (1983). Turnover in the transferrin iron pool during the hypoferremic phase of experimental *Neisseria meningitidis* infection in mice. *Infection and Immunity*, **39**, 50–59.

Letendre, E.D., and Holbein, B.E. (1984). Mechanism of impaired iron release by the reticuloendothelial system during the hypoferremic phase of experimental *Neisseria meningitidis* infection in mice. *Infection and Immunity*, **44**, 320–325.

Lynch, S.R., Simon, M., Bothwell, T.H., and Charlton, R.W. (1973). Circadian variation in plasma iron concentration and reticuloendothelial iron release in the rat. *Clinical Science and Molecular Medicine*, **45**, 331–336.

McFarlane, H., Reddy, S., Adcock, K.J., Adeshina, H., Cooke, A.R., and Akene, A.R. (1970). Immunity, transferrin and survival in kwashiorkor. *British Medical Journal*, **4**, 268–270.

MacLennan, J.D., and MacFarlane, R.Y. (1945). Toxin and antitoxin studies of gas gangrene in man. *Lancet*, **2**, 301–305.

Maskell, J.P., and Miles, A.A. (1984). The variable response of bacteria to free haemoglobin in the tissue. *Journal of Medical Microbiology*, **18**, 377–384.

Medical Research Council's Working Party on Leukaemia in Adults (1974). Treatment of acute myeloid leukaemia with daunorubicin, cystosine arabinoside, mercaptopurine, L-asparaginase, prednisone and thioguanine: results of treatment with five multiple-drug schedules. *British Journal of Haematology*, **27**, 373–389.

Melby, K., Slørdahl, S., Gutteberg, T.J., and Nordø S.A. (1982). Septicaemia due to *Yersinia enterocolitica* after oral doses of iron. *British Medical Journal*, **285**, 467–468.

Mizel, S.B., and Farrar, J.J. (1979). Revised nomenclature for antigen-nonspecific T-cell proliferation and helper factors. *Cellular Immunology*, **48**, 433–443.

Muller, D., Edwards, M.L., and Smith, D.W. (1983). Changes in iron and transferrin levels and body temperature in experimental airborne legionellosis. *Journal of Infectious Diseases*, **147**, 302–307.

Muller-Eberhard, U. (1970). Hemopexin. *New England Journal of Medicine*, **283**, 1090–1093.

Murphy, P.A., Simon, P.L., and Willoughby, W.F. (1980). Endogenous pyrogens made by rabbit peritoneal exudate cells are identical with lymphocyte-activating factors made by rabbit alveolar macrophages. *Journal of Immunology*, **124**, 2498–2501.

Murray, M.J., Murray, A., and Murray, C.J. (1980). The salutory effect of milk on ameobiasis and its reversal by iron. *British Medical Journal*, **1**, 1351–1352.

Murray, M.J., Murray, A.B., Murray, N.J. and Murray, M.B. (1975). Refeeding-malaria and hyperferraemia, *Lancet*, I, 653–654.

Murray, M.J., Murray, A.B., Murray, M.B., and Murray C.J. (1978). The adverse effect of iron repletion on the course of certain infections. *British Medical Journal*, II, 1113–1115.

Nahas, G.G., Tannieres, M.L., and Lennon, J.F. (1971). Direct measurement of leukocyte motility: effects of pH and temperature. *Proceedings of the Society of Experimental Biology and Medicine*, **138**, 350–352.

Nauman, H.N., Diggs, L.W., Barreras, L., and Williams, B.J. (1971). Plasma haemoglobin and haemoglobin fractions in sickle-cell crisis. *American Journal of Clinical Pathology*, **56**, 137–147.

North, J.P. (1947). Clostridial wound infection and gas gangrene. *Surgery*, **21**, 364–372.

Oakley, C.L. (1954). Gas gangrene. *British Medical Bulletin*, **10**, 52–58.

Overturf, D.G., Powers, P., and Baraff, L.J. (1977). Bacterial meningitis and septicaemia in sickle cell disease. *American Journal of Diseases of Children*, **131**, 784–787.

Payne, S.M., and Finkelstein, R.A. (1978) The critical role of iron in host-bacterial interactions. *Journal of Clinical Investigation*, **61**, 1428–1440.

Pepys, M.B. (1981). C-reactive protein fifty years on. *Lancet*, **I**, 653–657.

Perry, R.D., and Brubaker, R.R. (1979). Accumulation of iron by Yersiniae. *Journal of Bacteriology*, **137**, 1290–1298.

Phelps, P., and Stanislaw, D. (1969). Polymorphonuclear leukocyte mobility *in vitro*. I. Effect of pH, temperature, ethyl alcohol and caffeine, using a modified Boyden chamber technique. *Arthritis and Rheumatism*, **12**, 181–188.

Pootrakul, P., Rugkiatsakul, R., and Wasi, P. (1980). Increased transferrin iron saturation in splenectomised thalassaemic patients. *British Journal of Haematology*, **46**, 143–145.

Powanda, M.C., and Canonico, P.G. (Eds.) (1981). *Infection: The Physiologic and Metabolic Responses of the Host*. Elsevier–North Holland, Amsterdam.

Powanda, M.C., and Beisel, W.R. (1982). Hypothesis: leukocyte endogenous mediator/endogenous pyrogen/lymphocyte-activating factor modulates the development of nonspecific and specific immunity and affects nutritional status. *American Journal of Clinical Nutrition*, **35**, 762–768.

Pruett, T.L., Rotstein, O.R., Fiegel, V.D., Sorensen, J.J., Nelson, R.D., and Simmons, R.L. (1984). Mechanism of adjuvant effect of hemoglobin in experimental peritonitis VIII. A leukotoxin is produced by *Escherichia coli* metabolism in hemoglobin, *Surgey*, **96**, 375–380.

Quastel, M.R., and Ross, J.F. (1966). The effect of acute inflammation on the utilization and distribution of transferrin-bound and erythrocyte radioiron. *Blood*, **28**, 738–757.

Rabson, A.R., Hallett, A.F., and Koornhof, H.J. (1975). Generalized *Yersinia enterocolitica* infection. *Journal of Infectious Diseases*, **131**, 447–451.

Rehg, J.E., Burek, J.D., Strandberg, J.D., and Montali, R.J. (1980). Hemochromatosis in the rock hyrax. In *Comparative Pathology of Zoo Animals* (Eds. R.J. Montali and G. Migaki), pp. 113–120. Smithsonian Institute, Washington, DC.

Roberts, Jr., N.J., and Steigbigel, R.T. (1977). Hyperthermia and human leukocyte functions: effects on response of lymphocytes to mitogen and antigen and bactericidal capacity of monocytes and neutrophils. *Infection and Immunity*, **18**, 673–679.

Robins-Browne, R.M., and Prpic, J.K. (1985). Effects of iron and desferrioxamine on infections with *Yersinia enterocolitica. Infection and Immunity*, **47**, (3), 744–779.

Robins-Browne, R.M., Rabson, A.R., and Koornhof, H.J. (1979). Generalised infection with *Yersinia enterocolitica* and the role of iron. *Contributions to Microbiology and Immunology*, **5**, 277–282 (Karger, Basel).

Roeser, H.P. (1980). Iron metabolism in inflamation and malignant disease. In "Iron in Biochemistry and Medicine." (Eds. A. Jacobs and W. Worwood), pp. 605–640. Academic Press, New York.

Rogers, H.J. (1967). Bacteriostatic effect of horse sera and serum fractions on *Clostridium welchii* type A and the abolition of bacteriostasis by iron salts. *Immunology*, **12**, 285–301.

Rogers, H.J., Bullen, J.J., and Cushnie, G.H. (1970). Iron compounds and resistance to infection: further experiments with *Clostridium welchii* type A *in-vivo* and *in-vitro*. *Immunology*, **19**, 521–538.

Rosenwaser, L.J., Dinarello, C.A., and Rosenthal, A.S. (1979). Adherent cell function in murine T-lymphocyte antigen recognition. IV. Enhancement of murine T-cell antigen recognition by human leukocytic pyrogen. *Journal of Experimental Medicine*, **150**, 709–714.

Sacks, T., Moldow, C.F., Craddock, P.R., Bowers, T.K., and Jacobs, H.S. (1978). Oxygen radicals mediate endothelial cell damage by complement-stimulated granulocytes. An *in vitro* model of immune vascular damage. *Journal of Clinical Investigation*, **61**, 1161–1167.

Sears, D.A. (1967). Plasma heme-binding in patients with hemolytic disorders. *Journal of Laboratory and Clinical Medicine*, **71**, (3), 484–494.

Sebag, J., Reed, W.R., and Williams, Jr., R.C. (1977). Effect of temperature on bacterial killing by serum and by polymorphonuclear leukocytes. *Infection and Immunity*, **16**, 947–954.

Smith, R.J., Bowman, B.J., and Speziale, S.C. (1985). Interleukin-1 stimulates granule exocytosis form human neutrophils. In *Proceedings of the Symposium: The Physiologic, Metabolic and Immunologic Actions of Interleukin-1*. (Eds. M.J. Kluger, J.J. Oppenheim and M.C. Powanda). In the series, *Progress in Leukocyte Biology*. Alan Liss, New York.

Soltys, H.D., and Brody, J.I. (1970). Synthesis of transferrin by human peripheral blood lymphocytes. *Journal of Laboratory and Clinical Medicine*, **75**, 250–257.

Stoner, H.B., Bullen, J.J., Cushine, G.H., and Batty, I. (1967). Fatal intraperitoneal infection with *Clostridium welchii* type A in passively immunised guinea pigs. The effect on vascular permeability. *British Journal of Experimental Pathology*, **48**, 309–316.

Stoner, H.B., and Green, H.N. (1948). Bodily reactions to trauma. The effect of ischaemia on muscle protein. *British Journal of Experimental Pathology*, **29**, 121–132.

Sztein, M.B., Voge, S.N., Sipe, J.D., Murphy, P.A., Mizel, S.B., Oppenheim, J.J. and Rosenstreich, D.L. (1981). The role of macrophages in the acute phase response: SAA inducer is closely related to lymphocyte activating factor and endogenous pyrogen. *Cellular Immunology*, **63**, 164–176.

Tacket, C.O., Brenner, F., and Blake, P.A. (1984). Clinical features of an epidemiological study of *Vibrio vulnificus* infections. *Journal of Infectious Diseases*, **149**, 558–561.

Thomas, A.N., Pattinson, C., and Serjeant, G.R. (1983). Cause of death in sickle-cell disease in Jamaica. *British Medical Journal*, **285**, 633–635.

Teisner, B., and Haahr, S. (1974). Poikilothermia and susceptibility of suckling mice to Coxsackie B1 virus. *Nature*, **247**, 568.

Tocco, R.J., Kahn, L.L., Kluger, M.J., and Vander, A.J. (1983). Relationship of trace metals to fever during infection: are prostaglandins involved? *American Journal of Physiology*, **244**, R368–R373.

Ucar, D.A., Tocco, R.J., and Kluger, M.J. (1983). Circadian variation in circulating pyrogen: possible role in resistance to infection. *Proceedings of the Society for Experimental Biology and Medicine*, **173**, 319–323.

van Heyningen, W.E. (1955). The role of toxins in pathology. *Symposium, Society for General Microbiology*, **5**, 17–39.

van Oss, C.J., Absolom, D.R., Moore, L.L., Park, B.H., and Humbert, J.R. (1980). Effect of temperature on the chemotaxis, phagocytic engulfment, digestion and O_2 consumption of human polymorphonuclear leukocytes. *Journal of the Reticuloendothelial Society*, **27**, 561–565.

Van Snick, J.L., Masson, P.L., and Heremans, J.F. (1974). The involvement of lactoferrin in the hyposideremia of acute inflammation. *Journal of Experimental Medicine*, **140**, 1068–1084.

Vaughn, L.K., Veale, W.L., and Cooper, K.E. (1980). Antipyresis: its effect on mortality rate of bacterially infected rabbits. *Brain Research Bulletin*, **5**, 69–73.

Walker, R.J., and Williams, R. (1974). Haemochromatosis and iron overload. In *Iron in Biochemistry and Medicine* (Eds. A. Jacobs and M. Worwood), pp. 589–612. Academic Press, London.

Ward, C.G., Hammond, J. and Bullen, J.J. (1986). Effect of iron compounds on the antibacterial function of human polymorphs and plasma. *Infection and Immunity*, **51**, 723–730.

Ward, P.S., Till, G.O., Kunkel, R., and Beauchamp, C. (1983). Evidence for the role of hydroxyl radical in complement and neutrophil dependent tissue injury. *Journal of Clinical Investigation*, **72**, 789–801.

Wever, R.A. (1979). *The Circadian System of Man*, p.4. Springer-Verlag, New York.

Whitten, C.F. (1962). Studies on serum haptoglobin—a functional enquiry. *New England Journal of Medicine*, **266**, 529–534.

Wood, D.D., Ihrie, E.J., Dinarello, C.A., and Cohen, P.L. (1983). Isolation of an interleukin-1-like factor from human joint effusions. *Arthritis and Rheumatism*, **26**, 975–983.

Worsham, P.L., and Konisky, J. (1984). Effect of growth temperature on the acquisition of iron by *Salmonella typhimurium* and *Escherichia coli*. *Journal of Bacteriology*, **158**, 163–168.

Wright, A.C., Simpson, L.M., and Oliver, J.D. (1981). Role of iron in pathogensius of *Vibrio vulnificus* infections. *Infection and Immunity*, **34**, 503–507.

Yamishiro, K.M., Goldman, R.H., Harris, D., and Uyeda, C.T. (1971). *Pasteurella pseudotuberculosis*; acute sepsis with survival. *Archives of Internal Medicine*, **28**, 605–608.

Yerushalmi, A., Tovey, M.G., and Gresser, I. (1982). Antitumor effect of combined interferon and hyperthermia in mice. *Proceedings of the Society of Experimental Biology and Medicine*, **169**, 413–415.

Yull, A.B., Abrahams, J.S., and Davis, J.H. (1962). The peritoneal fluid in strangulated obstruction. The role of the red blood cell and *E. coli* bacteria in producing toxicity. *Journal of Surgical Research*, **2** (4), 223–232.

Iron and Infection
Edited by J.J. Bullen and E. Griffiths

Chapter 8

Iron and infection: future prospects

E. GRIFFITHS
National Institute for Biological Standards and Control,
Holly Hill, Hampstead,
London, NW3 6RB, England

J.J. BULLEN
Department of Surgery,
University of Miami School of Medicine,
Jackson Memorial Medical Center,
PO Box 016310, Miami,
Florida 33101, USA

1. INTRODUCTION

It is well known that bacterial pathogenicity and resistance of the host involve a large number of interacting factors. For this reason it is unwise to be dogmatic about the supposed importance of individual components of the systems concerned. For example, it is often said that the phagocytic cells are the most important defence against invading bacteria. It is true that in some instances it can be shown that phagocytic cells, such as polymorphs, are essential for defence, and this can be demonstrated quite easily by the use of an antipolymorphonuclear leucocyte serum (Bullen, Wallis and Griffiths, 1976). On the other hand, if the plasma transferrin is saturated with iron, the extracellular bacteria may grow twice as fast as normal and the polymorphs are overwhelmed, with fatal results for the host (Bullen, Ward and Wallis, 1974). In this instance it is the unsaturated iron-binding capacity of the transferrin that is essential for defence.

The truth is that both phagocytic cells and the bactericidal or bacteriostatic power of plasma, as well as other factors, have an essential part to play, and our purpose should be to define exactly the role of each. This can be quite difficult, and in spite of considerable progress, we still have much to discover about bacterial pathogenicity and host resistance, even with a single organism. One thing seems certain. The influence of iron metabolism, both of the invading bacterial pathogen and in the host, is widespread and often appears to be crucial in deciding the outcome of an infection. In the present chapter we consider how this knowledge is contributing to our understanding of infections in general and also to the development and use of new therapeutic and prophylactic measures.

2. IRON-RELATED CHANGES AND BACTERIAL VIRULENCE

The ability of an invading pathogen to proliferate successfully *in vivo* is essential for any infection, and the ability of certain virulent bacteria to resist the bactericidal action of serum or polymorphonuclear leukocytes or to resist phagocytosis has been known for a long time (Glynn, 1972; Olling, 1977; Björksten and Kaijser, 1978). Some of the determinants that endow them with this ability have been studied in considerable detail (Moll, Manning and Timmis, 1980; Robbins *et al.*, 1980; Opal, Cross and Gemski, 1982; Binns, Mayden and Levine, 1982; Ogata, Wintens and Levine, 1982; Agüero *et al.*, 1984; Montenegro *et al.*, 1985). More recently, bacterial pathogens which initiate infection on mucosal surfaces have been found to produce a protease that specifically destroys human IgA_1 (Mestecky *et al.*, 1980; Kornfeld and Plaut, 1981; Kilian *et al.*, 1983; Plaut, 1983; Mulks, 1985). The finding that certain closely related but non-pathogenic species do not produce an IgA_1 protease has led to the suggestion that the enzyme may be a factor in pathogenicity. However, not all mucosal pathogens produce IgA_1 proteases; *Bordetella pertussis*, a well-known mucosal pathogen, does not appear to express an IgA_1 protease, at least not *in vitro* (McPheat and Redhead, personal communication).

Generally, the study of bacterial virulence determinants has been carried out with organisms grown *in vitro*, in rich iron-replete culture media. It is known, however, that the growth of bacteria *in vivo* considerably affects their ability to resist certain host defences (Smith, 1980, 1983). For example, *Neisseria gonorrhoeae* isolated from urethral pus is more virulent for human volunteers than the same strain grown *in vitro*, and also more resistant to the killing action of human serum (Penn *et al.*, 1978). The discovery that bacteria undergo specific phenotypic changes both in their metabolism and in the composition of their outer membrane proteins to enable them the multiply in the iron-restricted environment of host tissues (Chapter 3) adds another dimension to the complex pattern of virulence determinants already found in the iron-replete pathogen. Possible connections between these iron-related changes, which are known to take place *in vivo*, and other bacterial properties such as resistance to phagocytosis or to the bactericidal action of serum now need to be explored, as does the effect of iron restriction on the synthesis of toxins and colonization factors. The presence of certain plasmid encoded proteins in the outer membrane of *Escherichia coli*, like the products of the *tra*T and *iss* genes, has been correlated with increased virulence in *E. coli* (Moll, Manning and Timmis, 1980; Binns, Mayden and Levine, 1982; Agüero *et al.*, 1984; Griffiths, 1985; Montenegro *et al.*, 1985). This, it has been suggested, could be due to an increased resistance of organisms expressing such proteins to the bactericidal effects of serum or to phagocytosis. Whether or not the expression of an iron-regulated outer membrane protein also confers resistance to such host defences remains to be seen. If it does, then *E.coli* would become more resistant to these particular host defence mechanisms, and therefore more virulent, as they adapt to and multiply in host tissues. It has already been reported that a large increase in virulence occurs in *Neisseria meningitidis* after growth under iron-restricted conditions at low pH (Brener, DeVoe and Holbein, 1981). In this case, the effect of iron restriction or of low pH (pH 6.6) alone on virulence was relatively small, although both independently induced the expression of a new outer membrane protein with a molecular mass of 69 kDa. Together, however, they induced not only large quantities of the 69 kDa protein in the outer membrane of the meningococcus but also another protein with an apparent molecular mass of 31 kDa. Growth at pH 6.6 had a pronounced effect on colony morphology and selected for a colonial type which, when combined with the effect of iron restriction, greatly increased the virulence of the organism for mice. Iron levels and the pH of the growth medium similarly affect the surface charge and colonial types of *N.gonorrhoeae* (Magnusson *et al.*, 1979a, 1979b). Since the inflammatory process characteristically involves a local decrease in pH as well as an increase in the level of lactoferrin, such changes may well be relevant to conditions *in vivo*.

It is known that in addition to the direct phenotypic changes induced in pathogens by the host environment, several bacterial species and protozoa are capable of altering their cell surface more permanently during growth *in vivo*, but at rates too high to be explained by ordinary mutations. Many of these phase variations are bidirectional and thus cannot be explained by high frequencey loss of a phage or plasmid. Examples of such phase changes are provided by *Salmonella* flagellar antigens (Zieg *et al.*, 1977; Simon *et al.*, 1980), trypanosomal surface antigens (Donelson and Rice-Ficht, 1985), *E.coli* type 1 pili (fimbriae) (Eisenstein, 1981; Nowicki *et al.*, 1985), *N.gonorrhoeae* type 1 pili (Meyer,

Mlawer and So, 1982) and *N.gonorrhoeae* outer membrane protein II (Mayer, 1982). The selection of particular bacterial types, or phases, *in vivo* is believed to play a part in enabling these pathogens to proliferate, but the genetic mechanisms responsible for the changes can be complex, as, for example, are those in *N.gonorrhoeae*. It is well known that *N.gonorrhoeae* can undergo alterations in cell surface characteristics during natural infection and on laboratory subculture (James and Swanson, 1978; Penn *et al.*, 1978; Swanson, 1978a; Lambden *et al.*, 1979; Draper *et al.*, 1980). These changes include the reversible loss of the ability to produce pili and changes in opacity. Fresh clinical isolates are invariably pilated and opaque organisms predominate in male urethral cultures; gonococci isolated from fallopian tubes form transparent colonies. During subculture pilated forms can give rise to non-pilated forms and vice versa. Similarly, opaque colonies can give rise to transclucent variants and vice versa. Variations in these characteristics may be important in permitting the gonococcus to colonize different sites in the human host during the course of natural infection and also to proliferate at these sites by helping the pathogen to evade host defences. Meyer, Mlawer and So (1982) have shown that the expression of pili is determined by rearrangements of the gonococcus chromosome. However, variations in pili involve not only an 'on–off' variation, but also changes between numerous antigenically distinct forms of pili (Lambden *et al.*, 1981). It has been shown that the protein subunit of gonococcal pili, pilin, consists of constant and variable regions (Edwards *et al.*, 1984; Rothbard, Fernandez and Schoolnik, 1984) and antigenic variation has been explained by chromosomal rearrangements resulting from intragenic recombination between a repertoire of cassettes of different pilin genes (Hagblom *et al.*, 1985; Segal *et al.*, 1985). However, there appear to be other mechanisms operating too, possibly at the post transcriptional level (Swanson *et al.*, 1985). A similar complexity exists among the alteration of gonococcal outer membrane protein designated PII; this appears to consist of a family of six or more closely related heat-modifiable proteins which are associated with differences in pathogenicity (James and Swanson, 1978; Swanson, 1978b; Saunders, 1982, 1985). Simpler chromosomal rearrangements seem to be responsible for antigenic variation in the flagella of *Salmonella typhimurium* (Simon *et al.*, 1980) and in the fimbriation of *E.coli* (Eisenstein, 1982). In *Salmonella*, a 970 base pair DNA segment containing a promoter for a flagella gene can invert reversibly by site-specific recombination at the ends of the segment. When the DNA segment is positioned in one particular direction, the promoter orientation is such that it will permit transcription (Silverman and Simon 1980; Simon *et al.*, 1980).

Phase variation shifts occur at much higher frequency than mutations and a slight selective advantage of one phase over another in a given environment results in the rapid outgrowth of a single phenotype. The selective pressures involved in most of these phase shifts are generally unkown and are likely to vary from case to case. Low pH, accompanied by iron restriction, may select certain variants of the gonococcus and meningococcus, but whether or not iron restriction affects any other phase shifts remains to be seen. There is a suggestion that iron restriction may exercise a selective pressure in the case of mucoid strains of *Pseudomonas aeruginosa*. Mucoid strains of *Pseudomonas* are frequently isolated from the lungs of individuals suffering from cystic fibrosis. These mucoid strains appear to be more stable under conditions of iron limitation and, in competition experiments, only under iron limitation were mucoid strains able to replace the wild type (Jones *et al.*, 1977; Ombaka, Cozens and Brown 1983). It has, of course, already been shown that *Pseudomonas* grows under iron-restricted conditions in the cystic fibrosis lung (Brown, Anwar and Lambert, 1984).

In addition to the various alterations which occur in pathogenic bacteria during growth under iron restriction, the production of some classical virulence determinants is also affected. Certain bacterial toxins, such as diphtheria toxin, are expressed optimally only during iron-restricted growth, and these are discussed in Chapter 4. The hydrolytic enzymes of *Pseudomonas* are also produced in optimal amounts only in a low-iron environment (Bjorn, Sokol and Iglewski, 1979). More recently there has been considerable interest in Shiga toxin, one of the most toxic biological agents known. This toxin has risen from relative obscurity to fame over a relatively short period of time and Shiga toxin, or Shiga-like toxins, have now been implicated not only in the pathogenesis of dysentry due to *Shigella* species, but also in haemorrhagic colitis and haemolytic ureamic syndrome caused by *E.coli*, as well as in infections with entero-pathogenic *E. coli* and other diarrhoeal diseases (Cantey, 1985). Oedema disease in pigs is thought to be similar to haemolytic ureamic syndrome in humans and is caused by *E.coli* which elaborate a Vero cell cytotoxin (Smith, Green and Parsell, 1983); Vero cell toxin is considered to be similar to the Shiga-like toxins (O'Brien *et al.*, 1982, 1983a, 1983b; Scotland, Smith and Rowe, 1985; Willshaw *et al.*, 1985; Karmali *et al.*, 1986). These toxins probably form a group of distinct cytotoxins which show varying degrees of antigenic relationships to each other. Although Shiga toxin was discovered over eighty years ago, it is interesting to speculate why Shiga-toxin-like activity has only recently been detected among so many new bacterial strains and species. Cantey (1985) believes that the answer lies in the observation of Dubos and Geiger in 1946 that inorganic iron in the culture medium suppresses Shiga toxin synthesis. Only when iron is removed from culture media, as was done by O'Brien and her colleagues (O'Brien and LaVeck, 1982, 1983; O'Brien *et al.*, 1982), can toxin synthesis be easily detected. Little is known at present about the organization of the genes necessary for synthesis of Shiga-like toxin, but the structural genes have now been cloned (Newland *et al.*, 1985). Furthermore, it is known that the ability to synthesize the toxin is transferred among certain strains of *E.coli* by a family of Shiga toxin-converting phages (Smith, Green and Parsell, 1983; O'Brien *et al.*, 1984; Smith *et al.*, 1984b). There are, of course, examples of other bacterial species carrying phages that determine toxin production. The structural genes for diphtheria toxin (Barksdale, Garmise and Rivera, 1961; Murphy, Pappenheimer and de Broms, 1974), erythrogenic toxin of *Streptococcus pyogenes* (Zabriskie, 1974; Weeks and Ferretti, 1984), the structural or regulatory genes of botulinum toxins C and D (Inoue and Iida, 1971) and staphylococcal enterotoxin A (Betley and Mekanolos, 1985) are all encoded by temperate phages.

The changes that bacteria may undergo when multiplying under the iron-restricted conditions found in host tissues have been discussed here and elsewhere in this book in some detail. However, it should be remembered that the ability of an organism to multiply in the iron-restricted environment of the host is only one factor, albeit an essential one, in the processes that decide the outcome of an infection. Other features of the host environment must also be considered and these are numerous and complex. It is therefore important to show, as far as is possible, that bacterial characteristics studied in isolation *in vitro* really reflect features of the bacteria when multiplying in host tissues during infection. Here we must consider not only specific phenotypic changes in bacteria resulting from transcriptional or translational events, but also from genotypic changes involving chromosomal rearrangements. The proliferation of bacteria *in vivo* depends on two bacterial qualities that are not always easy to separate, i.e. the ability to multiply *in vivo* and the ability to evade host antibacterial defences. As our understanding of the changes that occur in bacteria when they multiply *in vivo* increases, especially our understanding at the molecular level, then perhaps the contribution that various changes make to the capability of a pathogen to grow in host tissues will become clearer.

Factors that might be expected to influence bacterial multiplication *in vivo*, in addition to the restricted availability of iron, include temperature, pH, osmolarity, oxygen tension, and the availability of other nutrients. There is some evidence to suggest that the availability of phosphate may, like iron, be limiting in host tissues in certain instances and that the ability *Pseudomonas aeruginosa* to acquire phosphate via a specific transport system may be essential for establishing an infection (Vasil *et al.*, 1985). Furthermore, special nutritional conditions occurring only in certain tissues might be expected to lead to the localization of bacteria, or at least to their more rapid multiplication, at specific body sites. This has been shown to occur in brucellae where the carbohydrate erythritol, a preferred metabolite and growth stimulant for certain strains of this organism and present in significant amounts in the placental tissues of ungulates, promotes an intense placentitis with brucella which leads to abortion of the foetus (Smith *et al.*, 1962; Keppie *et al.*, 1965). In many other animals brucellosis is a relatively mild and chronic infection and the bacteria do not have a marked affinity for any particular tissue. Differences in host biochemistry and variations in bacterial nutritional requirements may also sometimes account for differences in host susceptibility to infection (Burrows and Gillett, 1971), as also may the condition of the host at the time of infection. Future studies must, therefore, not forget to take into account the condition of the host and the effect that this may have on the environment encountered by potentially pathogenic bacteria *in vivo*.

3. AVAILABILITY OF IRON DURING CLINICAL DISEASE AND TRAUMA

Throughout this book the emphasis has been on the necessity of iron for bacterial growth and the need of the host to sequestrate iron and make it unavailable. During clinical disease or trauma, host iron metabolism may alter and, quite clearly, infection of a compromised patient is likely to differ significantly from that in a healthy host. There is evidence already that some of the serum proteins that bind iron compounds can be reduced significantly in certain clinical conditions. A few examples include the reduction or disappearance of haptoglobin and the appearance of albumin–haem complexes (methaemalbumin) in sickle cell anaemia (Muller-Ebberhard, 1970; Naumann *et al.*, 1971) and the reduction in the level of transferrin in leukaemia (Hunter *et al.*, 1983) and in kwashiorkor (McFarlane *et al.*, 1970). In all these conditions there is an increased incidence of infection. The possibility that iron may be made more readily available to some pathogens by an increase in the degree of saturation of transferrin, such as occurs in leukaemia (Hunter *et al.*, 1983), should be considered. More knowledge is also required about the ability of pathogenic bacteria to utilize iron in haptoglobin–haemoglobin, haemopexin–haem or albumin–haem (methaemalbumin) complexes.

In the clinical field much advantage could be gained by assessing the levels of free haemoglobin, haem and iron in tissue fluids and finding out if the levels of haptoglobin, haemopexin and transferrin are sufficient for binding the appropriate iron compound. The presence or absence of methaemalbumin would also be important (see Chapter 7). In many cases there is a good case for carrying out bactericidal and bacteriostatic tests on patients' plasma. Controls should be plasma from normal individuals and the tests should be carried out for relatively long periods under controlled conditions of temperature and pH. It is essential to titrate the bacteria since the size of the inoculum can greatly influence the result. Tests with phagocytic cells are also useful and may eventually be considered essential (Ward, Hammond and Bullen, 1986).

In addition to the alterations which take place during various clinical disorders, trauma of several kinds may lead to the release of haem, the saturation of transferrin with iron, the lowering of transferrin levels or to an increase in the metabolites which could mobilize iron from transferrin, such as citrate. The best-known example is strangulated obstruction of the intestine (see Chapter 7) where a mixture of blood and intestinal contents provide an ideal medium for the growth of intestinal bacteria like *E.coli*. Experimental work with *E.coli* suggests that the concentration of haemoglobin released probably exceeds the binding capacity of the haptoglobin, but no measurements of this have been made in natural cases, or of the level and saturation of any locally derived transferrin or lactoferrin. In severe injury, such as that caused by extensive burns, the loss of red cells may be as high as 25 per cent (Davies, 1982). This could supply a large amount of iron but little is known about its availability to potential pathogens.

Perhaps the biggest gap in our knowledge is the effect of physical conditions on the availability of iron in clinical disease. The role of *Eh* in gas gangrene has been discussed in Chapter 7 and there is already evidence in the clinical literature that the level of oxygen tension can affect the likelihood of infection in tissues. Border, La Duca and Seibel (1978) point out that a fall in arterial oxygen tension predisposes to infection from contaminated wounds and they consider that increasing tissue O_2 tension is important in aiding resistance. The reasons for this are not entirely clear but could involve the availability of iron. That a fall in *Eh* and pH enhance infection should come as no surprise since at an *Eh* lower than -140mV (pH 7.5) the Fe^{3+} on transferrin is reduced to Fe^{2+} and is no longer bound by the protein. This abolishes the bacteriostatic effect of sera on certain organisms. Similar effects result from a fall in pH. There seems, therefore, to be a good case for more observations in patients on the consequences of altered physical conditions caused by trauma. However, any results should be combined with studies *in vitro* and in experimental infections since it is likely that the interrelationship between phagocytic cells, plasma, the pH, *Eh* and the level of available iron are complex.

4. IRON RESTRICTION AND THE SENSITIVITY OF BACTERIA TO ANTIMICROBIAL AGENTS

The changes in the metabolism of bacterial pathogens, and especially in the composition of their envelope, which occur as organisms adapt to and multiply *in vivo* have been discussed in this book in terms of enhancing a pathogen's ability to surivive and proliferate. Our increasing knowledge of the remarkable plasticity of the bacterial cell envelope may, however, also have important implications regarding the sensitivity of pathogens to antimicrobial agents used in therapy. Clinical isolates are typically subcultured *in vitro* several times before being tested for sensitivity and as a result may no longer have the same properties as the bacteria grown *in vivo*. The predictive value of *in vitro* tests in antibiotic research are therefore now being questioned (Mattie, 1984; Brown and Williams, 1985a), although the implications of this new knowledge are uncertain. However, in the case of both mucoid and non-mucoid strains of *Ps aeruginosa*, it is known that growth rate and iron limitation profoundly affect the production of penicillin-binding proteins, and alter the sensitivity of the organisms to the action of β-lactam antibiotics (Turnowsky *et al.*, 1983; Brown and Williams, 1985b). These antibiotics kill bacteria by binding to one or more penicillin-binding proteins located in the cytoplasmic membrane and inhibit their function in peptidoglycan synthesis (Spratt, 1977). Alterations in major membrane proteins, which appear to be involved in cephalosporin permeation, also affect the susceptibility of bacteria to β-lactam antibiotics (Sawai *et al.*, 1982; Kaneko, Yamaguchi and Sawai, 1984; Werner *et al.*, 1985). Brown and Williams (1985a) conclude that *in vitro* systems designed to predict the performance of antimicrobial agents *in vivo* should include iron-depleted test organisms. They also make the point that the effects of other host factors on bacteria, such as temperature, osmolarity and other nutrient limitations, all of which may vary from site to site in the body, should not be overlooked. Growth conditions also affect the production of penicillin-binding proteins of the Gram-positive bacterium *Staphylococcus aureus* (Reynolds and Brown, 1985).

In addition to the possible effects of iron limitation on the susceptibility of bacterial pathogens to antimicrobial agents, subinhibitory concentrations of antibiotics may themselves alter the surface properties of the bacterial cell, as well as affecting bacterial iron metabolism. Recently, Kadurugamuwa *et al.* (1985a, 1985b,) found that subinhibitory concentrations of several cephalosporins led to a reduction in enterobactin production by *Klebsiella pneumoniae* growing under iron-depleted conditions and also to a reduction in capsule formation, regardless of the availability of iron. The reduction in capsule formation resulted in the exposure on the bacterial cell surface of a number of outer membrane proteins, including the iron-regulated membrane proteins (Kadurugamuwa *et al.*, 1985b). Whether these effects have any bearing on the ability of organisms exposed to subinhibitory levels of cephalosporins to survive *in vivo* remains to be seen. In the presence of the subinhibitory concentrations of cephalosporin the iron-regulated proteins did, however, become readily accessible to antibodies, and antibodies reacting with the iron-regulated proteins of *E.coli* are already known to exist in the serum of human adults and in animals (Griffiths *et al.*, 1985; Kadurugamuwa *et al.*, 1985b). It is also known that subinhibitory concentrations of certain antibiotics can alter the morphology and virulence of bacterial species (Lorian, 1980; Shibil, 1983; Lorian and Atkinson, 1984; Dahlhoff and Stubner, 1985). Since antibiotics may not always achieve minimum inhibitory concentrational levels in tissues, the specific effects of subinhibitory concentrations might explain their clinical efficacy.

5. NEW THERAPEUTIC AND PREVENTIVE MEASURES

5.1 Antimicrobial agents

The better understanding of the environment encountered by bacterial pathogens in host tissues and of the ways they adapt to such conditions are leading not only to a radically different view of the behaviour of pathogens *in vivo* but also to ideas concerning the development of new antibacterial agents.

One interesting idea concerns the production of antibacterials based on siderophores. Since the siderophore enterobactin is produced by a number of enterobacterial pathogens during iron restriction (see Chapter 3), and indeed has been shown to be produced by pathogenic *E.coli* during growth *in vivo* in infection (Griffiths and Humphreys, 1980), it was reasoned that it might be possible to use complexes of enterobactin with ions other than Fe^{3+} as antimetabolites to Fe^{3+}– enterobactin (Rogers, Synge and Woods, 1980). Enterobactin forms complexes with a number of group III and transitional metal ions, but only the complexes of scandium (Sc^{3+}) and indium (In^{3+}) have shown any significant antibacterial activity. Rogers, Synge and Woods (1980) showed that the Sc^{3+} and In^{3+} complexes of enterobactin each exerted a bacteriostatic effect on *Klebsiella pneumoniae* in serum as well as on a number of pathogenic strains of *E.coli* including those carrying a $ColV^{+}$ plasmid known to produce aerobactin in addition to enterobactin (Rogers, Woods and Synge, 1982); the inhibition occurred only in an iron-restricted environment. The Sc^{3+}–enterobactin complex also exerted a significant therapeutic effect on *K.pneumoniae* and on *E.coli* infections *in vivo* in mice. However, the mechanism by which Sc^{3+}–enterobactin exerts its antibacterial effect is not known (Plaha and Rogers, 1983). Experiments have shown that the Sc^{3+}–enterobactin complex enters the bacterial cell where it is then probably degraded. Whether Sc^{3+} then exerts a general toxic effect of its own or whether the Sc^{3+}–enterobactin complex interferes specifically with the transport of Fe^{3+}–enterobactin is not clear. The fact that the complex inhibits an aerobactin-producing strain of *E.coli* suggests that, in this case at least, Sc^{3+} interfered with cellular functions in addition to those involved with the transport of Fe^{3+}–enterobactin; if Sc^{3+}–enterobactin interfered only with the enterobactin-mediated iron uptake then these bacteria should still have been able to acquire iron via the aerobactin system and multiplied.

Although it is too early to say how successful these or similar compounds might be for therapeutic purposes in man, an investigation of the mechanisms involved in their antibacterial action might suggest further possibilities for the synthesis of new compounds. One of the problems with the Sc^{3+}–enterobactin complex is the general toxicity of Sc^{3+}, and the development of antibacterials based on this metal could be difficult. Furthermore, there are also problems with antibacterials based on enterobactin because of the instability of the molecule itself (see Chapter 3). If such antibacterial compounds have a future then they are likely to be based on more stable enterobactin analogues or other siderophores. Several analogues of enterobactin have already been synthesized chemically (Harris, Weitl and Raymond, 1979, Venuti, Rastetter and Neilands, 1979; Weitl and Raymond, 1979, 1981; Harris, Raymond and Weitl, 1981; Pecoraro, Weitl and Raymond, 1981). Unlike enterobactin these compounds have stable central rings which lack the labile ester linkages, and they have been analysed in some detail with a view to making potential antimicrobial agents and for use in treating iron-overload diseases (see Section 4.4) (Heidinger *et al.*, 1983) (Fig. 1). The possibility of attaching a toxic ligand to such compounds, which then convey it into the bacterial cell via the high affinity, and highly specific, iron-uptake system, is an alternative option to the use of toxic metals. Indeed, two exisiting antibiotics, albomycin and ferrimycin, seem to function in this way. These sideromycins are homologues of ferrichrome and ferrioxamine B respectively (Benz *et al.*, 1982; Muller, Matzonke and Raymond, 1984). Albomycin is taken up by *E.coli* via the ferrichrome-transport system (Hantke and Braun, 1978). Theoretically, the bacterial outer membrane protein receptors should be able to take up the siderophore analogues at very low concentrations *in vivo*.

5.2 Vaccines

Since surface components play such an important part in host-bacteria interactions, the alterations induced in the bacterial cell envelope by iron-binding proteins are clearly of interest, especially now it has been shown that the iron-regulated outer membrane proteins are actually expressed by bacterial pathogens *in vivo* during infection (see Chapters 3 and 4). Some of the iron-regulated outer membrane proteins are exposed on the surface of pathogenic strains of *E.coli* and can interact *in situ* with large protein molecules in solution (Griffiths, Stevenson and Joyce, 1983; Griffiths *et al.*, 1985; Chart and Griffiths, unpublished data). Naturally occurring antibodies which react with the iron-regulated outer membrane proteins have been detected in the sera of human adults and of animals (Griffiths *et al.*, 1985). Of course, it is very likely that the iron-regulated proteins of different bacteria and bacterial strains will vary in their accessibility to proteins in solution; the fact that a protein is accessible in one strain does not necessarily mean that it will be so in another. The capsular polysaccharide, which is produced by some pathogens, certainly masks the iron-regulated proteins in at least one case, that of *K.pneumoniae* (Kadurugamuwa *et al.*, 1985b). However, the possibility that the receptors for ferric siderophores, or indeed any other iron-regulated determinants, are important protective antigens is worth exploring. Such antigens would, of course, only appear during growth and multiplication of the bacteria *in vivo* or *in vitro* in iron-restricted media. Whole cell vaccines made from iron-replete organisms would lack these proteins and might therefore have an imcomplete set of antigenic determinants. Iron-deficient media have been used for many years for growing *Corynebacterium diphtheriae* for the preparation of toxoid vaccines; such a medium is essential to allow expression of the iron-regulated tox genes (see Chapter 4).

The manner in which antibodies reacting with the iron-regulated outer membrane proteins might confer protection is not clear. Antibodies which react with the ferric siderophore receptor proteins have, so far, not been found to interfere with the uptake of iron nor with bacterial multipliction (Coulton,

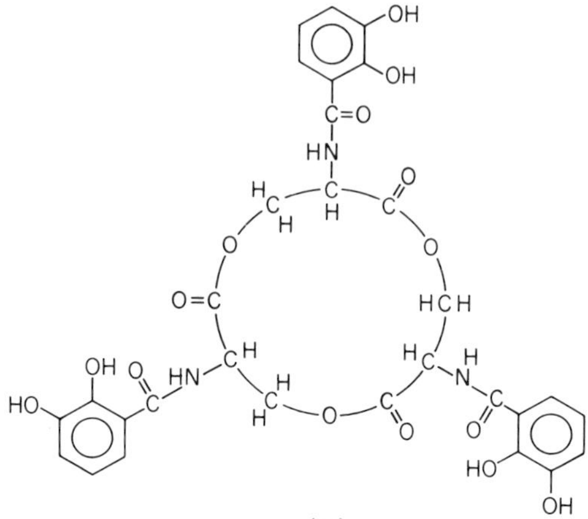

(a)

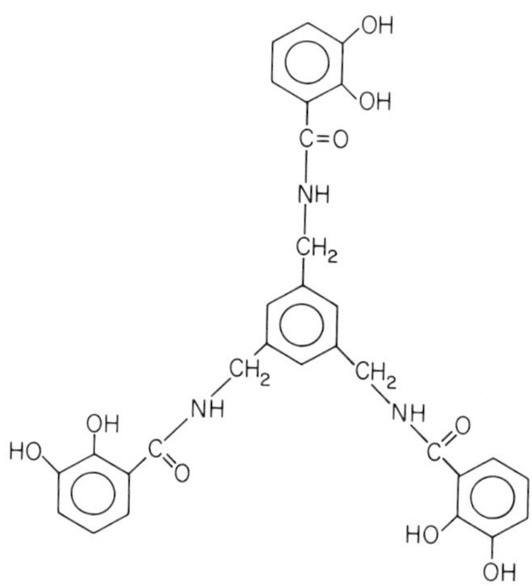

(b)

1982; Dimoudis, Komischke and Braun, 1984; Chart and Griffiths, unpublished data); some of these antibodies did, however, block the adsorption of certain phages to the receptor proteins, an observation which has been taken to indicate that the phages and antibodies in question bind to a region of the receptor protein distinct from the adsorption site of the ferric siderophore. The possibility that the affinity of the ferric siderophore for the receptor might be much larger than that of the antibodies, so that the latter cannot compete efficiently, must also be considered. Also, some of these results have been obtained with monoclonal antibodies, which are clearly highly specific for certain epitopes, and more work is needed before one can conclude that anti-siderophore receptor antibodies in general do not interfere with siderophore-mediated iron uptake. In addition, serum antibodies reacting with

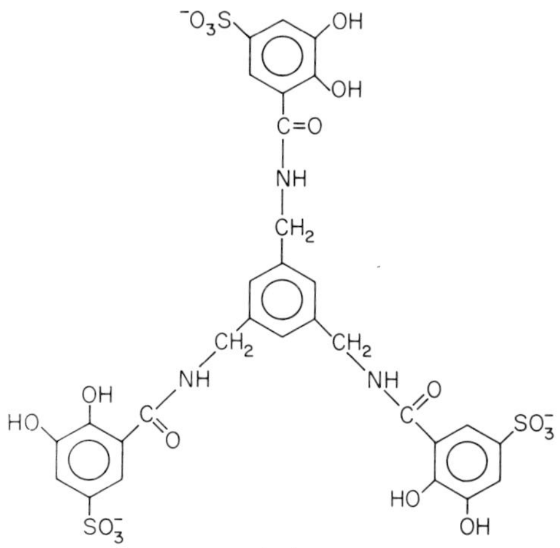

(c)

Figure 1 The structure of the siderophore enterobactin and of two synthetic enterobactin analogues: (a) enterobactin: (b) 1,3,5-*NN'N''*-tris-(2,3-dihydroxybenzoyl)-triaminomethylbenzene (MECAM) : (c) 5-sulphonated derivative of MECAM. From Heidinger *et al.* (1983)

the iron-regulated outer membrane proteins may be essential for the bactericidal effect of plasma or in phagocytosis. They could protect the host against bacterial invasion even if they do not block iron uptake and inhibit multiplication directly.

An interesting approach to the development of new vaccines has been made by Hoiseth and Stocker (1981). They made use of the fact that the siderophore enterobactin appeared to be essential for the virulence of *Salmonella typhimurium*. Yancey, Breeding and Lankford (1979) had shown that the loss by mutation of the ability to synthesize enterobactin reduced the virulence of *S.typhimurium* for mice and inhibited the ability of the organism to grow in human serum. In *Salmonella*, as well as in *E.coli*, enterobactin is synthesized from chorismate, the final product of the common aromatic (aro) biosynthetic pathway (Fig. 2). Using the tetracycline resistance transposon Tn10 inserted into the *aro*A gene, Hoiseth and Stocker (1981) produced non-reverting aromatic-requiring avirulent derivatives of virulent *S.typhimurim*. This block in the aromatic pathway made the organism auxotrophic for two compounds that are not available in mammalian tissues, enterobactin and *p*-aminobenzoic acid; enterobactin is needed by the organism for the uptake of iron in an iron-restricted environment and *p*-aminobenzoic acid is a precursor of folic acid, which is essential for C1 metabolism. Presumably, a lesion in the *p*-aminobenzoic acid pathway alone would also reduce considerably the virulence of *Salmonella*. However, the elimination of both metabolites, enterobactin and *p*-aminobenzoic acid, by the deletion of *aro*A, would seem to be

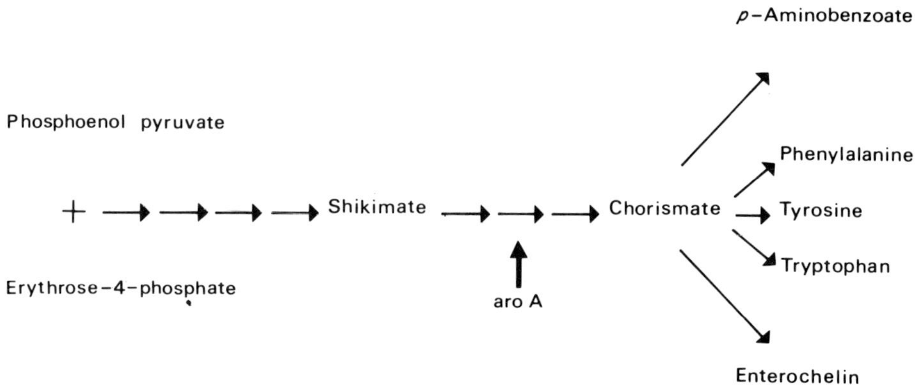

Figure 2 Relationship of the common aromatic amino acid biosynthetic pathway to the synthesis of enterobactin and to *p*-amino-benzoic acid. *From Griffiths (1985). Reproduced by permission of the Society for General Microbiology*

more satisfactory and such *Salmonella* derivatives have been found to be effective as live vaccines in mice and also in calves (Hoiseth and Stocker, 1981; Robertsson *et al.*, 1983; Smith *et al.*, 1984a). Very recently, the results of experiments carried out by Benjamin *et al.* (1985) suggest that enterobactin is not, after all, required for the virulence of *S.typhimurium* in mice. This is thought to be due to the fact that *Salmonella* is an intracellular pathogen and may not need siderophores for growth in this location (See Chapter 3). Although the results of Benjamin *et al.* (1985) imply that the avirulence of the *aro*A$^-$ strains of *Salmonella* for mice may be due solely to their inability to produce *p*-aminobenzoic acid, more work is needed to define precisely the nature of the lesion or lesions leading to the loss of virulence in general. Furthermore, the mechanism whereby such strains confer immunity needs to be better characterized, although work to date does suggest that cellular immunity plays an important role (Killar and Eisenstein, 1985).

It appears that in many cases live vaccines offer considerable advantages over killed vaccines since they are capable of eliciting effective and long-lasting immunity. There is, therefore, much interest in the possible use of live attenuated organisms, such as *aro*A strains, not only as vaccines themselves, but also as carriers for cloned antigens from a variety of other pathogens, bacterial, viral and protozoal. However, a major consideration with any live vaccine is safety and this depends on its inability to revert to a virulent form. Detailed genetic analysis of non-reverting *aro*A strains is therefore being carried out in order to understand the nature of any mutations which have occurred in addition to the inactivation of the *aro*A gene and which lead to the inability of the strains to revert (Hoiseth and Stocker, 1985). Armed with such knowledge steps can be taken to improve the genetic stability of such strains. So far only *aro*A derivatives of *Salmonella typhimurium* and *S.dublin* have been made and used as vaccines, although similar genetically constructed vaccine strains with lesions in the aromatic pathway are being constructed in other organisms, such as *Salmonella typhi* (Hoiseth and Stocker, 1985).

5.3 Treatment of iron overload

Coincidental with investigations into the role of siderophores and membrane protein receptors in microbial iron metabolism has been the development of drugs for use in iron-chelation therapy. These are used to treat patients with primary and secondary iron overload (Hoffbrand, 1980). So far, naturally occurring siderophores derived from various microorganisms, or closely related synthetic analogues of these siderophores, have proved to be the most useful. Currently, desferrioxamine B is the drug of choice and its administration leads to the elimination of the chelated iron via the urine. Desferrioxamine B is produced by *Streptomyces pilosus* (Muller and Raymond, 1984) and is available commercially as the methane sulphonate salt, 'Desferal', from Ciba-Geigy, Basel. Although it is generally well tolerated in humans it is, unfortunately, not absorbed from the gastrointestinal tract and it must therefore be given parenterally, either by injection or infusion. Furthermore, it is not particularly efficient and does not easily remove iron from transferrin. There is evidence that ascorbic acid increases the effectiveness of Desferal as an iron chelator, possibly by increasing the mobilization of iron (Propper *et al.*, 1977; Hoffbrand, 1980), and so the chelator is sometimes used in conjunction with low doses of vitamin C.

Experiments *in vitro* have shown that desferrioxamine inhibits the growth of a number of bacteria by depriving them of iron (Calver, Kenny and Kushner, 1979; Finkelstein and Yancey, 1981; van Asbeck *et al.*, 1983a, 1983b). Desferrioxamine has also been used as an iron chelator for inducing the expression of iron-regulated outer membrane proteins in *E.coli* (Chart *et al.*, 1986). It might be expected, therefore, that in individuals suffering form iron overload, where the excess iron increases susceptibility to infection (see Chapters 5 and 7), the use of desferrioxamine to chelate iron would lead to a decrease in the susceptibility of the host to infection by lowering the concentration of iron available to invading pathogens. Calver, Kenny and Kushner (1979) have suggested that Desferal may have a chemotherapeutic role in severe neisserial disease, even in individuals with a normal iron load.

However, there is evidence that infection with certain other organisms may be aggravated by Desferal. It has been shown that desferrioxamine can, in fact, increase the virulence of *S.typhimurium* in mice (Jones *et al.*, 1977) and promote the growth of *Staphylococcus aureus* and *Yersinia enterocolitica in vitro* (Perry and Brubaker, 1979; Brock and Ng, 1983). Exogenously supplied desferrioxamine can also enhance infections caused by *Klebsiella* (Khimji and Miles, 1978). Furthermore, Melby *et al.* (1982) have reported two cases of septicaemia due to *Y.enterocolitica* in infants treated with Desferal to relieve acute iron overload caused by accidental overdoses of iron tablets; these authors proposed that the iron chelator used in treatment contributed to the development of systemic yersiniosis. The effect of desferrioxamine on *Y.enterocolitica* has been investigated in detail by Brock and Ng (1983) and more recently by Robins-Browne and Prpic (1985). Their work shows that *Y.enterocolitica* lacks a high affinity iron-chelating system of its own but that it is able to utilize siderophores produced by other organisms, including desferrioxamine; Desferal therefore enhances the growth of the pathogen *in vivo*. It is interesting to note that although *Y.enterocolitica* is an important cause of enteritis and mesenteric adenitis (Battone, 1977; Perry and Brubaker, 1979), systemic involvement is unusual and when it does occur it is usually in individuals with underlying disease, commonly cirrhosis or iron overload (Rabson, Hallett and Koornhof, 1975; Butzler *et al.*, 1978; Bouza *et al.*, 1980). The close relationship between systemic yersiniosis and haemosiderosis is believed to reflect the ease with which the organism might acquire iron in such instances and the difficulty it has in obtaining iron from normal tissues (Robins-Browne and Prpic, 1985). It is not known how the bacterium obtains sufficient iron for growth during enteric infections.

Vibrio vulnificus is an organism which can make use of the freely available iron found in patients suffering from iron-overload disease, such as haemochromatosis, and can, in such cases, produce septicaemias (see Section 5.4 below). This organism, too, can make use of iron bound to desferrioxamine (Wright, Simpson and Oliver, 1981). Thus, although iron-chelating agents are available and can be used for binding 'free' iron in the serum of patients with haemochromatosis and for chelating and eliminating iron in other iron-overload conditions, caution must be taken in the choice of chelator to be used. Currently, only Desferal is in widespread clinical use, but there is considerable incentive for designing new therapeutically useful iron chelators, especially ones which can be administered orally (Heidinger *et al.*, 1983; Kontoghiorghes and Evans, 1985). Ideally, a chelator for treating iron-overload diseases should be designed not only to chelate iron effectively, to be capable both thermodynamically and kinetically of removing iron from host iron-binding proteins and to be removed readily from the host by excretion in urine, but also to be incapable of donating iron to potential pathogens.

Heidinger *et al.* (1983) have investigated a number of stable synthetic analogues of enterobactin in which certain sites on the molecule have been modified. In this way features of the molecule critical to the iron-uptake process in *E.coli* have been identified. They found that the tricatechol–iron portion of the molecule is specifically recognized by the FepA protein, the outer membrane receptor protein for ferric–enterobactin. Also, the analogue ferric–MECAM (Fig. 1b), but not the derivative of ferric–MECAM sulphonated at the 5 position of the benzene ring (Fig. 1c), can promote the growth in iron-limited medium of *E.coli* strains which are unable to synthesize their own enterobactin owing to a mutation in the *aro*B gene. Thus, sulphonated derivatives of enterobactin analogues which do not support the growth of *E.coli* are worth considering as candidate chelators for treating iron-overload syndromes. However, their ability to act as microbial siderophores should be checked with several potential bacterial pathogens, not simply with *E.coli*.

5.4 Antibacterial use of apotransferrin and haptoglobin

It has already been mentioned that systemic infections caused by *Y.enterocolitica* are unusual and that when they do occur it is in individuals suffering from underlying iron-overload diseases of one kind or another. Similarly, *V.vulnificus* usually causes only localized infections in humans but may give rise to lethal septicaemias in patients with idiopathic haemochromatosis or other disorders which result in elevated serum iron levels. In the case of haemochromatosis, it has been shown that it is the presence of low molecular weight, loosely bound iron complexes in the serum that is responsible for promoting *V.vulnificus* multiplication (Chart and Griffiths, 1985; Gutteridge *et al.*, 1985). Although iron-chelating agents are available which could be used to chelate the 'free' iron pool, care must be taken in selecting a chelator for therapeutic use. As discussed in Section 5.3, Desferal can actually be utilized both by *V.vulnificus* and by *Y.enterocolitica* as a vehicle for obtaining iron and clearly should not be used. Since *V.vulnificus* causes fulminating septicaemias that can lead to the death of the patient in a very short time, and since these infections are extremely difficult to control, it may be possible to exploit the ability of apotransferrin to bind excess iron as a means of treatment. *In vitro* experiments (Chart, Gutteridge and Griffiths, unpublished data) have suggested that the administration of apotransferrin, or normal human serum or plasma, which also have considerable unsaturated iron-binding capacity, may be useful as a form of immediate therapy for patients with iron-overload conditions and suspected of being infected with *V.vulnificus*. It must be pointed out, however, that although intravenous administration of transferrin has already been used in the treatment of atransferrinaemia (Goya *et al.*, 1972) its use clinically as a therapeutic measure in *V.vulnificus* septicaemia has not yet been tried.

The possible therapeutic use of haptoglobin, the naturally occurring haemoglobin-binding protein in serum, in treating potentially fatal haemoglobulin-induced bacterial infections (see Chapter 3) has also been proposed (Eaton *et al.*, 1982). Indeed, it has already been shown that the administration of haptoglobin protects against experimental *E.coli* infections promoted by haemoglobin in rats (Eaton *et al.*, 1982). From such experimental work it appears that haptoglobin not only accelerates the clearance of free haemoglobin but also blocks its utilization as a source of iron by *E.coli*. In man it is known that the haptoglobin–haemoglobin complex is rapidly cleared by the reticuloendothelial system and the administration of haptoglobin has been shown to have useful prophylactic and therapeutic effects on renal injury secondary to haemolysis (Ohshiro, Kosaki and Funakoshi, 1978; Ohshiro and Kosaki, 1978; Yoshioka *et al.*, 1985). Usually, intravascular haemolysis releases free haemoglobin into the plasma where it combines with free haptoglobin to form a tight complex which is carried to the liver where it is metabolized (Keene and Jandl, 1965). However, massive haemolysis, e.g. following a severe burn injury, results in the release of a great quantity of free haemoglobin which may overwhelm the binding capacity of the haptoglobin and result in the presence of free haemoglobin in plasma. This excess free haemoglobin passes through the glomerulus of the kidney where it causes degenerative necrosis of tubular cells, occlusion of renal tubes with haemoglobin casts and eventual renal failure (Goldberg, 1962). From the point of view of infection, Eaton *et al.*, (1982) consider that the administration of haptoglobin would have two beneficial effects; first, it would reduce the level of free haemoglobin and, second, the haemoglobin in the haptoglobin–haemoglobin complex formed would be unavailable for supplying iron directly to pathogenic bacteria. However, although this may apply in the case of *E.coli*, it seems not to apply in all cases. For example, *V.vulnificus* can use the haemoglobin in the haemoglobin–haptoglobin complex as a source of iron (Helms, Oliver and Travis, 1984).

6. IRON AND VIRULENCE OF FUNGAL AND PROTOZOAL PATHOGENS

Most of the work discussed in this book has been concerned with the role of iron in bacterial infections, especially in those caused by Gram-negative bacteria. This is because it is these particular infections which have been investigated in the greatest detail to date. However, non-bacterial pathogens in host tissues are faced with exactly the same iron-restricted environment as bacteria, and iron is an essential nutrient for these organisms too. Unfortunately, very much less is known about the ability of non-bacterial pathogens to sequester iron *in vivo*, and little is known about the effects that an iron-restricted environment may have on their structure and behaviour.

It has been known for a long time that the growth of several fungi, including *Candida albicans*, is inhibited *in vitro*, in the presence of iron-binding proteins or serum and that this inhibition can be abolished by adding iron (Caroline *et al.*, 1964; Esterly, Brammar and Crounse, 1967; Kirkpatrick *et al.*, 1971; Elin and Wolff, 1973). Elin and Wolff (1974) showed that the injection of *E.coli* endotoxin into mice resulted in a fall in the percentage saturation of the serum transferrin and that this was accompanied by an increased resistance to infection with *C.albicans*; this effect was overcome by injecting ferric ammonium sulphate. Abe *et al.* (1985) have shown that excess iron promotes the proliferation of *Candida* infection in mice and there is a suggestion that systemic candidiasis in patients with acute leukaemia might be related to the increased saturation of their serum transferrin with iron (Caroline, Rosner and Kozinn, 1969) (See Chapter 7). However, the mechanism whereby *C.albicans* normally acquires iron when growing in its human host is not known. Of course, it is well known that fungi in general do produce siderophores (Lankford, 1973; Neilands, 1981a, 1981b), but studies on the production of siderophores by pathogenic yeasts and fungi are limited. Investigations have shown that a number of opportunistic fungi, including *C.albicans*, can secrete siderophores of the hydroxamate type (Holzberg and Artis, 1983; Ismail, Bedell and Lupan, 1985), and it is thought that certain isolates may also produce a phenolate-type chelator (Ismail, Bedell and Lupan, 1985). The chemical structures of the *Candida* chelators are unknown, as is their role, if any, *in vivo* during infection. Similarly, there is no information concerning the effect of iron restriction on the properties of *C.albicans*. Whether or not changes occur in the envelope of *Candida* as a result of iron restriction is, similarly, not known.

It is, of course, known that the organism can exist in one of two forms, a yeast form and a filamentous fungal form (Epstein, Truelove and Izutzu, 1984). However, the significance of the yeast as compared with the filamentous form for pathogenicity is not clear (Kimura and Pearsall, 1980). There is some evidence that the yeast form of *Candida* may be the pathogenic form, but with clinical infection the altered microenvironment favours a change to the filamentous form (Epstein, Truelove and Izutzu, 1984). Whether iron restriction plays a part in such transformations remains to be seen. With the increasing importance of *Candida* and other fungi as opportunistic human pathogens, more work is clearly needed in order to gain a better understanding of the mechanisms involved with the pathogenicity of this organism with a view to improving therapy or instituting preventive measures.

As in the case of the pathogenic fungi, little is known about the way that protozoan parasites obtain iron *in vivo*, although there is now a growing interest in the role of iron in diseases caused by organisms such as *Plasmodium falciparum* and *Trypanosoma cruzi*. It would seem reasonable to expect the intraerythrocytic malaria parasite, *P.falciparum*, to use the iron in haemoglobin. The local availability of a large excess of iron would seem therefore to obviate any influence of iron deficiency or excess on the progress of the disease. Nevertheless, treatment of iron deficiency in Somali nomads caused recrudescent malaria in 13 out of 71 individuals at risk, as compared to 1 in 66 at risk in a placebo group (Murray *et al.*, 1978). Also, Masawe, Muindi and Swai (1974) found that in patients with iron deficiency, malaria flared up regularly following treatment with iron. Such observations led Nurse (1979) to suggest that malaria may be inhibited by iron deficiency (See also Chapter 7). The demonstration that desferrioxamine completely inhibited the growth of

P.falciparum, despite the approximately 1,000-fold excess or iron available to the organism in the form of haemogloblin, suggested that the aquisition of iron by the intraerythrocytic parasite might not be simply from degraded haem. It has been known for many years that in parasitized red cells the haemoglobin continues to be degraded but that the haem concentration remains unchanged (Ball *et al.*, 1948). Also, the malaria pigment, the material generated by the parasite during degradation of haemoglobin (Theakston, Fletcher and Malgraith, 1970) does not stain with Prussian blue (Morselt, Glastra and James, 1973), suggesting that the haem in that pigment has not been catabolized with the release of iron. Together, these results suggested that the parasite's iron supply comes not from haemoglobin but from elsewhere. In 1984, Pollack and Fleming suggested that red cells infected with *P.falciparum* take iron from transferrin and proposed that transferrin is the source of iron for this intracellular parasite. Though mature red cells have no transferrin receptors (Enns *et al.*, 1981), it is apparent that the parasite can insert its own protein into the red cell membrane (Howard, Barnwell and Kao, 1983) and it was possible that a transferrin receptor could be among these. However, more recent data (Peto and Thompson, 1986) is in conflict with this view and it is still not clear how the parasite obtains iron. It is very likely that more will become known about this fascinating problem in the near future, not merely bacause of its intrinsic biological interest but also because it may suggest new approaches to therapy or even preventive measures. The continual emergence of drug-resistant malaria throughout the world makes the availability of new control procedures a practical concern of some importance (Hurwitz, Johnson and Campbell, 1981).

The role of iron in the pathogenesis of *Trypanosoma cruzi* is also now under active investigation. *T.cruzi*, a haemoflagellate protozoan, causes Chagas' disease, which is a common debilitating disease in Latin America (Brener, 1973). Unlike the African trypanosomes, which cause trypanosomiasis in man and livestock, *T.cruzi* does not undergo the characteristic antigenic variations of the African strains (Donelson and Rice-Ficht, 1985) and it has an intracellular stage in the mammalian host. Infection of mice with *T.cruzi* provokes a hypoferraemic response in which the extracellular iron concentration in blood is reduced and the iron moved into the intracellular stores of the reticuloendothelial system (Lalonde and Holbein, 1984). During the course of experimental Chagas' disease, *T.cruzi* becomes lodged within mononuclear phagocytic cells (Brener, 1973) and it might be expected that they would not then be exposed to the decreasing supply of iron in the bloodstream. However, Loo and Lalonde (1984) believe that there is a possibility that such a hypoferraemic response may itself sustain an intracellular infection by transferring iron from the serum into the intracellular sites where *T.cruzi* replicates. A decrease in host iron stores certainly reduces the pathogenicity of *T.cruzi* for mice and it seems that it is the amount of intracellular iron that is responsible for this (Lalonde and Holbein, 1984); Loo and Lalonde (1984) have shown that the amount of iron within cultured cells affects the ability of *T.cruzi* to replicate within them. It is suggested that interventions which successfully decrease the iron content of macrophages or block the hypoferraemic response may favourably alter the course of infection with *T.cruzi*. As yet there is no information on the availability of the iron within macrophages nor on the mechanism whereby *T.cruzi* acquires iron intracellularly. There is no information either on how the African trypanosomes acquire iron for replication in the bloodstream.

A start at understanding the role of iron and iron-binding proteins in the host–parasite relationship of another protozoan pathogen, *Trichomonas vaginalis*, has, however, been made. *T. vaginalis* is perhaps the most frequently acquired human protazoan infestation and it is responsible for trichomonal vaginitis (Honigberg, 1978; Ackers, 1982). Trichomoniasis has now emerged as a major sexually transmitted disease, although the determinants of pathogenicity have not yet been clearly identified. Recent studies have shown that *T.vaginalis* may acquire iron in the infected host through a direct receptor-mediated process, much in the same way as do the *Neisseria* species (see Chapter 3). *T. vaginalis* possesses specific cell surfact receptors for human lactoferrin, and the binding of iron-loaded lactoferrin results in the intracellular accumulation of iron (Peterson and Alderete, 1984a, 1984b). It is not yet clear whether iron is removed from the lactoferrin at the parasite cell surface or whether lactoferrin is internalized before the iron is released; the release of lactoferrin after binding to the trichomonas receptors suggests that the former sequence of events is taking place, allowing for a turnover of exogenous lactoferrin. The specificity of the receptors for lactoferrin is particularly interesting. Transferrin does not bind to *T.vaginalis* with high affinity and fails to compete with labelled lactoferrin in binding to intact trichomonads. The ability of *T.vaginalis* to bind lactoferrin and to use this as a source of iron more effectively than serum transferrin may be a significant factor in the non-invasive nature of this pathogen. A similar specificity in the binding of these two iron-binding proteins has also been found in the case of *Neisseria gonorrhoeae* and *N.meningitidis* (see Chapter 3).

7. UPTAKE OF IRON BY MALIGNANT AND OTHER RAPIDLY PROLIFERATING CELLS

In addition to the growing interest in the way that parasites obtain iron *in vivo*, there is also now considerable interest in the mechanism whereby rapidly dividing cells, especially malignant cells, obtain sufficient iron to support their multiplication. Indeed, it is only recently that the critical role of iron in the growth of such cells has been generally appreciated (Trowbridge and Omary, 1981; Brock and Maniou-Fowler, 1983; Bowern *et al.*, 1984; Taetle *et al.*, 1985). As has been discussed elsewhere in this book, the delivery of iron to vertebrate cells is mediated by transferrin via specific cell surface receptors that reside on the cell surface, and there is now a considerable amount of information available about the structure and biosynthesis of these receptors (Testa, 1985). Initially, work on transferrin receptors focused on the maturing cells of the erythroid line, which have a high iron requirement for haem synthesis, and on the placental trophoblast, but in the last few years evidence has accumulated to show that many other cell types express this receptor. In particular, it has been shown that expression of the transferrin receptor on the cell surface correlates with the state of cell activation. Cells proliferating *in vitro* or *in vivo* express large quantities of the receptor, whereas most non-dividing cells express low or undetectable quantities (Sutherland *et al.*, 1981; Trowbridge and Omary, 1981; Newman *et al.*, 1982; Testa, 1985). For example, resting T and B lymphocytes do not produce the transferrin receptor but rapdily express this protein at high levels on their cell surfaces following activation by mitogens (Neckers and Cossman, 1983; Neckers, Jenokida and James, 1984). These findings explain why transferrin is usually a necessary additive for the growth of both normal and malignant cells in serum-free culture media (Barnes and Sato, 1980); it seems that normally cells can acquire iron only from transferrin and cannot use other sources of iron. However, certain cell lines have adapted *in vitro* to use other iron sources and they can multiply without transferrin (Okabe, Fujisawa and Takaku, 1984; Taetle *et al.*, 1985).

Since receptor-mediated uptake of iron from transferrin provides for the efficient uptake of iron by activated cells, including malignant cells, it might be expected that intefering with this process would lead to the inhibition of cell multiplication, much in the same way that interfering with bacterial iron uptake leads to the inhibition of bacterial growth (see Section 5.2 of this chapter and Chapter 5). During the last few years monoclonal antibodies directed against human transferrin receptors have been produced in several laboratories (Testa, 1985). These antibodies can be classified into two categories, those that block receptor function and those that do not. Thus, some antitransferrin-receptor monoclonal antibodies, such as OKT9 (Reinherz *et al.*, 1980; Goding and Burns, 1981), do not interfere significantly with receptor function. In contrast, others like monoclonal antibody 42/6, directed against the human receptor, and R17 208, which reacts with the rat transferrin receptor, bind to the receptors and block the binding of transferrin. These antibodies prevent iron uptake and inhibit the growth of tumour cells *in vitro* (Trowbridge and Lopez, 1982; Taetle, Honeysett and Trowbridge, 1983; Taetle *et al.*, 1985) and *in vivo* (Trowbridge *et al.*, 1984). Soluble iron can overcome the inhibitory effects of the monoclonal antibodies in some cases but not in all (Testa, 1985), suggesting that different cell types have different capabilities to take up iron from iron salts, or possibly that different mechanisms may exist by which anti-transferrin receptor antibodies can inhibit cell growth.

Much work is currently going on in this field since there is, clearly, considerable interest in the use of such antibodies as antitumour agents, either on their own or in 'drug targeting'. In the latter approach, a toxin such as the ricin 'A' chain is conjugated to the monoclonal antibody which then selectively delivers it to the required cells where the receptor–transferrin–toxin complex is internalized (Trowbridge and Domingo 1981, 1982; Fitzgerald *et al.*, 1983; Rass and Basala, 1984). There is also interest in the use of gallium complexes of transferrin as therapeutic antitumour agents, much along the same lines as the use of Sc^{3+}–enterobactin to inhibit bacterial growth (see Section 5.1 of this chapter; Chitomber, Massey and Seligman, 1983). A possible problem with some of these agents might be the fact that transferrin receptors are also expressed by other tissue cells and injection of antibody, especially as a drug conjugate, may induce unexpected deleterious effects. The fact that sites rich in transferrin receptors have been found in the brain (Hill *et al.*, 1985) means that the use of drug-targeting agents based on anti-transferrin-receptor antibodies will have to be particularly carefully evaluated. Nevertheless, many exciting results may be expected from this area of work in the next few years, as well as from the studies currently being carried out on the role of transferrin and lactoferrin in regulating lymphocyte transformation and lymphoid cell traffic (Bagby *et al.*, 1981; De Sousa 1981; Birgens *et al.*, 1983; Brock, 1984; Brown, Rickard and Kronenberg, 1985; see also Chapter 6).

8. CONCLUDING REMARKS

The investigation of the pathogenesis of infectious diseases at a molecular level is just beginning and it is hoped that a clearer understanding of the molecular basis of pathogenicity will suggest improved methods for the diagnosis, treatment and prevention of infections. Nevertheless, careful attention to biological and clinical aspects remains essential to ensure that individual studies are relevant to the problem as a whole. Studies on the role of iron in infection have been successful because they have, in general, integrated *in vivo* and *in vitro* investigations. Without a doubt, current developments are rapidly increasing our understanding of the critical part played by iron in bacterial, fungal and protozoal diseases, as well as in the growth of tumours and other rapidly proliferating cells. Although much remains to be discovered, the translation of this new knowledge into practical ways of diagnosing, treating and preventing infections of different kinds, and in controlling malignancies, is now beginning and should be encouraged.

REFERENCES

Abe, F., Tateyma, M., Shibuya, H., Azumi, N., and Ommura, Y. (1985). Experimental candidiasis in iron overload. *Mycopathologia*, **89**, 59–63.
Ackers, J.P. (1982). Immunology of amebas, giardia and trichomonads. In *Immunology*

of Human Infection, Volume 9, Part II, *Viruses and Parasites: Immunodiagnosis and Prevention of Infectious Diseases* (Eds. A.J. Nahmias and R.J. O'Reilly), pp. 403–443. Plenum Publishing Corporation, New York.

Agüero, M.E., Aron, L., DeLuca, A.G., Timmis, K.N., and Cabella, F.C. (1984). A plasmid-encoded outer membrane protein, TraT, enhances resistance of *Escherichia coli* to phagocytosis. *Infection and Immunity*, **46**, 740–746.

Bagby, Jr., G.C., Vasiliki, D.R., Bennet, R.M., Vandenbark, A.A., Garewal, H.S.,, Wilkinson, B., and Davis, J. (1981). Interaction of lactoferrin, monocytes and T-lymphocyte subsets in the regulation of steady-state granulopoiesis *in vitro*. *Journal of Clinical Investigation*, **68**, 56–63.

Ball, E.G., McKee, R.W., Anfinsen, G.B., Cruz, W.O., and Geiman, Q.M. (1948). Studies on malarial parasites IX: Chemical and metabolic changes during growth and multiplication *in vivo* and *in vitro*. *Journal of Biological Chemistry*, **175**, 547–571.

Barksdale, L., Garmise, L., and Rivera, R. (1961). Toxinogeny in *Corynebacterium diphtheriae*. *Journal of Bacteriology*, **81**, 527–540.

Barnes, D., and Sato, G. (1980). Serum-free cell culture: a unifying approach. *Cell*, **22**, 649–655.

Battone, E.J. (1977). *Yersinia enterocolitica*: a panoramic view of a charismatic microorganism. *Critical Reviews in Microbiology*, **5**, 211–241.

Benjamin, Jr., W.H., Turnbough, Jr., C.L., Posey, B.S., and Briles, D.E. (1985). The ability of *Salmonella typhimurium* to produce the siderophore enterobactin is not a virulence factor in mouse typhoid. *Infection and Immunity*, **50**, 392–397.

Benz, G., Schröder, T., Kurz, J., Wünsche, C., Karl, W., Steffens, G., Pfitzner, J., and Schmidt D. (1982). Constitution of the deferriform of the albomycins δ_1, δ_2 and ϵ. *Angewandte Chemie: International Edition in English*, **21**, 527–528.

Betley, M.J., and Mekalanos, J.J. (1985). Staphylococcal enterotoxin A is encoded by phage. *Science*, **229**, 185–187.

Binns, M.M., Mayden, J., and Levine, R.P. (1982). Further characterization of complement resistance conferred on *Escherichia coli* by the plasmid gene *tra*T of R100 and *iss* of ColV, I-K94. *Infection and Immunity*, **35**, 654–659.

Birgens, H.S., Hansen, N.E., Karle, H., and Kristensen, L.O. (1983). Receptor binding of lactoferrin by human monocytes. *British Journal of Haematology*, **54**, 383–391.

Björksten, B., and Kaijser, B. (1978). Interaction of human serum and neutrophils with *Escherichia coli* strains: differences between strains isolated from urine of patients with pyelonephritis or asymptomatic bacteruria. *Infection and Immunity*, **22**, 308–311.

Bjorn, M.J., Sokol, P.A., and Iglewski, B.H. (1979). Influence of iron on yields of extracellular products in *Pseudomonas aeruginosa* culture. *Journal of Bacteriology*, **138**, 193–200.

Border, J.R., La Duca, J., and Seibel, R. (1978). Acute susceptibility to infection in trauma and shock and its prevention. In *The Infection-Prone Hospital Patients* (Eds. J. F. Burke and G.Y. Hildick-Smith) pp. 209–225. Little, Brown and Company, Boston.

Bouza, A., Dominguez, A., Meseguer, M., Bujon, L., Bioxeda, D., Revillo, M.J., de Rafael, L., and Martinez-Beltran, J. (1980). *Yersinia entrocolitica* septicaemia. *American Journal of Clinical Pathology*, **74**, 404–409.

Bowern, N., Ramshaw, I.A., Badenoch-Jones, P., and Doherty, P.C. (1984). Effect of an iron-chelating agent on lymphocyte proliferation. *Australian Journal of Experimental Biology and Medical Science*, **62**, 743–754.

Brener, Z. (1973). Biology of *Trypanosoma cruzi*. *Annual Review of Microbiology*, **27**, 347–382.

Brener, D., DeVoe, I.W., and Holbein, B.E. (1981). Increased virulence of *Neisseria meningitidis* after *in vitro* iron-limited growth at low pH. *Infection and Immunity*, **33**, 59–66.

Brock, J.H. (1984). The role of transferrin in lymphocyte transformation. *Haematologia (Budapest)*, **17**, 187–198.

Brock, J.H., Mainou-Fowler, T. (1983). The role of iron and transferrin in lymphocyte transformation. *Immunology Today*, **4**, 347–351.

Brock, J.H., and Ng, J. (1983). The effect of desferrioxamine on the growth of *Staphylococcus aureus, Yersinia enterocolitica* and *Streptococcus faecalis* in human serum: uptake of desferrioxamine-bound iron. *FEMS Microbiology Letters*, **20**, 439–442.

Brown, M.R.W., Anwar, H., and Lambert, P.A. (1984). Evidence that mucoid *Pseudomonas aeruginosa* in the cystic fibrosis lung grows under iron-restricted conditions. *FEMS Microbiology Letters*, **21**, 113–117.

Brown, M.R.W., and Williams, P. (1985a). Influence of substrate limitation and growth phase on sensitivity to antimicrobial agents. *Journal of Antimicrobial Chemotherapy*, **15**, Supplement A, 7–14.

Brown, M.R.W., and Williams, P. (1985b). The influence of environment on envelope properties affecting survival of bacteria in infections. *Annual Review of Microbiology*, **39**, 527–556.

Brown, R.D., Rickard, K.A., and Kronenberg, H. (1985). Lactoferrin in the myeloproliferative disorders: a search for granulopoietic regulator defects. *British Journal of Haematology*, **59**, 617–626.

Bullen, J.J., Wallis, S.N., and Griffiths, E. (1976). The effect of antipolymorphonuclear leukocyte serum on *Pseudomonas aeruginosa* infection in rabbits. *Immunology*, **30**, 603–610.

Bullen, J.J., Ward, C.G., and Wallis, S.N. (1974). Virulence and the role of iron on the virulence of *Pseudomonas aeruginosa*. *Infection and Immunity*, **10**, 443–450.

Burrows, T.W., and Gillett, W.A. (1971). Host specificity of Brazilian strains of *Pasteurella pestis*. *Nature (London)*, **229**, 51–52.

Butzler, J.P., Alexander, M., Segers, A., Cremer, N., and Blum, D. (1978). Enteritis, abscess and septicaemia due to *Yersinia enterocolitica* in a child with thalassemia. *Journal of Pediatrics*, **93**, 619–621.

Calver, G.A., Kenny, C.P., and Kushner, D.J. (1979). Inhibition of the growth of *Neisseria meningitidis* by reduced ferritin and other iron-binding agents. *Infection and Immunity*, **25**, 880–890.

Cantey, J.R. (1985). Shiga toxin–an expanding role in the pathogenesis of infectious diseases. *Journal of Infectious Diseases*, **151**, 766–771.

Caroline, L., Rosner, F., and Kozinn, P.J. (1969). Elevated serum iron, low unbound transferrin and candidiasis in acute leukaemia. *Blood*, **34**, 441–451.

Caroline, L., Taschdjian, C.L., Kozinn, P.J., and Schade, A.L. (1964). Reversal of serum fungistasis by addition of iron. *Journal of Investigative Dermatology*, **42**, 415–419.

Chart, H., Buck, M., Stevenson, P., and Griffiths, E. (1986). Iron regulated outer membrane proteins of *Escherichia coli*: variations in expression due to the chelator used to restrict the availability of iron. *Journal of General Microbiology*, **132**, 1373–1378

Chart, H., and Griffiths, E. (1985). The availability of iron and the growth of *Vibrio vulnificus* in sera from patients with haemochromatosis. *FEMS Microbiology Letters*, **26**, 227–231.

Chitomber, C.R., Massey, E.J., and Seligman, P.A. (1983). Regulation of transferrin receptor expression on human leukemic cells during proliferation and induction of differentiation: effects of gallium and dimethylsulfoxide. *Journal of Clinical Investigation*, **72**, 1314–1325.

Coulton, J.W. (1982). The ferrichrome-iron receptor of *Escherichia coli* K12. Antigenicity of the *fhu*A protein. *Biochimica et Biophysica Acta*, **717**, 154–162.

Dahlhoff, A., and Stubner, G. (1985). Comparative analysis of the antimicrobial action of polymorphonuclear leucocytes *in vitro*, *ex vivo* and *in vivo*. *Journal of Antimicrobial Chemotherapy*, **15**, Supplement A, 283–291.

Davies, J.W.L. (1982). Anaemia and red cell disorders. In *Physiological Responses to Burning Injury* (Ed. J.W.L. Davies), pp. 393–423. Academic Press, London.

De Sousa, M. (1981). *Lymphocyte Circulation—Experimental and Clinical Aspects*. John Wiley and Sons Limited, New York.

Dimoudis, N., Komischke, K., and Braun, V. (1984). Monoclonal antibodies against the *Fhu*A (Ton A) protein of the *Escherichia coli* outer membrane. *FEMS Microbiology Letters*, **25**, 97–104.

Donelson, J.E., and Rice-Ficht, A.C. (1985). Molecular biology of trypanosome antigenic variation. *Microbiological Reviews*, **49**, 107–125.

Draper, D.L., James, J.F., Brooks, G.F., and Sweet, R.L. (1980). Comparison of virulence markers of peritoneal and fallopian tube isolates with endocervical *Neisseria gonorrhoeae* isolates from women with acute salpingitis. *Infection and Immunity*, **27**, 882–888.

Dubos, R.J., and Geiger, J.W. (1946). Preparation and properties of shiga toxin and toxoid. *Journal of Experimental Medicine*, **84**, 143–156.

Eaton, J.W., Brandt, P., Mahoney, J.R., and Lee, J.T. (1982). Haptoglobin: a natural bacteriostat. *Science*, **215**, 691–693.

Edwards, M., McDade, R.L., Schoolnik, G., Rothbard, J.B., and Gotschlich, E.C. (1984). Antigenic analysis of gonococcal pili using monoclonal antibodies. *Journal of Experimental Medicine*, **160**, 1782–1791.

Eisenstein, B.I. (1981). Phase variation of type I fimbriae in *Escherichia coli* is under transcriptional control. *Science*, **214**, 337–339.

Eisenstein, B.I. (1982). Operon fusion of the phase variation switch. A virulence factor in *Escherichia coli*. *Infection*, **10**, 112–115.

Elin, R.J., and Wolff, S.M. (1973). Effect of pH and iron concentration on growth of *Candida albicans* in human serum. *Journal of Infectious Diseases*, **127**, 705–708.

Elin, R.J., and Wolff, S.M. (1974). The role of iron in non-specific resistance to infection induced by endotoxin. *Journal of Immunology*, **112**, 737–754.

Enns, C.A., Shindelman, J.E., Tomik, S.E., and Sussman, H.H. (1981). Radioimmunochemical measurement of the transferrin receptor in human trophoblast and reticulocyte membranes with a specific antireceptor antibody. *Proceedings of the National Academy of Sciences (USA)*, **78**, 4222–4225.

Epstein, J.B., Truelove, E.L., and Izutzu, K.T. (1984). Oral candidiasis: pathogenesis and host defense. *Reviews of Infectious Diseases*, **6**, 96–105.

Esterly, N.B., Brammar, S.R., and Crounse, R.G. (1967). The relationship of transferrin and iron to serum inhibition of *Candida albicans*. *Journal of Investigative Dermatology*, **49**, 437–442.

Finkelstein, R.A., and Yancey, R.J. (1981). Effect of siderophores on virulence of *Neisseria gonorrhoeae*. *Infection and Immunity*, **32**, 609–613.

Fitzgerald, D.P.P., Trowbridge, I.S., Paston, I., and Willingham, M.C. (1983). Enhancement of toxicity of anti-transferrin receptor antibody—*Pseudomonas* exotoxin conjugates by adenovirus. *Proceedings of the National Academy of Sciences (USA)*, **80**, 4134–4138.

Glynn, A.A. (1972). Bacterial factors inhibiting host defence mechanisms. In *Microbial*

Pathogenicity in Man and Animals (Eds. H. Smith and J.H. Pearce), Society for General Microbiology Symposium No. 22, pp. 75–112.

Goding, J.W., and Burns, G.F. (1981). Monoclonal antibody OKT 9 recognises the receptor for transferrin on human acute lymphocytic leukamia cells. *Journal of Immunology*, **127**, 1256–1258.

Goldberg, M. (1962). Studies of the acute renal effects of hemolyzed red blood cells in dogs including estimations of renal blood flow with krypton. *Journal of Clinical Investigation*, **41**, 2112–2122.

Goya, N., Miyazaki, S., Kodate, S., and Ushio, B. (1972). A family of congenital atrasferrinaemia. *Blood*, **40**, 239–245.

Griffiths, E. (1985). Candidate virulence markers. In *The Virulence of Escherichia coli* (Ed. M. Sussman), Special publication of the Society for General Microbiology No. 13, pp. 193–226. Academic Press, London.

Griffiths, E., and Humphreys, J. (1980). Isolation of enterochelin from the peritoneal washings of guinea pigs lethally infected with *Escherichia coli. Infection and Immunity*, **28**, 286–289.

Griffiths, E., Stevenson, P., and Joyce, P. (1983). Pathogenic *Escherichia coli* express new outer membrane proteins when growing *in vivo*. *FEMS Microbiology Letters*, **16**, 95–99.

Griffiths, E., Stevenson, P., Thorpe, R., and Chart, H. (1985). Naturally occurring antibodies in human sera that react with the iron-regulated outer membrane proteins of *Escherichia coli. Infection and Immunity*, **47**, 808–813.

Gutteridge, J.M.C., Rowley, D.A., Griffiths, E., and Halliwell, B. (1985). Low-molecular weight complexes and oxygen radical reactions in idiopathic haemochromatosis. *Clinical Science*, **68**, 463–467.

Hagblom, P., Segal, E., Billyard, E., and So, M. (1985). Intragenic recombination leads to pilus antigenic variation in *Neisseria gonorrhoeae. Nature*, **315**, 156–158.

Hantke, K., and Braun, V. (1978). Functional interaction of the *ton*A/*ton*B receptor system in *Escherichia coli. Journal of Bacteriology*, **135**, 190–197.

Harris, W.R., Raymond, K.N., and Weitl, F.L. (1981). Ferric iron sequestering agents 6; the spectrophotometric and potentiometric evaluation of sulfonated tricatecholate ligands. *Journal of the American Chemical Society*, **103**, 2667–2675.

Harris, W.R., Weitl, F.L., and Raymond, K.N. (1979). Synthesis and evaluation of an enterobactin model compound. 1,3, 5-tris-(2,3-dihydroxybenzoyl aminomethyl) benzene and its iron (III) complex. *Journal of the Chemical Society, Chemical Communications*, 177–178.

Heidinger, S., Braun, V., Pecoraro, V.L., and Raymond, K.N. (1983). Iron supply to *Escherichia coli* by synthetic analogs of enterochelin. *Journal of Bacteriology*, **153**, 109–115.

Helms, S.D., Oliver, J.D., and Travis, J.C. (1984). Role of heme compounds and haptoglobin in *Vibrio vulnificus* pathogenicity. *Infection and Immunity*, **45**, 345–349.

Hill, J.M., Ruff, M.R., Weber, R.J., and Pert, C.B. (1985). Transferrin receptors in rat brain: neuropeptide-like pattern and relationship to iron distribution. *Proceedings of the National Academy of Sciences (USA)*, **82**, 4553–4557.

Hoffbrand, A.V. (1980). Transfusion siderosis and chelation therapy. In *Iron in Biochemistry and Medicine* (Eds. A. Jacobs and M. Worwood) Vol. II, pp. 499–527. Academic Press, New York.

Hoiseth, S.K., and Stocker, B.A.D. (1981). Aromatic-dependent *Salmonella typhimurium* are non-virulent and effective as live vaccines. *Nature*, **291**, 238–239.

Hoiseth, S.K., and Stocker, B.A.D. (1985). Genes *aro*A and *ser*C of *Salmonella typhimurium* constitute an operon. *Journal of Bacteriology*, **163**, 355–361.

Holzberg, M., and Artis, W.M. (1983). Hydroxamate siderophore production by opportunistic and systemic fungal pathogens. *Infection and Immunity*, **40**, 1134–1139.

Honigberg, B.M. (1978). Trichomonads of importance in human medicine. In *Parasitic Protozoa* (Ed. J.P. Kreier), Vol. II, pp. 275–392. Academic Press, New York.

Howard, R.J., Barnwell, J.W., and Kao, V. (1983). Antigenic variation in *Plasmodium knowlesi* malaria; identifictaion of the variant antigen on infected erythrocytes. *Proceedings of the National Academy of Sciences (USA)*, **80**, 4129–4133.

Hunter, R.L., Bennett, B., Towns, M., and Vogler, W.R. (1983). Transferrin and disease I: Defects in the regulation of transferrin saturation with iron contribute to susceptibility to infection. *American Journal of Clinical Pathology*, **81**, 748–753.

Hurwitz, E.S., Johnson, D., and Campbell, C.C. (1981). Resistance of *P.falciparum* malaria to sulfadoxine-pyremethamine (Fansidor) in a refugee camp in Thailand. *Lancet*, **I**, 1068–1070.

Inoue, K., and Iida, H. (1971). Phage-conversion of toxigenicity in *Clostridium botulinum* types C and D. *Japanese Journal of Medical Sciences and Biology*, **24**, 53–56.

Ismail, A., Bedell, G.W., and Lupan, D.M. (1985). Siderophore production by the pathogenic yeast *Candida alibcans. Biochemical and Biophysical Research Communications*, **130**, 885–891.

James, J.F., and Swanson, J. (1978). Studies on gonococcus infection XIII. Occurrence of color/colonial variants in clinical cultures. *Infection and Immunity*, **19**, 332–340.

Jones, R.L., Peterson, C.M., Grady, R.W., Kumbaraci, T., Cerami, A., and Graziano, J.H. (1977). Effects of iron chelators and iron overload on *Salmonella* infection. *Nature*, **267**, 63–64.

Kadurugamuwa, J.L., Anwar, H., Brown, M.R.W., and Zak, O. (1985a). Effect of sub-inhibitory concentrations of cephalosporins on surface properties and siderophore production in iron-depleted *Klebsiella pneumoniae. Antimicrobial Agents and Chemotherapy*, **27**, 220–223.

Kadurugamuwa, J.L., Anwar, H., Brown, M.R.W., and Zak, O. (1985b). Protein antigens of encapsulated *Klebsiella pneumoniae* surface exposed after growth in the presence of sub-inhibitory concentrations of cephalosporins. *Antimicrobial Agents and Chemotherapy*, **28**, 195–199.

Kaneko, M., Yamaguchi, A., and Sawai, T. (1984). Purification and characterization of two kinds of porins from *Enterobacter cloacae* outer membrane. *Journal of Bacteriology*, **158**, 1171–1181.

Karmali, M.A., Petric, M., Louie, S., and Cheung, R. (1986). Antigenic heterogeneity of *Escherichia coli* verotoxins. *Lancet*, **I**, 164–165.

Keene, W.R., and Jandl, J.H. (1965). The site of hemoglobin catabolism. *Blood*, **26**, 705–718.

Keppie, J., Williams, A.E., Witt, K., and Smith,H. (1965). The role of erythritol in the tissue localization of the brucellae. *British Journal of Experimental Pathology*, **46**, 104–108.

Khimji, P.L., and Miles, A.A. (1978). Microbial iron-chelators and their action on *Klebsiella* infections in the skin of guinea pigs. *British Journal of Experimental Pathology*, **59**, 137–147.

Kilian, M., Thomsen, B., Petersen, T.E., and Bleeg, H.S. (1983). Occurrence and nature of bacterial IgA proteases. *Annals of the New York Academy of Sciences*, **409**, 612–624.

Killar, L.M., and Eisenstein, T.K. (1985). Immunity to *Salmonella typhimurium* infection in C3H/HeJ and C3H/HeNCr1BR mice: studies with an aromatic-dependent live *S.typhimurium* strain as a vaccine. *Infection and Immunity*, **47**, 605–612.

Kimura, L.H., and Pearsall, N.N. (1980). Relationship between germination of *Candida albicans* and increased adherence to human buccal epithelial cells. *Infection and Immunity*, **28**, 464–468.

Kirkpatrick, C.H., Green, I., Rich, R.R., and Schade, A.L. (1971). Inhibition of growth of *Candida albicans* by iron-unsaturated lactoferrin: relation to host-defense mechanisms in chronic mucocutaneous candidiasis. *Journal of Infectious Diseases*, **124**, 539–544.

Kontoghiorghes, G.J., and Evans, R.W. (1985). Site specificity of iron removal from transferrin by α-ketohydroxy-pyridine chelators. *FEBS Letters*, **189**, 141–144.

Kornfeld, S.J., and Plaut, A.G. (1981). Secretory immunity and the bacterial IgA proteases. *Reviews in Infectious Diseases*, **3**, 521–534.

Lalonde, R.G., and Holbein, B.E. (1984). Role of iron in *Trypanosoma cruzi* infection of mice. *Journal of Clinical Investigation*, **73**, 470–476.

Lambden, P.R., Heckels, J.E., James, L.T., and Watt, P.J. (1979). Variations in surface protein composition associated with virulence properties in opacity types of *Neisseria gonorrhoeae*. *Journal of General Microbiology*, **114**, 305–312.

Lambden, P.R., Heckels, J.E., McBride, H., and Watt, P.J. (1981). The identification and isolation of novel pilus types produced by variants of *Neisseria gonorrhoeae* P9 following selection *in vivo*. *FEMS Microbiology Letters*, **10**, 339–341.

Lankford, C.E. (1973). Bacterial assimilation of iron. *CRC Critical Reviews in Microbiology*, **2**, 273–331.

Loo, V.G., and Lalonde, R.G. (1984). Role of iron in intracellular growth of *Trypanosoma cruzi*. *Infection and Immunity*, **45**, 726–730.

Lorian, V. (1980). Effects of sub-minimum inhibitory concentrations of antibiotics on bacteria. In *Antibiotics in Laboratory Medicine* (Ed. V. Lorian), pp. 342–408. The Williams and Wilkins Company, Baltimore.

Lorian, V., and Atkinson, B.A. (1984). Bactericidal effects of polymorphonuclear neutrophils on antibiotic-induced filaments of Gram-negative bacilli. *Journal of Infectious Diseases*, **149**, 719–727.

McFarlane, H., Reddy, S., Adcock, K.J., Adesina, H., Cooke, A.R., and Akene, A.R. (1970). Immunity, transferrin and survival in kwashiokor. *British Medical Journal*, **4**, 268–270.

Magnusson, K.E., Kihlstrom, E., Norlander, L., Norqvist, A., Davies, J., and Normark, S. (1979a). Effect of colony type and pH on surface charge and hydrophobicity of *Neisseria gonorrhoeae*. *Infection and Immunity*, **26**, 397–401.

Magnusson, K.E., Kihlstrom, E., Norqvist, A., Davies, J., and Normark, S. (1979b). Effect of iron on surface charge and hydrophobicity of *Neisseria gonorrhoeae*. *Infection and Immunity*, **26**, 402–407.

Masawe, A.E.J., Muindi, J.M., and Swai, G.R.B. (1974). Infection in iron deficiency and other types of anaemia in the tropics. *Lancet*, **II**, 314–317.

Mattie, H. (1984). Animal models in antibacterial drug research. *Journal of Antimicrobial Chemotherapy*, **14**, 101–104.

Mayer, L.W. (1982). Rates of *in vitro* changes of gonococcal colony opacity phenotypes. *Infection and Immunity*, **37**, 481–485.

Melby, K., Slordahl, S., Guttenberg, T.J., and Nordbo, S.A. (1982). Septicaemia due to *Yersinia enterocolitica* after oral doses of iron. *British Medical Journal*, **285**, 467–468.

Mestecky, J., McGhee, J.R., Crago, S.S., Jackson, S., Kilian, M., Kryono, H., Babb, J.U., and Michalek, S.M. (1980). Molecular–cellular interactions in the secretory IgA response. *Journal of the Reticuloendothelial Society*, **28** (Supplement), 45–60, S.

Meyer, T.F., Mlawer, N., and So, M. (1982). Pilus expression in *Neisseria gonorrhoeae* involves chromosomal rearrangements. *Cell*, **30**, 45–52.

Moll, A., Manning, P.A., and Timmis, K.N. (1980). Plasmid-determined resistance to serum bactericidal activity: a major outer membrane protein, the *tra* T gene product, is responsible for plasmid-specified serum resistance in *Escherichia coli*. *Infection and Immunity*, **28**, 359–367.

Montenegro, M.A., Bitter-Suermann, D., Timmis, J.K., Agüero, M.E., Cabello, F.C., Sanyal, S.C., and Timmis, K.N. (1985). *Tra* T gene sequences, serum resistance and pathogenicity-related factors in clinical isolates of *Escherichia coli* and other Gram-negative bacteria. *Journal of General Microbiology*, **131**, 1511–1521.

Morselt, A.F.W., Glastra, A., and James, J. (1973). Micro-spectrophotometric analysis of malaria pigment. *Experimental Parasitology*, **33**, 17–22.

Mulks, M.H. (1985). Microbial IgA proteases. In *Bacterial Enzymes and Virulence* (Ed. I.A. Holder), pp. 82–104, CRC Press Inc., Florida.

Muller, G., Matzonke, B.F., and Raymond, K.N. (1984). Iron transport in *Streptomyces pilosus* mediated by ferrichrome siderophores, rhodotorulic acid and enantio-rhodotorulic acid. *Journal of Bacteriology*, **160**, 313–318.

Muller, G., and Raymond, K.N. (1984). Specificity and mechanism of ferrioxamine-mediated iron transport in *Streptomyces pilosus*. *Journal of Bacteriology*, **160**, 304–312.

Muller-Ebberhard, U. (1970). Hemopexin. *New England Journal of Medicine*, **283**, 1090–1093.

Murphy, J., Pappenheimer, Jr., A.M., and de Broms, S.T. (1974). Synthesis of diphtheria *tox*-gene products in *Escherichia coli* extracts. *Proceedings of the National Academy of Sciences (USA)*, **71**, 11–15.

Murray, M.J., Murray, A.B., Murray, M.B., and Murray, C.J. (1978). The adverse effect of iron repletion on the course of certain infections. *British Medical Journal*, **II**, 1113–1115.

Naumann, H.N., Diggs, L.W., Barreras, L., and Williams, B.J. (1971). Plasma haemoglobin and haemoglobin fractions in sickle cell crisis. *American Journal of Clinical Pathology*, **56**, 137–147.

Neckers, L.M. and Cossman, J. (1983). Transferrin receptor induction in mitogen-stimulated human T-lymphocytes is required for DNA synthesis and cell division and is regulated by interleukin 2. *Proceedings of the National Academy of Sciences (USA)*, **80**, 3494–3498.

Neckers, L.M., Yenokida, G., and James, S.P. (1984). The role of the transferrin receptor in human B lymphocyte activation. *Journal of Immunology*, **133**, 2437–2441.

Neilands, J.B. (1981a). Microbial iron compounds. *Annual Review of Biochemistry*, **50**, 715–731.

Neilands, J.B. (1981b). Iron absorption and transport in microorganisms. *Annual Review of Nutrition*, **1**, 27–46.

Newland, J.W., Strockline, N.A., Miller, S.F., O'Brien, A.D., and Holmes, R.K. (1985). Cloning of Shiga-like toxin structural genes from a toxin converting phage of *Escherichia coli*. *Science*, **230**, 179–181.

Newman, R., Schneider, C., Sutherland, R., Vodinelich, L.A., and Greaves, M. (1982). The transferrin receptor. *Trends in Biochemical Sciences*, **7**, 397–400.

Nowicki, B., Rhen, M., Väisänen-Rhen, V., Pere, A., and Korhonen, T.K. (1985). Kinetics of phase variation between S and type-1 fimbriae of *Escherichia coli*. *FEMS Microbiology Letters*, **28**, 237–242.

Nurse, G.T. (1979). Iron, the thalassemias and malaria. *Lancet*, **II**, 314–317.

O'Brien, A.D., and LaVeck, G.D. (1982). Immunochemical and cytotoxic activities of *Shigella dysenteriae* (Shiga) and shiga-like toxins. *Infection and Immunity*, **35**, 1151–1154.

O'Brien, A.D., and LaVeck, G.D. (1983). Purification and characterization of a *Shigella dysenteriae* 1-like toxin produced by *Escherichia coli*. *Infection and Immunity*, **40**, 675–683.

O'Brien, A.D., LaVeck, G.D., Thompson, M.R., and Formal, S.B. (1982). Production of *Shigella* dysenteriae type 1-like cytotoxin by *Escherichia coli*. *Journal of Infectious Diseases*, **146**, 763–769.

O'Brien, A.D., Lively, T.A., Chang, T.W., and Gorbach, S.L. (1983a). Purification of *Shigella dysenteriae* 1 (Shiga)-like toxin from *Escherichia coli* 0157:H7 strain associated with haemorrhagic colitis. *Lancet*, **II**, 573.

O'Brien, A.D., Lively, T.A., Chen, M.E., Rothman, S.W., and Formal, S.B. (1983b). *Escherichia coli* 0157 H7 strains associated with haemorrhagic colitis in the United States produce a *Shigella dysenteriae* 1 (Shiga)-like cytotoxin. *Lancet*, **1**, 702.

O'Brien, A.D., Newland, J.W., Miller, S.F., Holmes, R.K., Williams Smith, H., and Formal, S.B. (1984). Shiga-like toxin-converting phages from *Escherichia coli* strains that cause hemorrhagic colitis or infantile diarrhoea. *Science*, **226**, 694–696.

Ogata, R.T., Wintens, C., and Levine, R.P. (1982). Nucleotide sequence analysis of the complement resistance gene from plasmid R100. *Journal of Bacteriology*, **151**, 819–827.

Ohshiro, T., and Kosaki, G. (1978). Clinical study of haptoglobin therapy for prevention of hemoglobinuria. *Medical Journal of Osaka University*, **29**, 151–161.

Ohshiro, T., Kosaki, G., and Funakoshi, S. (1978). Haptoglobin therapy: effect on prevention and treatment of hemaglobinuria. *Medical Journal of Osaka University*, **29**, 269–279.

Okabe, T., Fujisawa, M., and Takaku, F. (1984). Long-term cultivation and differentiation of human erythroleukemic cells in a protein-free chemically defined medium. *Proceedings of the National Academy of Sciences (USA)*, **81**, 453–455.

Olling, S. (1977). Sensitivity of Gram-negative bacilli to the serum bactericidal activity: a marker of the host–parasite relationship in acute and persisting infections. *Scandinavian Journal of Infectious Diseases Supplement*, **10**, 1–10.

Ombaka, E.A., Cozens, R.M., and Brown, M.R.W. (1983). Influence of nutrient limitation of growth on stability and production of virulence factors of mucoid and non-mucoid strains of *Pseudomonas aeruginosa*. *Reviews of Infectious Diseases*, **5**, 5880–5888.

Opal, S., Cross, A., and Gemski, P. (1982). K antigen and the serum sensitivity of rough *Escherichia coli*. *Infection and Immunity*, **37**, 956–960.

Pecoraro, V.L., Weitl, F.L., and Raymond, K.N. (1981). Ferric ion-specific sequestering agents 7; synthesis, iron exchange kinetics and stability constants of N-substituted sulfonated catecholamide analogues of enterobactin. *Journal of the American Chemical Society*, **103**, 5133–5140.

Penn, C.W., Parsons, N.J., Rittenberg, S.C., Sanyal, S.C., Veale, D.R., and Smith, H. (1978). Gonococci grown *in vivo* and *in vitro*: selection and phenotypic change in relation to pathogenesis and immunity. In *Immunobiology of Neisseria gonorrhoeae* (Eds. G.F. Brooks, E.C. Gotschlich, K.K. Holmes, W.D. Sawyer and F.E. Young), pp. 356–359. American Society for Microbiology, Washington DC.

Perry, R.D., and Brubaker, R.R. (1979). Accumulation of iron by Yersiniae. *Journal of Bacteriology*, **137**, 1290–1298.

Peterson, K.M., and Alderete, J.F. (1984a). Selective acquisition of plasma proteins by *Trichomonas vaginalis* and human lipoproteins as a growth requirement for this species. *Molecular and Biochemical Parasitology*, **12**, 37–48.

Peterson K.M., and Alderete, J.F. (1984b). Iron uptake and increased intracellular enzyme activity follow host lactoferrin binding by *Trichomonas vaginalis* receptors. *Journal of Experimental Medicine*, **160**, 398–410.

Peto, T.E.A. and Thompson, J.L. (1986). A reappraisal of the effects of iron and desferrioxamine on the growth of *Plasmodium falciparum* "*in vitro*": the unimportance of serum iron. *British Journal of Haematology*, **63**, 273–280.

Plaha, D.S., and Rogers, H.J. (1983). Antibacterial effect of the scandium complex of enterochelin; studies on the mechanism of action. *Biochimica et Biophysica Acta*, **760**, 246–255.

Plaut, A.G. (1983). The IgA1 proteases of pathogenic bacteria. *Annual Review of Microbiology*, **37**, 603–622.

Pollack, S., and Fleming, J. (1984). *Plasmodium falciparum* takes up iron from transferrin. *British Journal of Haematology*, **58**, 289–293.

Propper, R.D., Cooper, B., Rufo, R.R., Nienhuis, A.W., Anderson, W.F., Bunn, H.F., Rosenthal, A., and Nathan, D.G. (1977). Continuous subcutaneous administration of deferrioxamine in patients with iron overload. *New England Journal of Medicine*, **297**, 418–422.

Rabson, A.R, Hallett, A.F., and Koornhof, H.J. (1975). Generalized *Yersinia enterocolitica* infection. *Journal of Infectious Diseases*, **131**, 447–451.

Rass, V., and Basala, M. (1984). A highly cytotoxic human transferrin-ricin A conjugate used to select receptor-modified cells. *Journal of Biological Chemistry*, **259**, 1143–1149.

Reinherz, E.L., Kung, P.C., Goldstein, G., Levey, R.H., and Schlossman, S.F. (1980). Discrete stages of human intrathymic differentiation: analysis of normal thymocytes and leukemic lymphoblasts of T-cell lineage. *Proceedings of the National Academy of Sciences (USA)*, **77**, 1588–1592.

Reynolds, P.E., and Brown, D.F.J. (1985). Penicillin-binding proteins of β-lactam-resistant strains of *Staphylococcus aureus*. *FEBS Letters*, **192**, 28–32.

Robbins, J.B., Schneerson, R., Egan, W.B., Vann, W., and Liu, D.T. (1980). Virulence properties of bacterial capsular polysaccharide—unanswered questions. In *The Molecular Basis of Microbial Pathogenicity* (Eds. H. Smith, J.J. Skehel and M.J. Turner), pp. 115–132. Dahlem Konferenzen, Weinheim, Verlag Chemie GmbH.

Robertsson, J.A., Lindberg, A.A., Hoiseth, S., and Stocker, B.A.D. (1983). *Salmonella typhimurium* infection in calves: protection and survival of virulent challenge bacteria after immunization with live or inactivated vaccines. *Infection and Immunity*, **41**, 742–750.

Robins-Browne, R.M., and Prpic, J.K. (1985). Effects of iron and desferrioxamine on infections with *Yersinia enterocolitica*. *Infection and Immunity*, **47**, 774–779.

Rogers, H.J., Synge, C., and Woods, V.E. (1980). Antibacterial effect of scandium and indium complexes of enterochelin on *Klebsiella pneumoniae*. *Antimicrobial Agents and Chemotherapy*, **18**, 63–68.

Rogers, H.J., Woods, V.E., and Synge, C. (1982). Antibacterial effect of the scandium and indium complexes of enterochelin on *Escherichia coli*. *Journal of General Microbiology*, **128**, 2389–2394.

Rothbard, J.B., Fernandez, R., and Schoolnik, G.K. (1984). Strain-specific and common epitopes of gonococcal pili. *Journal of Experimental Medicine*, **160**, 208–221.

Saunders, J.R. (1982). Chromosomal rearrangements in gonococcal pathogenicity. *Nature*, **299**, 781–782.

Saunders, J.R. (1985). Antigenic variation in gonococcal pili explained. *Nature*, **315**, 100–101.

Sawai, T., Hiruma, R., Kawana, N., Kaneko, M., Taniyasu, F., and Inami, A. (1982). Outer membrane permeation of β-lactam antibiotics in *Escherichia coli*, *Proteus mirabilis* and *Enterobacter cloacae*. *Antimicrobial Agents and Chemotherapy*, **22**, 585–592.

Scotland, S.M., Smith, H.R., and Rowe, B. (1985). Two distinct toxins active on vero cells from *Escherichia coli* 0157. *Lancet*, **II**, 885–886.

Segal, E., Billyard, E., So, M., Storzbach, S., and Meyer, T.F. (1985). Role of chromosomal rearrangment in *N.gonorrhoeae* pilus phase variation. *Cell*, **40**, 293–300.

Shibil, A.M. (1983). Effects of antibiotics on production of enzymes and toxins by microorganisms. *Reviews in Infectious Diseases*, **5**, 865–875.

Silverman, M., and Simon, M. (1980). Phase variation: genetic analysis of switching mutants. *Cell*, **19**, 845–854.

Simon, M., Zieg, J., Silverman, M., Mondel, G., and Doolittle, R. (1980). Phase variation: evolution of a controlling element. *Science*, **209**, 1370–1374.

Smith, B.P., Reina-Guerra, M., Hoiseth, S.K., Stocker, B.A.D., Habasha, F., Johnston, E., and Merritt, F. (1984a). Aromatic-dependent *Salmonella typhimurium* as modified live vaccines for calves. *American Journal of Veterinary Research*, **45**, 59–66.

Smith, H. (1980). The effect of environmental conditions *in vivo* and *in vitro* on the determinants of microbial pathogenicity. In *The Molecular Basis of Microbial Pathogenicity* (Eds. H. Smith., J.J. Skehel and M.J. Turner), pp. 159–172. Dahlem Konferenzen, Weinheim, Verlag Chemie GmbH.

Smith, H. (1983). The elusive determinants of bacterial intereference with non-specific host defences. *Philosophical Transactions of the Royal Society, London*, Series B, **303**, 99–113.

Smith, H., Williams, A.E., Pearce, J.H., Keppie, J., Harris-Smith, P.W., Fitzgeorge, R.B., and Witt, K. (1962). Foetal erythritol: a cause of the localization of *Brucella abortus* in bovine contagious abortion. *Nature*, **193**, 47–49.

Smith, H.R., Day, N.P., Scotland, S.M., Gross, R.J., and Rowe, B. (1984b). Phage determined production of Vero cytotoxin in strains of *Escherichia coli* serogroup 0157. *Lancet*, **II**, 1242–1243.

Smith, H.W., Green, P., and Parsell, Z. (1983). Vero cell toxins in *Escherichia coli* and related bacteria: transfer by phage and conjugation and toxic action in laboratory animals, chickens and pigs. *Journal of General Microbiology*, **129**, 3121–3127.

Spratt, B.G. (1977). Properties of penicillin-binding proteins of *Escherichia coli* K12. *European Journal of Biochemistry*, **72**, 341–352.

Sutherland, R., Delia, D., Schneider, C., Newman, R., Kemshead, J., and Greaves, M. (1981). Ubiquitous cell-surface glycoprotein on tumour cells is proliferation-associated receptor for transferrin. *Proceedings of the National Academy of Sciences (USA)*, **78**, 4515–4519.

Swanson, J. (1978a). Studies in gonococcus infection XII. Colony color and opacity variants of gonococci. *Infection and Immunity*, **19**, 320–331.

Swanson, J. (1978b). Studies on gonococcus infection XIV. Cell wall protein differences among color/opacity colony variants of *Neiserria gonorrhoeae*. *Infection and Immunity*, **21**, 292–302.

Swanson, J., Bergström, S., Barrera, O., Robbins, K., and Corwin, D. (1985). Pilus-gonococcal variants: evidence for multiple forms of piliation control. *Journal of Experimental Medicine*, **162**, 729–744.

Taetle, R., Honeysett, R.J.M., and Trowbridge, I.S. (1983). Effects of anti-transferrin receptor antibodies on growth of normal and malignant myeloid cells. *International Journal of Cancer*, **32**, 343–349.

Taetle, R., Rhyner, K., Castagnola, J., To, D., and Mendelsohn, J. (1985). Role of transferrin, Fe, and transferrin receptors in myeloid leukemia cell growth: studies with an antitransferrin receptor monoclonal antibody. *Journal of Clinical Investigation*, **75**, 1061–1067.

Testa, U. (1985). Transferrin receptors: structure and function. In *Current Topics in Hematology*, (Eds. S. Piomelli and S. Yachnin), Vol. 5, pp. 127–161. Alan R. Liss Inc., New York.

Theakston, R.D.G., Fletcher, K.A.,and Maegraith, B.G. (1970). The use of electron microscope autoradiography for examining the uptake and separation of haemoglobin by *Plasmodium berghei*. *Annals of Tropical Medicine and Parasitology*, **64**, 63–77.

Trowbridge, I.S., and Domingo, D.L. (1981). Effects on growth of human tumour cells of anti-transferrin receptor antibody and toxin-antibody conjugates. *Nature,* **294**, 171–173.

Trowbridge, I.S., and Domingo, D.L. (1982). Prospects for the clinical use of cytotoxic monoclonal antibody conjugates in the treatment of cancer. *Cancer Surveys*, **1**, 543–556.

Trowbridge, I.S., and Lopez, F. (1982). Monoclonal antibody to transferrin receptor blocks transferrin binding and inhibits human tumor cell growth *in vitro*. *Proceedings of the National Academy of Sciences (USA)*, **79**, 1175–1179.

Trowbridge, I.S., Newman, R.A., Domingo, D.L., and Sauvage, C. (1984). Transferrin receptors: structure and function. *Biochemical Pharmacology*, **33**, 925–932.

Trowbridge, I.S., and Omary M.B. (1981). Human cell surface glycoprotein related to cell proliferation is the receptor for transferrin. *Proceedings of the National Academy of Sciences (USA)*, **78**, 3039–3043.

Turnowsky, F., Brown, M.R.W., Anwar, H., and Lambert, P.A. (1983). Effect of iron limitation of growth rate on the binding of penicillin G to the penicillin binding proteins of mucoid and non-mucoid strains of *Pseudomonas aeruginosa*. *FEMS Microbiology Letters*, **17**, 243–245.

van Asbeck, B.S., Marcelis, J.H., Marx, J.J.M., Struyrenberg, A., van Kats, J.H., and Verhoef, J. (1983a). Inhibition of bacterial multiplication by the iron chelator deferroxamine: potentiating effect of ascorbic acid. *European Journal of Clinical Microbiology*, **2**, 426–431.

van Asbeck, B.S., Marcelis, J.H., van Kats, J.H., Jaarsma, E.Y., and Verhoef, J. (1983b). Synergy between the iron chelator deferroxamine and the antimicrobial agents gentamicin, chloramphenicol, cefalothin, cefotiam and cefsulodin. *European Journal of Clinical Microbiology*, **2**, 432–438.

Vasil, M.L., Berka, R.M., Gray, G.L., and Pavlouskis, O.R. (1985). Biochemical and genetic studies of iron-regulated (exotoxin A) and phosphate-regulated (hemolysin phospholipase C) virulence factors of *Pseudomonas aeruginosa*. *Antibiotics and Chemotherapy*, **36**, 23–39.

Venuti, M.C., Rastetter, W.H., and Neilands, J.B. (1979). 1,3,5-tris(N, N^1,N^{11}-2,3-dihydroxybenzoyl) aminomethyl benzene, a synthetic iron chelator related to enterobactin. *Journal of Medicinal Chemistry*, **22**, 123–124.

Ward, C.G., Hammond, J.S., and Bullen, J.J. (1986). Effect of iron compounds on the antibacterial function of human polymorphs and plasma. *Infection and Immunity*, **51**, 723–730.

Weeks, C.R., and Ferretti, J.J. (1984). The gene for type A streptococcal exotoxin (erythrogenic toxin) is located in bacteriophage T12. *Infection and Immunity*, **46**, 531–536.

Weitl F.L. and Raymond K.N. (1979). Ferric ion sequestering agents I. Hexadentate O-bonding N,N^1,N^{11}-tris(2,3-dihydroxybenzoyl) derivatives of 1,5,9-triazacyclotridecane and 1,3,5-triaminomethylbenzene. *Journal of the American Chemical Society*, **101**, 2728–2731.

Weitl, F.L., and Raymond, K.N. (1981). Lipophilic enterobactin analogues. Terminally N-alkylated spermine/spermidine catecholcarboxamides. *Journal of Organic Chemistry*, **46**, 5234–5237.

Werner, V., Sanders, C.C., Sander, Jr., W.E., and Goering, R.V. (1985). Role of β-lactamases and outer membrane proteins in multiple β-lactam resistance to *Enterobacter cloacae*. *Antimicrobial Agents and Chemotherapy*, **27**, 455–459.

Willshaw, G.A., Smith, H.R., Scotland, S.M., and Rowe, B. (1985). Cloning of genes determining the production of Vero cytotoxin by *Escherichia coli*. *Journal of General Microbiology*, **131**, 3047–3053.

Wright, A.C., Simpson, L.M., and Oliver, J.D. (1981). Role of iron in the pathogenesis of *Vibrio vulnificus* infections. *Infection and Immunity*, **34**, 503–507.

Yancey, R.J., Breeding, S.A.L., and Lankford, C.E. (1979). Enterochelin (enterobactin): virulence factor for *Salmonella typhimurium*. *Infection and Immunity*, **24**, 174–180.

Yoshioka, T., Sugimoto, T., Ukai, T., and Oshiro, T. (1985). Haptoglobin therapy for possible prevention of renal failure following thermal injury: a clinical study. *The Journal of Trauma*, **25**, 281–287.

Zabriskie, J.B. (1974). The role of temperate bacteriophage in the production of erythrogenic toxin by group A streptococci. *Journal of Experimental Medicine*, **119**, 761–779.

Zieg, J., Silverman, M., Hilmen, M., and Simon, M. (1977). Recombinational switch for gene expression. *Science*, **196**, 170–172.

Index